Nurturing Indonesia

Hans Pols proposes a new perspective on the history of colonial medicine from the viewpoint of indigenous physicians. Members of the Indonesian medical profession in the Dutch East Indies actively participated in political affairs by joining and leading nationalist associations, by publishing in newspapers and magazines, and by being elected to city councils and the colonial parliament. Indonesian physicians were motivated by their medical training, their experiences as physicians, and their subordinate position within the colonial health care system to organise, lead, and join social, cultural, and political associations. Opening with the founding of Indonesia's first political association in 1908 and continuing with the initiatives of the Association of Indonesian Physicians, Pols describes how the Rockefeller Foundation's projects inspired the formulation of a nationalist health program. Tracing the story through the Japanese annexation, the war of independence, and independent Indonesia, Pols reveals the relationship between medicine and decolonisation, and the role of physicians in Asian history.

HANS POLS is Associate Professor in the School of History and Philosophy of Science at the University of Sydney. He helped found the Indonesian Association of the History of Medicine (PERSEKIN) in 2009.

Global Health Histories

Series Editor:
Sanjoy Bhattacharya, University of York

Global Health Histories aims to publish outstanding and innovative scholarship on the history of public health, medicine and science worldwide. By studying the many ways in which the impact of ideas of health and well-being on society were measured and described in different global, international, regional, national and local contexts, books in the series reconceptualise the nature of empire, the nation state, extra-state actors and different forms of globalisation. The series showcases new approaches to writing about the connected histories of health and medicine, humanitarianism and global economic and social development.

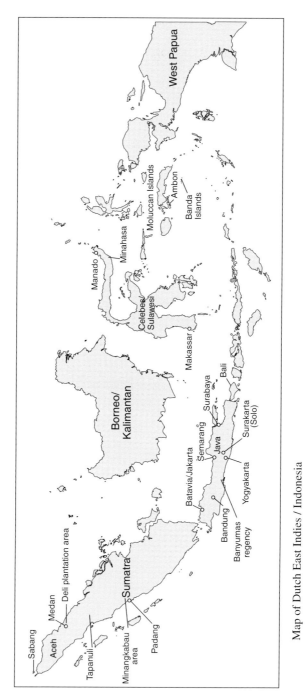

Map of Dutch East Indies / Indonesia

Nurturing Indonesia

Medicine and Decolonisation in the Dutch East Indies

Hans Pols

University of Sydney

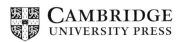

CAMBRIDGE
UNIVERSITY PRESS

University Printing House, Cambridge CB2 8BS, United Kingdom

One Liberty Plaza, 20th Floor, New York, NY 10006, USA

477 Williamstown Road, Port Melbourne, VIC 3207, Australia

314–321, 3rd Floor, Plot 3, Splendor Forum, Jasola District Centre, New Delhi – 110025, India

79 Anson Road, #06-04/06, Singapore 079906

Cambridge University Press is part of the University of Cambridge.

It furthers the University's mission by disseminating knowledge in the pursuit of education, learning, and research at the highest international levels of excellence.

www.cambridge.org
Information on this title: www.cambridge.org/9781108424578
DOI: 10.1017/9781108341035

First published 2018

Printed in the United Kingdom by TJ International Ltd. Padstow Cornwall

A catalogue record for this publication is available from the British Library.

ISBN 978-1-108-42457-8 Hardback

Christophina Georgina Sigismunda ('Noenie') van
Bosse-Remmert
(* Bintaran, Yogyakarta, 26 November 1880–25
November 1974, The Hague, The Netherlands)

Hermine Jeanne Christine ('Hamie') Cramer-van Bosse
(* Bintaran, Yogyakarta, 24 November 1908–15 July
1995, Ede, The Netherlands)

Anna Christina ('Anneke') Pols-Cramer
(* Menteng, Batavia, 14 September 1938–23 January
1974, Assen, The Netherlands)

Contents

Figures

Acknowledgements

This book is dedicated to three generations of women born in the Dutch East Indies: my great-grandmother, my grandmother, and my mother. The first two women were born in Bintaran in Yogyakarta. This neighbourhood is close to Yogyakarta's smaller sultanate (Paku Alam) where Wahidin Soedorohoesodo served as court physician. It also was the home of Soewardi Soerjaningrat; the first Taman Siswa school he founded after he changed his name to Ki Hadjar Dewantara is a mere ten-minute walk away (as is a former prison) from the family home. The largest house in the neighbourhood was occupied by the wealthy Weijnschenck family, which owned the sugar factory Padokan (today: Madukismo) where my great-great-grandfather worked as managing director. In 1943, the house was taken over by General Sudirman (today it houses the Sudirman Museum). Soegija (Albertus Soegijapranata), a priest who sided with the Indonesian revolution, preached in the Catholic church in the same neighbourhood, and embittered Dutch physician Isaac Groneman lived there too.

This book has a long history, and over the years I have accrued many intellectual debts, too numerous to mention. I wish to single out several individuals who played crucial roles when this project was taking shape.

Through Herman Keppy, I found out about the Tehupeiory brothers and many other Indonesian physicians who studied in the Netherlands. Hiskia Coumou shared his extensive insights about J. H. F. Kohlbrugge. With Frances Gouda, I discussed many issues related to the Dutch East Indies. Bart Luttikhuis has been very helpful in thinking about the predicament of Indonesian social climbers in the archipelago. With Liesbeth Hesselink, I fruitfully discussed the STOVIA and its graduates. I have been very fortunate to spend several summers at the Royal Netherlands Institute of Southeast Asian and Caribbean Studies (KITLV). The discussions I had there with Henk Schulte Nordholt, Gary van Klinken, Harry Poeze, Marieke Bloembergen, Tom van den Berge, Leo van Bergen, and David Henley have all contributed to this book.

When I visited Indonesia in 2005, Loka Tjahjana, former director of the mental hospital in Bogor, kindly showed me around that institution. Irmansyah, the head of the Department of Psychiatry, invited me to give a presentation.

Soon after, I met Rushdy Hoesein, Firman Lubis, and Dodi Partomihardjo, three physicians with an interest in the history of medicine in Indonesia. In 2008, we organised a symposium entitled 'One Hundred Years of National Awakening' in the old STOVIA building and then founded the Indonesian Association of the History of Medicine (PERSEKIN) the following year. In Surabaya I met Indropo Agusni, the founder of the NIAS museum, and his wife, Thalca Hamid, who hosted me during several visits. In Yogyakarta, I discussed Sardjito, and several others who were central to the history of medicine in Indonesia, with Soenarto Sastrowijoto, his wife, Yati (whose grandfather Goembrek was a co-founder of Boedi Oetomo), and Sutaryo. In Cambridge, MA, and Yogyakarta, I had many conversations with Byron Good and Mary-Jo DelVecchio Good about nationalism and medicine before and after Indonesian independence. Discussions with James Bourk Hoesterey have been extremely helpful.

In Australia, I owe heartfelt thanks to Terry Hull, whose encouragement in the beginning of this project made all the difference. He provided me with valuable items from his collection of historical materials and introduced me to Indonesian physicians interested in the history of medicine. The many discussions at Warwick Anderson's Centre for Race and Ethnicity in the Global South at the University of Sydney provided ample inspiration. Alison Bashford was always willing to offer encouragement and support. Several colleagues at the University of Sydney, including Robert Aldrich, James Dunk (whose phenomenal copy-editing skills made this manuscript much more readable), Daniela Helbig, Max Lane, Ricardo Roque, Adrian Vickers, and Sarah Walsh, have provided support along the way.

Over the years, I have conducted several interviews, which all contained valuable insights. In Surabaya, I spoke with Sentot Soeatmadji, who also let me consult his collection of NIAS materials; in Jakarta, with ninety-eight-year-old Gré Soetopo-van Eijbergen (Soetopo's widow) and Ilya Waleida (Tita) Soeprapto (Bahder Djohan's daughter); and, in Bandung, with Koestedjo, who fondly recalled his days at the Batavia Medical School. In the Netherlands, I met Anton Amir (the son of Mohamad Amir), W. de Vogel (the daughter-in-law of W. T. de Vogel), and Ine Glastra van Loon-de Mol van Otterloo (the daughter of F. H. Glastra van Loon). In Glen Ellen, CA, I met with John S. Wellington to discuss the association of the Faculty of Medicine at the University of Indonesia with the University of California at San Francisco.

Several friends read the whole manuscript and provided helpful feedback: Claire Edington, Liesbeth Hesselink, Jan Pols, Jeannette Pols, and Jean Gelman Taylor.

I have had several wonderful research assistants: Eline Sepers, Self Rumbewas, Vivek Neelakantan, Claire Kennedy, and Gemma Smart.

Two individuals stand out for their contributions. Starting in 1991, when we met at the University of Pennsylvania, I have had many conversations with the extraordinary Warwick Anderson. His suggestion to study the history of colonial psychiatry in the Dutch East Indies led, eventually, to this book. His patience in reading all chapters, and his numerous suggestions, have immeasurably increased its quality.

I owe more thanks than I could ever express to my wife, Stephanie, who has encouraged me for years to start writing, to continue writing, and to revise. She patiently read everything, time and time again, making this book possible.

Medical Institutions

Medical Education in Batavia/Jakarta

Dokter Djawa School (1851–1901)	Javanese Doctors' School Degree: Dokter Djawa [Javanese Physician]
School ter Opleiding van Inlandsche Artsen; STOVIA (1902–13)	School for the Education of Native Physicians (also referred to as: Batavia Medical College) Degree: Inlandsch Arts [Native Physician]
School ter Opleiding van Indische Artsen; STOVIA (1913–33)	School for the Education of Indies Physicians (also referred to as: Batavia Medical College) Degree: Indisch Arts [Indies Physician]
Geneeskundige Hoogeschool (1927–42)	Batavia Medical School Degree: Arts [Physician] Degree after dissertation: Docter in de Geneeskunde [Doctor in Medical Science]
Jakarta Ika Daigaku (1943–45)	Jakarta Medical School, during the Japanese annexation
Balai Perguruan Tinggi, RI (1945–49)	Indonesian Institute of Higher Education
Pendidikan Tinggi Kedoktoran (1945–49)	Faculty of Medicine
Fakultas Kedoktoran, Universitas Indonesia (1950–)	Faculty of Medicine, University of Indonesia

Medical Education in Surabaya

Nederlandsch-Indische Artsen School; NIAS (1913–42)	Surabaya Medical College Degree: Indisch Arts [Indies Physician]

The Main Hospital in Batavia/Jakarta

(Batavia) Centraal Burgelijk Ziekenhuis; CBZ (1919–42)	(Batavia) Central Civic Hospital
Ika Daigaku Byongin (1943–45) or Rumah Sakit Perguruan Tinggi	Jakarta University Hospital
Rumah Sakit Perguruan Tinggi (1945–48)	Jakarta University Hospital
Rumah Sakit Umum Pusat (1950–64)	Central General Hospital
Rumah Sakit Umum Pusat Cipto Mangunkusumo (1964–)	Cipto Mangunkusumo Central General Hospital

A Note on Spelling, Pronunciation, and Names

Indonesian spelling has changed over the years, even though these changes have not been uniformly applied, in names in particular. For the names of the characters in this book, I use the way their names were spelled at the time. For example, I refer to Tjipto Mangoenkoesoemo instead of Cipto Mangunkusumo. For geographical indications, I use today's spelling, referring to, for example, Surabaya rather than Soerabaja.

Most Indonesian names do not follow the common Western convention of using a first name or names, followed by a family name, although many currently use names according to Western conventions by passing the last element of their name on to their children. Many Indonesians only have one name (e.g. Sukarno). In some regions, clan names function as last names (e.g. in the Batak name Parada Harahap). Menadose and Moluccan families adopted the Western pattern of naming early on: the brother of Moluccan physician Willem Karel Tehupeiory was Johannes Everhardus Tehupeiory; they shared their last name with their father. These conventions were not followed elsewhere: the name of Abdul Rivai's father, who came from the Minangkabau area in Sumatra, was Abdul Karim. In general, persons are named using the more unique part of their names (Mohamad Amir was generally called 'Amir'; Abdul Rivai 'Rivai'). The Javanese generally call someone by the first part of their name: Professor Sarwono Prawirohardjo was generally called Professor Sarwono – using the first name did not indicate any disrespect.

Several areas in Indonesia have great varieties of noble and aristocratic titles. The most common Javanese titles are Mas, Raden, and Raden Mas, which precede the first name (and are often abbreviated as 'M.', 'R.', and 'R. M.'), although the use of these honorific titles is optional. The last element of the names of upper-level Javanese aristocrats ends with –*ningrat*: for example: R. M. Soewardi Soerja*ningrat*). Indonesians could change their names during their lifetime (Soewardi renamed himself Ki Hadjar Dewantara in 1922, when he turned forty) or when aristocratic titles were bestowed upon them (Radjiman Wediodipoero's name became *Kanjeng Raden Tumenggung* Radjiman Wediodi*ningrat*; the first three elements of the name are honorifics). Sumatra also bestows a great number of aristocratic titles, which generally follow the last element of one's name and title [*gelar*]. Abdul Rasjid's full name was Abdul Rasjid *gelar* Maharadja Mahkota Soangkoepon. Some Indonesians make up a short version of their name for general use. Abdurrahman Wahid, the fourth president of Indonesia, for example, is generally known as Gus Dur.

The legal system in the Dutch East Indies divided the population into three categories: Europeans, foreign Orientals (mostly Chinese and Arab traders), and natives. These categories map imperfectly onto social and anthropological categories with the same name. When, in this book, I use the term 'native', I follow common usage in colonial discourse and generally refer to the legal category.

All translations of Indonesian and Dutch sources are mine, unless otherwise indicated.

Introduction: Colonial Dreams, National Awakenings, and Cosmopolitan Aspirations

On 20 May 2008, I stood outside Jakarta's Museum of National Awakening, located at the premises of the former Batavia Medical College, about to attend a symposium commemorating the centenary of Indonesia's 'National Awakening'. A large banner reading 'Indonesia Can' ['*Indonesia Bisa*'] featured two historical figures, the physicians Soetomo and Wahidin Soedirohoesodo, with the colonial medical college in the background (Figure 0.1).[1] Adjacent were pictures of Indonesia's then president and vice president waving Indonesian flags. Other images depicted the country's proud embrace of modernity: skyscrapers, highways, fighter jets, an electric train, a navy ship, an airport, a large harbour, and students working at computers. Smaller images portrayed people wearing traditional attire and sportsmen holding an impressive trophy. The event celebrated the founding of Boedi Oetomo [Noble Endeavour] in the medical college's main lecture hall by a group of medical students led by Soetomo and Wahidin.[2] Boedi Oetomo advocated access to modern education for all Javanese

---

[1] The suffix *–hoesodo* indicates 'healer' in Javanese. The slogan 'Indonesia Bisa!' appears to have been inspired by Barack Obama's slogan for the 2008 American presidential election: 'Yes, we can!'

[2] The leading role of physicians and medical students in the Indonesian nationalist movement has been observed in passing by several historians. M. C. Ricklefs mentions that the STOVIA was 'one of the most important institutions producing the lesser *priyayi* [clerks and lower functionaries in the colonial administration]' and discusses the leading role of medical students in the Indonesian youth movement and the political activities of a number of Indonesian physicians. Colin Brown, in his *Short History of Indonesia*, attributes the involvement of medical students in the founding of Boedi Oetomo to their commitment to education: 'These students represented the new emerging Indonesian professional elite, people making their way in the world not through reliance on birth or family connections but through their own efforts, and particularly through education.' George McTurnan Kahin, in his path-breaking study on the Indonesian revolution, commented that a 'surprising number of Indonesian nationalist leaders ... have been and are doctors' but does not explore why this might be the case. Bruce Grant, in his introductory *Indonesia*, states that 'physicians had an unusual influence in the nationalist movement [and] the number of medical doctors in responsible political positions shortly after independence was noticeable.' The authors of the standard *National History of Indonesia*, used in most Indonesian high schools, stated that the 'spirit of nationalism started blooming' at the Batavia Medical College. See M. C. Ricklefs, *A History of Modern Indonesia: c. 1200 to the Present*, 3rd edn (Stanford, CA: Stanford University Press, 2001), 197; Colin Brown, *A Short History of Indonesia: The Unlikely Nation?* (Sydney: Allen & Unwin, 2003), 118; George McTurnan

1

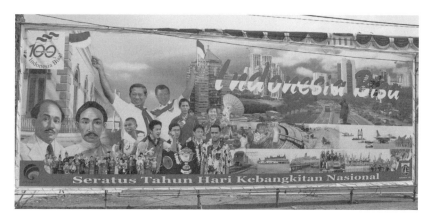

Figure 0.1 Banner outside the Museum of National Awakening, Jakarta, on the occasion of the symposium commemorating 100 years of national awakening on 20 May 2008. Figure by author

and is widely viewed as Indonesia's first nationalist organisation.[3] Wahidin has been called the 'spiritual father of the entire Indies movement' and 'the figure who separate[d] our past from our future'.[4] Many Indonesians view the former medical college as a place where a new form of political awareness emerged which, eventually, led to today's Indonesia. In March 2014, Joko Widodo, later Indonesia's seventh president, launched his election campaign in the same building.[5] 'This is the place where Indonesia's … national awakening began',

Kahin, *Nationalism and Revolution in Indonesia* (Ithaca, NY: Cornell University Press, 1952), 58; Bruce Grant, *Indonesia*, 3rd edn (Melbourne: Melbourne University Press, 1996), 21; Marwati Djoened Poesponegoro and Nugroho Notosusanto, *Zaman Kebangkitan Nasional dan Masa Hindia Belanda* [*The Era of National Awakening and Dutch Colonial Times*], 6 vols., vol. 5, Sejarah Nasional Indonesia (Jakarta: Balai Pustaka, 2008), 113.

[3] See, for example, Goenawan Mangoenkoesoemo and Soewardi Soeryaningrat in Sosro Kartono, Noto Soeroto, and Soewardi Soeryaningrat, eds., *Soembangsih: Gedenkboek Boedi Oetomo, 1908–1918* (Amsterdam: Tijdschrift Nederlandsch Indië Oud & Nieuw, 1918); Soewardi Soeryaningrat, *Levensschets van Wahidin Soedirohoesodo* (The Hague: Hadi Poestaka, 1922), 5, 7, 9. This honour was bestowed upon Boedi Oetomo for many reasons. It was a Javanese movement, it embraced education and other ideas of the Ethical Policy, and it was silent on the role of Islam, to mention a few. The Sarekat Islam [Islamic Association, founded in 1912] has been proposed as alternative first nationalist movement in the Indies; see, for example, Achmad Mansur Suryanegara, *Api Sejarah: Buku yang Akan Mengubah Drastis Pandangan Anda tentang Sejarah Indonesia* (Bandung: Salamadani Pustaka Semesta, 2009). For the history of Boedi Oetomo, see Akira Nagazumi, *The Dawn of Indonesian Nationalism: The Early Years of the Budi Utomo, 1908–1918* (Tokyo: Institute of Developing Economies, 1972); and Bambang Eryudhawan, ed. *100 Tahun Kebangkitan Nasional: Jejak Boedi Oetomo, Peristiwa, Tokoh dan Tempat* (Jakarta: Badan Pelestarian Pusaka Indonesia, 2009).

[4] Soeryaningrat, *Levensschets Wahidin*, 4, 9.

[5] Michael Bachelard, 'Red-Hot Favourite Joko Widodo Launches Presidential Campaign in Indonesia', *Sydney Morning Herald*, 17 March 2014, www.smh.com.au/world/redhot-favourite-joko-widodo-launches-presidential-campaign-in-indonesia-20140316-hvjdc.html, accessed on 17 March 2014.

the cradle of Indonesian nationalism, and therefore, he declared, the most suitable place to announce Indonesia's next mental revolution: 'We hope that with a new national awakening, [the era] of [a] Great Indonesia will begin.'[6]

The metaphor of Indonesia's national awakening originated in colonial times with the founding of Boedi Oetomo. It was first articulated by Conrad Theodor van Deventer, a lawyer, Member of Parliament, prolific writer of opinion pieces, and one of the leading advocates of the so-called Ethical Policy – the Dutch equivalent of the British 'white man's burden' and the French *mission civilatrice* – which was inaugurated as the official colonial policy of the Netherlands in 1901. Rather than viewing the colonies purely as opportunities for profit, advocates of the Ethical Policy urged the citizens of the Netherlands to accept their God-given guardianship over the Indies. Colonial profits were to be reinvested in the colony itself, with a view to elevate the indigenous population through modern education, technological innovation, agricultural reform, and economic development. As with the imperial discourses of England and France, however, there was an element of darkness within the Ethical Policy. Historian Elsbeth Locher-Scholten has analysed the enmeshment of Dutch imperialism, colonial expansion, and the subjugation of the indigenous population with its ideals, which amounted to 'acquiring *de facto* political control of the entire archipelago and the development of both country and people under Dutch leadership and after Western example'.[7] The Ethical Policy, then, entailed extensive military campaigns, the subordination or displacement of local rulers, and the forceful suppression of opposition. Those who promoted the Policy had faith that modern civilisation would supplant primitive and tribal communities following the full subjugation of the archipelago.

Dutch politicians gave admirable motives for their colonial initiatives. The *Pax Neerlandica*, they argued, 'liberated' the indigenous population from pointless tribal warfare, headhunting, barbarism, and exploitation by warlords and power-hungry sultans. Direct intervention in the economy and in society through irrigation projects, new agricultural methods, modern infrastructure, a banking system providing small credits, subsidies for indigenous industry and

---

[6] From the speech Joko Widodo held at the Museum Kebangkitan Nasional, as quoted in 'Indonesian Political Parties Mark Start of Campaign Season', *Jakarta Globe*, 16 March 2014, www.thejakartaglobe.com/news/indonesia-political-parties-mark-start-campaign-season/, accessed on 17 March 2014. On Joko Widodo's promise of a mental revolution, see also Hans Nicholas Jong, 'Jokowi Wants to Start "Mental Revolution"', *Jakarta Post*, 12 May 2014, www.thejakartapost.com/news/2014/05/12/jokowi-wants-start-mental-revolution.html, accessed on 3 March 2017.

[7] Elsbeth Locher-Scholten, *Ethiek in Fragmenten: Vijf Studies over Koloniaal Denken en Doen van Nederlanders in de Indonesische Archipel, 1877–1942* (Utrecht: H&S, 1981), 212–13. Other important sources on the Dutch Ethical Policy are Suzanne Moon, *Technology and Technical Idealism: A History of Development in the Netherlands East Indies* (Leiden: CNWS, 2007) and Robert Cribb, 'Development Policy in the Early 20th Century', in *Development and Social Welfare: Indonesia's Experiences under the New Order*, ed. Jan-Paul Dirkse, Frans Hüsken, and Mario Rutten (Leiden: KITLV Press, 1993).

arts, transmigration programs, and expanded educational opportunities would result in previously unknown levels of prosperity. In 1904, lieutenant-general J. B. van Heutsz – nicknamed the butcher of Aceh – claimed victory in the brutal warfare against the Acehnese that had lasted more than forty years. This is the symbolic marker of the subjugation of all rebellious groups in the archipelago.[8] That same year, van Heutsz was appointed Governor-General, and became widely known for his 'Ethical' initiatives, particularly in the field of education. With military control established, such initiatives sought to produce a mental transformation among the indigenous population, instilling true affection for and genuine allegiance to the Dutch queen. After establishing military control, the Dutch wanted to colonise the Indonesian mind.[9]

The Dutch considered education the most suitable method for transforming supposedly ignorant, primitive, and restive indigenous 'natives' into obedient, civilised, and productive colonial subjects.[10] At the founding of Boedi Oetomo, van Deventer waxed poetic, evoking Plato's allegory of the cave and a well-known European fairy tale:

The miracle has happened. Insulinde, sleeping beauty, has awoken. Half dreaming still she raises herself from her resting place … and moves her hand to cover her eyes to avoid the bright sunlight. She directs her gaze to the West, as if she expects to find there the answer to the question of what is going to happen to her.[11]

How had this miracle come to pass? Was it a loving kiss from a fair Western prince, or had the long-term burden of economic exploitation become unbearable? Did her awakening echo Japan's victory over Russia in 1905, or had the wind conveyed the sounds of other Asian voices to her? Perhaps it was simply time to wake.[12] All these factors had played a role, suggested van Deventer. Something had changed in the Indies, and new aspirations, new ways of life, and new ways of feeling, thinking, and behaving were emerging – the many

---

[8] For the way the brutality of the Aceh war registered, or failed to register in Dutch national memory, see Paul Bijl, *Emerging Memory: Photographs of Colonial Atrocity in Dutch Cultural Remembrance* (Amsterdam: Amsterdam University Press, 2015).

[9] The terms 'Indonesia' and 'Indonesian' were not commonly used until around 1925. When they were introduced, they carried a distinct political loading. In this chapter, I use these phrases to describe the indigenous population of the Dutch East Indies. In the remainder of this book, I follow the usage common at the time.

[10] In this book, I use the word 'native' despite its current derogatory meaning. My reasons for this are twofold: first, I do not want to 'clean up' the discourse of colonial Europeans; second, in the Dutch East Indies, the term 'native' referred to a legal category to which all individuals indigenous to the Indies belonged. The two other legal categories were 'foreign Orientals' (for Chinese-Indonesians and Arab-Indonesians) and Europeans.

[11] Conrad Theodor van Deventer, 'Insulinde's Toekomst', *De Gids* 72, no. 3 (July 1908), 69. Van Deventer's 1899 article 'Een Eereschuld [A Debt of Honour]' is generally considered the founding document of the Ethical Policy. See Conrad Theodor van Deventer, 'Een Ereschuld', *De Gids* 63 (1899), 205–57.

[12] Van Deventer, 'Insulinde's Toekomst', 69, paraphrased.

promises of modernity. The medical students who founded Boedi Oetomo, recipients of the most advanced form of education available in the Indies, had banded together to bring education, progress, and the fruits of modern science, technology, and medicine to Java and then to the archipelago as a whole. It was a colonial dream come true for van Deventer: Indonesians had embraced the ideals of the Ethical Policy and made them their own.

In this book, I explore the relationship between medicine, colonial modernity, and decolonisation in the Dutch East Indies. I investigate why a number of outspoken Indonesian medical students and physicians embraced Western ideals of science and progress, and how this inspired them to participate in the nationalist movement. I look at the roles they played in the various associations, unions, and political parties that, together, formed the Indonesian nationalist movement. I analyse how they imagined the future of the Indies, why many of them came to support independence, and how they participated in building the Indonesian nation after independence had been achieved.[13] I investigate how the multiple and at times conflicting commitments of Indies physicians and medical students to the colonial state, Western modernity, the cosmopolitan medical profession, and their ethnic traditions and cultural heritage inspired them to articulate new personal and professional identities, to formulate new scientific ideals, to shape social and political associations, and eventually to push for independence. Finally, I examine how Indonesia's physicians viewed their changing relationship with the state as their identity shifted from *nationalist* physicians in a colonial state to *national* physicians in an independent one.

In the past three decades it has become commonplace to portray medicine as a tool of empire.[14] This book instead investigates the role of medicine in the process of decolonisation. Medicine inspired Indonesian physicians to criticise the colonial administration for the high prevalence of disease among the indigenous population and the colony's inadequate health care provisions. It offered methods, styles of thinking, and biological and physiological metaphors, for evaluating colonial society and diagnosing its ills. Indonesian physicians were ideally placed to diagnose the colonial social body, to prescribe therapeutic interventions, and to determine how colonial realities impeded the

---

[13] For a different analysis of the role of science, Western-style education, and modernity in the Indonesian nationalist movement, see Andrew Goss, *The Floracrats: State-Sponsored Science and the Failure of the Enlightenment in Indonesia* (Madison: University of Wisconsin Press, 2011), 96–116.

[14] For historians who analysed medicine as a tool of empire, see Daniel R. Headrick, *The Tools of Empire: Technology and European Imperialism in the Nineteenth Century* (New York: Oxford University Press, 1981); Roy MacLeod, 'Introduction', in *Disease, Medicine, and Empire: Perspectives on Western Medicine and the Experience of European Expansion*, ed. Roy MacLeod and Milton Lewis (London: Routledge, 1988), 1–18.

natural process of social evolution. It was their commitment to medicine that inspired several of these young men to imagine a new, independent, and healthy nation. Individually and through their professional association, these physicians actively articulated their scientific identity, which included views on the potential and actual roles of medicine in colonial society, and ideas on the nature of that society itself. This motivated them first to criticise colonial health provisions and then to formulate medical policies that would serve all Indonesians. Throughout the first part of the twentieth century, Indonesian physicians retained their dedication to science and medicine as well as to progress and development but became increasingly disenchanted with the strictures of colonial society and its Dutch rulers who continued to portray themselves as benefactors. After independence, they found themselves in a very different political context, where these strictures no longer pertained. Unfortunately, Indonesian physicians were not able to realise their medical ideals fully in an independent Indonesia.

Medicine and the Ethical Policy

Until the late nineteenth century, Dutch military offices, merchants, and soldiers feared the East Indies as one of the unhealthiest places in the world. There were periods when all soldiers of new regiments perished within three years of arrival; it was not unusual for a third of the European population to die each year. Batavia was widely known as the Europeans' graveyard.[15] The colonies were rife with diseases hardly known in Europe, and Dutch physicians did not know how to treat them. Malaria was endemic in coastal settlements, near swamps, and on recently established plantations; dysentery and various other intestinal ailments were common as were dengue fever and typhoid. Cholera, influenza, tuberculosis, and nutritional deficiencies such as beriberi also caused problems for Europeans. Before the 1870s, physicians attributed the high mortality rate of Europeans in the tropics to a mismatch between race and climate, and argued that whites could never flourish there. Medical investigation focused on the process of acclimatisation, and the factors that accelerated or impeded it.[16] European physicians were not particularly concerned about

---

[15] Hans Pols, 'Notes from Batavia, the Europeans' Graveyard: The 19th Century Debate on Acclimatization in the Dutch East Indies', *Journal of the History of Medicine and Allied Sciences* 67, no. 1 (2012), 120–48.

[16] For medical theories on acclimatisation, see Philip D. Curtin, ' "The White Man's Grave": Image and Reality, 1780–1850', *Journal of British Studies* 1, no. 1 (1961), 94–110; Dane Kennedy, 'The Perils of the Midday Sun: Climatic Anxieties in the Colonial Tropics', in *Imperialism and the Natural World*, ed. John M. MacKenzie (Manchester: Manchester University Press, 1990), 118–40; Mark Harrison, *Climates and Constitutions: Health, Race, Environment and British Imperialism in India, 1600–1850* (New Dehli: Oxford University Press, 1999); Warwick Anderson, *Colonial Pathologies: American Tropical Medicine, Race, and Hygiene in the*

the health of indigenous people who were, by the same logic, ideally adjusted to the tropical environment and, by definition, in good health. Early in the nineteenth century, the colonial administration established a medical service to provide care to soldiers, officers, and administrative officials. Although keeping these officials in good health was necessary to maintain colonial rule, the medical service was chronically underfunded and had a poor reputation. The indigenous population came to its attention only when epidemics that might threaten Europeans broke out, providing the rationale for extensive smallpox vaccination campaigns.

In the 1880s, European and North American physicians who saw the significance of the recent discoveries of Louis Pasteur and Robert Koch on the role of microbes in disease transmission advocated broad sanitary measures to improve health. These included establishing sewers, supplying fresh drinking water, improving food production, institutionalising building codes, and making health care available to all.[17] Individual behaviour was also targeted: washing hands and cooking food were encouraged, and spitting in public discouraged.[18] Around the turn of the twentieth century, medical research in parasitology inspired new ways of framing tropical disease by relating ailments to parasites, other microorganisms, and disease vectors, rather than to a mismatch between climate and constitution.[19] European physicians working in the colonies advocated environmental measures to promote health, such as clearing swamps to deprive mosquito larvae of places to grow, and supplementary changes in individual behaviour, including the use of mosquito nets and personal hygiene. Despite profound changes in medical theory, European physicians continued to see the Indies as an essentially unhealthy place, but they had acquired some optimism that Europeans could adopt strategies to circumvent, manage, and alleviate tropical diseases. The once reassuring idea that indigenous people were more or less healthy was shattered as it became clear that they in fact suffered from the conditions which affected Europeans, and in greater numbers,

---

Philippines (Durham, NC: Duke University Press, 2006); and David N. Livingstone, 'Tropical Climate and Moral Hygiene: The Anatomy of a Victorian Debate', *British Journal for the History of Science* 32, no. 1 (1999), 93–110.

[17] See Nancy Tomes, *The Gospel of Germs: Men, Women, and the Microbe in American Life* (Cambridge, MA: Harvard University Press, 1998) and Michael Worboys, *Spreading Germs: Disease Theories, and Medical Practice in Britain, 1865–1900* (New York: Cambridge University Press, 2000).

[18] Tomes, *The Gospel of Germs*.

[19] Laurence Monnais and Hans Pols, 'Health and Disease in the Colonies: Medicine in the Age of Empire', in *The Routledge History of Western Empires*, ed. Robert Aldrich and Kirsten McKenzie (New York: Routledge, 2014), 270–84. For the notion of framing disease, see Charles E. Rosenberg and Janet Golden, eds., *Framing Disease: Studies in Cultural History, Health and Medicine in American Society* (New Brunswick, NJ: Rutgers University Press, 1992).

and also from yaws, infestations with hookworm and other parasitic intestinal worms, trachoma, and smallpox. The colonists had simply not noticed.

Inspired by these recent developments in medical science, pioneering physician W. T. de Vogel, future director of the Indies Civil Medical Service, introduced measures of urban sanitation and *kampong* [indigenous neighbourhood] improvement in Semarang around the turn of the twentieth century.[20] He successfully guided the expanding city away from the malarious coast to the salubrious hills. At the same time, German physician and future professor of tropical medicine at the University of Amsterdam W. A. P. Schüffner was implementing a systematic public health program in the Deli plantation area around Medan, on the east coast of Sumatra, which led to a significant reduction in illness and premature death among indentured plantation workers.[21] Schüffner's initiatives were the medical counterpart of the 'Deli miracle', the development of vast and immensely profitable plantations in Deli. In this sparsely populated area, 'coolies' (indentured labourers) were recruited in China and Java, and a premium was placed on their productivity – and therefore on their health. Schüffner's initiatives were so successful that the plantation owners who had employed him became convinced that the Indies needed more, and more affordable, physicians. In 1899, three wealthy plantation owners who were known as 'welfare capitalists' in the Netherlands donated funds for a new building for the Batavia Medical School (Figure 0.2). They believed that modern medical science could make the Indies safe for European habitation and transform natives into energetic workers for Dutch mines and plantations. Western medicine could also convince natives of the superiority of European civilisation and instil gratitude towards the colonisers. Moreover, they expected that locally trained and modestly waged indigenous physicians would be eager to provide the needed services. The enormous growth of the privately run plantation economy in the Indies was therefore the main driver of medical education.

In the 1880s, Indonesian intellectuals began to identify progress and development as ways to realise modern conditions in the colonies. Modernist idealism was highly appealing to Indies physicians (the degree conferred by the Batavia Medical Colleges was Indies Physician [*Indisch Arts*]), who were convinced that medical science was of tremendous potential benefit to Indonesians. Modern medicine, which they believed had powerful tools to

---

[20] De Vogel was assisted by pharmacist-turned millionaire H. F. Tillema. For a biography of the latter, including the public health initiatives both undertook, see Ewald Vanvugt, *Een Propagandist van het Zuiverste Water: H. F. Tillema (1870–1952) en de Fotografie van Tempo Doeloe* (Amsterdam: Jan Mets, 1993).

[21] See Jan Peter Verhave, *The Moses of Malaria: Nicolaas H. Swellengrebel (1885–1970) Abroad and at Home* (Rotterdam: Erasmus Publishing, 2011).

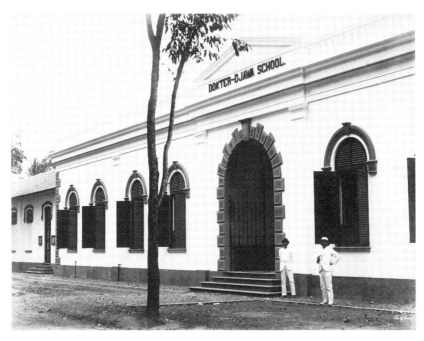

Figure 0.2 The Dokter Djawa School around the turn of the twentieth century, just after the new building had been completed. In 1902 it was renamed as the School for the Education of Native Physicians [School ter Opleiding van Inlandsche Artsen] (STOVIA). Figure: University of Leiden library, KITLV collection (35810)

eradicate disease, appeared far superior to the age-old medical traditions of the Indies. It constituted a novel site of authority which enabled young educated men to question traditional medicine and, subsequently, tradition in general and traditional hierarchies. Their dedication to science and medicine became part of a broader social program – a political commitment to emancipation, equality, and progress. 'Progress' and 'modernity' may imply science, learning, and education, but also, as Henk Schulte Nordholt has argued, a modern lifestyle characterised by consumption, fashion, hygiene, and the conveniences of new technologies, including modern transport and communications.[22] The

---

[22] Henk Schulte Nordholt, 'Modernity and Cultural Citizenship in the Netherlands Indies: An Illustrated Hypothesis', *Journal of Southeast Asian Studies* 42, no. 3 (2011) 435–57. See also Henk Schulte Nordholt, 'Modernity and Middle Classes in the Netherlands Indies: Cultivating Cultural Citizenship', in *Photography, Modernity and the Governed in Late-Colonial*

protagonists of modernity were the middle classes, who came to distinguish themselves through their education, new skills, and new knowledge. The small group of educated Indonesians slowly grew after the turn of the twentieth century. Its members articulated their distinct, modern identity through their educational accomplishments and their belief in the powers of science, medicine, and technology. In the words of David Scott, they were conscripts of modernity: their adherence to these ideals was neither voluntary nor accidental, but the foundation of their modern identities.[23]

Advocates of modernity worldwide questioned tradition, religion, and hierarchies; they renounced the past and embraced the future.[24] They promoted personal liberation, freedom, and equality, all to be achieved through the elevation of reason. Some applied evolutionary models to human societies, and came to hold an intense faith in social development. It was driven by economic rationalisation, agricultural reform, industrialisation, urbanisation, secularisation, and human migration, and its markers were scientific, technological, and economic progress. Others viewed modernity politically, and saw its realisation in democracy, educational institutions, and efficient state bureaucracies. The foundational idea of modernism is that human society is open to human intervention, and may be moulded to suit the needs of humankind. The pursuit of modernity led to the rise of cosmopolitanism – the discounting of racial, ethnic, and cultural distinctions, and the heralding of a global community transcending national boundaries. For cosmopolitans, all peoples were members of the same human family, and all were striving towards the common good.[25] The scientific and medical communities exemplified cosmopolitanism: they were inherently egalitarian, and dedicated to the common good, to progress and to social evolution through the application of scientific findings. To Indies physicians, the egalitarian nature of the imagined cosmopolitan medical profession provided a distinct contrast to the realities of colonial life, where racial and ethnic distinctions were paramount and educational accomplishment signified little, despite repeated promises to the contrary.

Indonesia, ed. Susie Protschky (Amsterdam: Amsterdam University Press, 2015), 223–54; and Tom Hoogervorst and Henk Schulte Nordholt, 'Urban Middle Classes in Colonial Java (1900–1942): Images and Language', *Bijdragen tot de Taal-, Land- en Volkenkunde* 173 (2017), 442–74.

23 David Scott, *Conscripts of Modernity: The Tragedy of Colonial Enlightenment* (Durham, NC: Duke University Press, 2004).

24 See, for example, Marshall Berman, *All That Is Solid Melts into Air: The Experience of Modernity* (New York: Simon & Schuster, 1982), in particular the introduction, as most of the rest of the book applies more to Europe and North America than the rest of the world.

25 Kwame Anthony Appiah, *Cosmopolitanism: Ethics in a World of Strangers* (New York: Penguin, 2007), 10–18.

Medicine, Politics, Nationalism, and Decolonisation

In Asia, it was not uncommon for physicians to be involved in politics, and their political activism has received some historical attention.[26] In *Doctors within Borders*, Ming-Cheng M. Lo analysed how Taiwanese physicians articulated their identity as physicians of the nation on the basis of their professional training and in opposition to the Japanese colonial powers.[27] Warwick Anderson has detailed the political activities of physicians in the Philippines, starting with José Rizal.[28] Vincanne Adams has examined the role of physicians in Nepal's democratic revolution in the early 1990s.[29] Pheng Cheah has analysed literary sources from Indonesia and other Southeast Asian countries, and concluded that the many biological, physiological, and evolutionary metaphors used in political discourse are traces of the central roles that physicians have played in political movements.[30] Dealing with another continent, Marcos Cueto and Steven Palmer have observed that many Latin American medical leaders became politicians during the first part of the nineteenth century when most colonies won independence.[31] John Iliffe has analysed the development of the medical profession in Uganda, Tanzania, and Kenya. In each, medicine played an important role in the history of nationalism and decolonisation.[32] Medical anthropologist Claire Wendland has described how physicians in poverty-stricken Malawi were confronted with hospitals and clinics virtually devoid of medical equipment and necessary medications because of bureaucratic failures, economic mismanagement, misappropriation of funds, outright corruption, and lack of political commitment to health. Empathising with their patients, they engaged in political activism, calling for incremental improvement.[33] Additional observations suggests that physicians from various countries and continents have embraced political activism: Sun Yat Sen, Ramon Betances, and Che Guevara were all physicians, as are Mahathir Mohamad, Radovan Karadžić, and Bashar al-Assad.

---

[26] See also Warwick Anderson and Hans Pols, 'Scientific Patriotism: Medical Science and National Self-Fashioning in Southeast Asia', *Comparative Studies in Society and History* 54, no. 1 (2012), 93–113.

[27] Ming-Cheng M. Lo, *Doctors within Borders: Profession, Ethnicity, and Modernity in Colonial Taiwan* (Berkeley: University of California Press, 2002).

[28] Anderson, *Colonial Pathologies*.

[29] Vincanne Adams, *Doctors for Democracy: Health Professionals in the Nepal Revolution* (Cambridge: Cambridge University Press, 1998).

[30] Pheng Cheah, *Spectral Nationality: Passages of Freedom from Kant to Postcolonial Literatures of Liberation* (New York: Columbia University Press, 2003).

[31] Marcos Cueto and Steven Palmer, *Medicine and Public Health in Latin America: A History* (Cambridge: Cambridge University Press, 2014), 51.

[32] John Iliffe, *East African Doctors: A History of the Modern Profession* (Cambridge: Cambridge University Press, 1998).

[33] Claire Wendland, *A Heart for the Work: Journeys through an African Medical School* (Chicago: University of Chicago Press, 2010).

Starting in the late nineteenth century, physiological metaphors became increasingly common in political discourse. Philosopher Auguste Comte had already connected science, progress, and social evolution, and nominated sociology as the science most suitable for analysing the social body. Ernest Gellner, one of the foremost scholars of nationalism, has argued that during the late nineteenth century the discourse of nationalism shifted 'from history to biology as the main mythopoetic science'.[34] Organic metaphors and evolutionary theory came to permeate nationalist ideas, and societies came to be described as social bodies suffering from a range of diseases, which were represented as impediments to the organic process of social evolution. In a similar vein, Indonesian intellectuals have viewed the emergence of nationalist sentiment as the inevitable, organic outcome of social evolution, which necessarily prevails over whatever obstacles it encounters. Evolutionary theory, particularly Herbert Spencer's social Darwinism, reinforced the tendency to analyse social processes as biological ones. In colonial regions it was physicians who were conversant in these sciences, uniquely placing them to diagnose the pathologies of colonialism, identify the nature and pressures inherent in the process of social evolution, and prescribe therapeutic interventions for social arrangements gone awry.

The everyday experiences of physicians and medical students also inspired the development of political awareness. During their residential training, medical students are readily sensitised to cultural, social, economic, and political issues because they are regularly in contact with a broad cross-section of society. More than most professionals, physicians are consistently confronted with the human suffering of members of all social classes and ethnic groups. In the Dutch East Indies, they were exposed to the unhygienic conditions and poverty of *kampongs* and *desas* [rural villages]. Some of them came to realise that their patients suffered not only from disease but also from poverty, malnutrition, and, at times, adverse working conditions, abuse, cruelty, and the impact of military interventions. In their medical practice, Indies physicians witnessed these realities of colonial life, which were unusually conducive to the spread of disease and the incidence of injuries. They also observed that the colonial administration allocated insufficient funds for the medical care of the indigenous population, and came to express these complaints publicly.

During the nineteenth and twentieth centuries, a handful of European physicians participated in politics, as the work of the brilliant and influential nineteenth-century German biomedical scientist Rudolf Virchow illustrates. During 1848, the year of revolution, Virchow wrote that 'medicine is a

---

[34] Ernest Gellner, *Nationalism* (New York: New York University Press, 1997), 74.

social science, and politics is nothing else but medicine on a large scale.' He saw physicians as 'the natural attorney of the poor'.[35] Virchow developed his radical political ideas while investigating a typhus epidemic in Upper Silesia – a poor, predominantly Polish area under Prussian control. Rather than recommending sending more physicians, opening more hospitals, and distributing medicines, Virchow advocated democratic self-government, using Polish as the official language, separating church and state, and organising agricultural cooperatives: he prescribed political change, not medicine, to treat underlying etiological conditions. This same argument appeared in the Dutch East Indies. In 1847, a year before Virchow presented his ideas, Willem Bosch, head of the colonial Medical Service from 1845 to 1854, criticised the appalling state of health of the indigenous population while investigating a typhoid fever epidemic in Central Java.[36] The cultivation system, he argued, which required Javanese farmers to produce export crops on 20 per cent of their land, had produced widespread poverty, hunger, and malnutrition. Bosch was likely the first European physician in the Indies whose commitment to medicine inspired a critique of colonial governance.

The ambiguous social status of Indies physicians provided an additional spur for their political engagement. The status Indonesian physicians enjoyed was a source of both pride and perpetual discontent. Having received the most advanced form of education in the colony, Indies physicians became the first indigenous group that could claim entry into the European sphere.[37] They supported this claim in their dress, palates, and social manners, but despite their qualifications and aspirations, their hopes of social advancement were rarely fulfilled. The medical degree available in the Indies was considered inferior to European ones, so Indies physicians received less than half the salary of their European colleagues and were placed in less desirable positions in the colonial medical service. Colonial Europeans generally regarded Indies physicians and other educated Indies individuals as overly

---

[35] Rudolf Virchow, cited in Rex Taylor and Annelie Rieger, 'Rudolf Virchow on the Typhus Epidemic in Upper Silesia: An Introduction and Translation', *Sociology of Health and Illness* 6, no. 2 (1984), 202; and in Theodore M. Brown and Elizabeth Fee, 'Rudolf Carl Virchow: Medical Scientist, Social Reformer, Role Model', *American Journal of Public Health* 96, no. 12 (2006), 2104. Throughout the twentieth century, many physicians embraced social medicine and explored the ways its mandates could be implemented. See Iris Borowy and Anne Hardy, *Of Medicine and Men: Biographies and Ideas in European Social Medicine between the World Wars* (Frankfurt am Main: Peter Lang, 2008).

[36] See Liesbeth Hesselink, *Healers on the Colonial Market: Native Doctors and Midwives in the Dutch East Indies* (Leiden: KITLV Press, 2011), 58–67; A. H. Borgers, *Doctor Willem Bosch (1798–1874) en zijn Invloed op de Geneeskunde in Nederlandsch Oost-Indië* (Utrecht: Kemink en Zoon, 1941), 95–121.

[37] This aspirational entry in the European social sphere in the Indies was already noted in colonial times. See, for example, I. J. Brugmans, *Geschiedenis van het Onderwijs in Nederlandsch-Indië* (Groningen, Batavia: J. B. Wolters, 1938), 287.

ambitious mimics who had forgotten their place in colonial society. European physicians harboured an especially strong and forthright hostility towards them, which issued from their own social and professional frustrations and their own discontent with their (much higher) salaries. Indies physicians would become the poster children of the successes, failures, and misconceptions of the Ethical Policy.

Halfway through the nineteenth century, several national governments participated in the founding of international agencies to compile statistical information on epidemics, disease outbreaks, the international transfer of disease, and quarantine measures.[38] Around the turn of the twentieth century, newly established international health organisations began compiling epidemiological information and population measures, and making information available worldwide. Alison Bashford has argued that 'world health bodies created new communication circuits, and brought new global biopolitical ambitions for epidemiological intelligence.'[39] These new international organisations also started to address issues related to health and medicine outside the Western world by establishing trans-colonial networks. In particular the Far Eastern Association of Tropical Medicine, which was founded in 1908 and held its first meeting in Manila in 1910, became a meeting point for physicians in Southeast Asia; in 1921, its fourth meeting was held in Batavia.[40] The League of Nations Health Organisation and the International Health Board of the Rockefeller Foundation also commenced operations in Southeast Asia at this time. Sunil Amrith has argued that 'the problems of Asia's health emerged, during the inter-war years, in an increasingly transnational arena of debate and exchange.'[41] As a consequence, the 'field of public health in mid-twentieth-century Asia was, irreducibly, both transnational and international.'[42] Amrith emphasises the importance of indigenous physicians in these international and trans-colonial networks, as they participated in innovative health demonstrations and articulated ideas about international health. Their symbolic and actual participation in the

---

[38] Alison Bashford, *Imperial Hygiene: A Critical History of Colonialism, Nationalism, and Public Health* (Basingstoke: Palgrave MacMillan, 2004); Paul Weindling, ed. *International Health Organizations and Movements, 1918–1939* (New York: Cambridge University Press, 1995).

[39] Alison Bashford, 'Global Biopolitics and the History of World Health', *History of the Human Sciences* 19, no. 1 (2006), 75.

[40] Deborah Neill, *Networks in Tropical Medicine: Internationalism, Colonialism, and the Rise of a Medical Specialty, 1890–1930* (Stanford, CA: Stanford University Press, 2012). On the occasion of the fourth meeting, held in Batavia, the following book was published: L. S. A. M. von Römer, *Historical Sketches: An Introduction to the Fourth Congress of the Far Eastern Association of Tropical Medicine, to be Held at Batavia from 6th to 13th August 1921* (Batavia: Javasche Boekhandel en Drukkerij, 1921).

[41] Sunil S. Amrith, *Decolonizing International Health: India and Southeast Asia, 1930–1965* (Basingstoke: Palgrave Macmillan, 2006), 1.

[42] Amrith, *Decolonizing International Health*, 11.

international and global world of medicine strengthened their identification with the cosmopolitan medical profession.

Medical students in the Indies participated symbolically in the international and cosmopolitan world of medicine by reading medical textbooks from the Netherlands, Germany, France, the United Kingdom, and the United States. Through their participation in international networks of health and medicine, leading Indies physicians helped shape new discourses on health beyond national and colonial boundaries, the organisation of medicine, and the relationship between health, social conditions, and political realities. During the 1930s, Indies physicians' criticism of the colonial health service was bolstered by their knowledge of health conditions and health arrangements elsewhere in Southeast Asia. Their participation in the health demonstration programs of the Rockefeller Foundation made them familiar with alternative ways of organising health care, and Indonesian physicians began participating in the international debates fostered by international health organisations. In the 1950s, the recently founded World Health Organization [WHO] formulated initiatives to stimulate the economies of non-Western nations – initiatives that dealt with economic and political development combined with health. Indonesian physicians took part in these discussions and initiatives and in doing so, they became participants in global medical networks. Even though they no longer lived in a colonial society, they remained, to a certain extent, subordinate to medical experts in international health organisations who provided advice and assistance in the development of Indonesia's health care system.

Chapter Overview

In this book, I highlight the ideas, initiatives, and careers of a specific group of Indonesian physicians and medical students in the Dutch East Indies and then free Indonesia. This group was defined by their views on the political responsibilities of physicians and the role of medicine in society, as well as their readiness to participate in the Indonesian nationalist movement. W. K. Tehupeiory, Jeremias Kaijadoe, and Abdul Rasjid, for example, all played active roles in the Association of Indies Physicians while Rasjid often discussed medical issues as a member of the Volksraad, the proto-parliament of the Dutch East Indies created in 1918. All of them participated in political associations. I focus less on well-known physician-nationalists such as Tjipto Mangoenkoesomo and Raden Soetomo, because their activities have received much historical attention, although without, unfortunately, elaborating upon their medical background.

The origins of the Indonesian nationalist movement were tentative. An Indies vernacular press, considered by historians and political scientists as essential to the formation of nationalist sentiments, appeared in the Indies in the 1880s and featured frequent discussions on progress, development, and education.[43] Around the turn of the twentieth century, a number of Indies physicians and medical students became active as journalists, authors, and editors. In 1902, Abdul Rivai founded the biweekly illustrated magazine *Bintang Hindia* [*Star of the Indies*], which informed readers about everyday life in the Netherlands, the importance of education, and the benefits of modern civilisation. Chapter 1 follows Rivai's activities as a physician, journalist, and politician. Most members of the first generation of nationalist Indies physicians believed that progress could best be realised by working within the framework of the colonial state. The promises of the Ethical Policy Dutch government reinforced their optimism.

The Batavia Medical College and its counterpart in Surabaya, founded in 1913, were theatres for young men (and an increasing but relatively small group of young women) to articulate and perform modern and Western identities (Figure 0.3). As detailed in Chapter 2, during their training they were socialised as members of the cosmopolitan medical profession, which subordinated family ties and ethnic affiliations. Following the well-known arguments of Benedict Anderson, this professional identity became a model for their identification with Indonesia, a country that did not yet exist, but with boundaries that coincided with those of the colony.[44] Through their education, students acquired a medical, biological, and physiological approach to disease, the body, and society. Because biological and physiological metaphors were increasingly used to describe the process of evolution and the diseases that plagued the social body, Indies physicians realised that they were well placed to analyse and diagnose the social and political condition of colonial society.

Although many physicians and medical students accepted their calling as doctors of the nation, they held very different opinions about its current state, its prognosis, and what interventions were necessary. At the first congress of Boedi Oetomo, medical students and other participants expressed various political views, anticipating those articulated later by Indonesian nationalists. Some speakers advocated modernisation on a Western model and the jettisoning of moribund cultural traditions. Others saw in Indonesia's rich cultural heritage the basis for an alternate, Eastern modernity emphasising spirituality and

---

[43] For newspapers, periodicals, and nationalism, see Benedict R. O'G. Anderson, *Imagined Communities: Reflections on the Origin and Spread of Nationalism*, rev. and extended edn (London: Verso, 2006 [1983]), 61–65. For the origins of the vernacular press in the Indies, see Ahmat B. Adam, *The Vernacular Press and the Emergence of Modern Indonesian Consciousness* (Ithaca, NY: Southeast Asia Program, Cornell University, 1995). For a fascinating analysis of the early indigenous press in the Dutch East Indies, see Ulbe Bosma, 'Citizens of Empire: Some Comparative Observations on the Evolution of Creole Nationalism in Colonial Indonesia', *Comparative Studies in Society and History* 46, no. 4 (1004), 646–81.

[44] Anderson, *Imagined Communities*, 119–23.

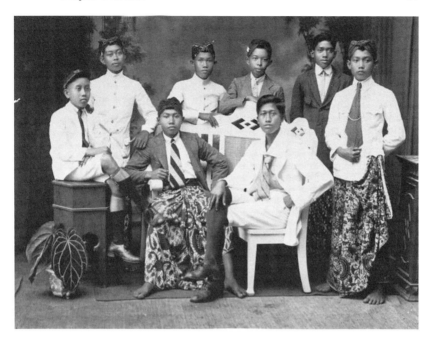

Figure 0.3 Medical students at the Batavia Medical College (STOVIA) in 1919. Figure courtesy of the Dutch National Museum of Ethnology, Leiden (TM-60047128)

communitarianism. Soon after the congress, two participants joined the board of the first political party in the Dutch East Indies advocating independence, though it was shortly afterwards outlawed and its founders exiled. After traditional regents came to dominate Boedi Oetomo's board, medical students founded several youth associations on the basis of ethnic affiliation, which served to prepare them, covertly, for later political action. Boedi Oetomo and its various legacies are the topic of Chapter 3.

Graduates of the Indies medical colleges occupied an ambiguous and at times even paradoxical social position. Because of their advanced education, they aspired to be recognised as equals by their European colleagues. This rarely happened. The Association of Indies Physicians was founded in 1909, and its history is explored in Chapter 4. The emancipatory impulse of the Association was clear from the outset, with a key aim of bringing equality between Indies and European physicians. The Association's activities provide insights into the way members articulated their professional identity. Initially, activities were limited to polite requests to the colonial administration for better working conditions and higher salaries, but by 1919 members had grown sufficiently radical to organise a physicians' strike. At this time, several nationalist leaders identified the inferior professional position of Indies physicians as evidence of the racial discrimination inherent in colonial society, and rallied to their cause.

After 1920, the political climate in the Dutch East Indies became increasingly repressive. Indies physicians were furious when two Dutch colonial psychiatrists publicised theories on the primitive nature of normal Indonesian minds. The fallout of this debate is covered in Chapter 5. The Association of Indies Physicians transformed itself into a scientific society by publishing research conducted by its members and by pursuing and promoting scientific neutrality. Its members decided to forgo political action and to focus instead on training a cadre of physicians capable of staffing the medical institutions of the future, independent nation. This shift in strategy reflected the increasing importance of the small but growing medical elite of Indonesian physicians holding European medical qualifications. Despite vast political changes over the next forty years, the composition of this elite was relatively stable.

The Great Depression devastated the export-based economy of the Dutch East Indies, and the Association of Indies Physicians became inactive. In the late 1930s, Volksraad member Abdul Rasjid reinvigorated it, and from 1938 to 1942 it was more vigorous than ever before. Rasjid formulated a social philosophy employing biological and physiological metaphors to analyse the development of indigenous society and the leading position of Indies physicians within it. Inspired by Rockefeller Foundation health demonstration projects in poor, rural areas – projects which they had participated in – Indies physicians articulated idealistic policies detailing a health care plan for the Indonesian population as a whole. These policies contrasted markedly with existing health provisions, which emphasised hospital-based interventions in large urban areas mostly benefitting Europeans and only a handful of wealthy Indonesians.

The Japanese annexation of the archipelago in 1942, part of the creation of the Greater East Asia Co-Prosperity Sphere, resulted in dramatic political changes. The new political reality after the annexation provided unprecedented opportunities for Indonesia's physicians, which are discussed in Chapter 7. The small medical elite improved its position when its members came to lead the archipelago's medical institutions. The larger group of Indies physicians embraced Japanese medical ideals which closely resembled those of Rasjid. Most Indonesians were quickly disenchanted with the Japanese. In 1943, a large group of medical students actively opposed the new colonial power by covertly organising resistance activities among youth groups. These youths [*pemuda*] came to play a significant role during the Indonesian revolution.

Indonesia declared independence on 17 August 1945. After the Netherlands prepared its armed forces to recolonise the archipelago, conflict broke out and hostilities continued until the end of 1949. With increasing hostilities between the Dutch and the Indonesians, the dormitory of the resurrected

Jakarta Medical School became an important site of resistance. After the Dutch took full control of Jakarta, most Indonesian medical instructors relocated to the heartland of the Republic of Indonesia around Yogyakarta, where they continued to teach medicine. Their commitment to the young republic transformed them into national heroes. At the same time, many young physicians and medical students opted for careers in the military, business, and government, engaging in different types of nation-building. They were badly needed by the new republic, but their decisions left the Indonesian medical profession in a state of disarray.

After the transfer of sovereignty from the Netherlands to Indonesia on 27 December 1949, Indonesian physicians faced the massive task of building a national health care system from the remains of the colonial structures. As Chapter 9 narrates, *nationalist* physicians opposing the colonial state now became *national* physicians working in the state's medical institutions. A variety of international health organisations supported Indonesia's government in this task, strengthening the position of the medical profession. During Sukarno's rule, physicians safeguarded the medical domain by retreating from political activity. Suharto's dictatorial regime required them to relinquish all forms of political involvement. Consequently, political engagement, one of the defining characteristics of the Indonesian medical profession during colonial times, disappeared.

During the second part of the twentieth century, international health organisations assisted governments of developing nations in building national health care systems, thereby strengthening the position of Indonesia's physicians. Beginning with the international AIDS epidemic, and increasingly after the turn of the twenty-first century, new approaches to health threats became dominant, generally clustered under the rubric of 'global health'. Advocates of global health tend to favour vertical, disease-specific programs and pharmaceutical, and vaccine innovation to counter the threats posed by infectious diseases such as tuberculosis, malaria, and AIDS, severe acute respiratory syndrome (SARS), Ebola, and bird and swine influenza, problems that generally exceed national boundaries. Global health initiatives often bypass national governments and rarely depend on, or even interact with, national health care systems. As a consequence of the rise of global health, the status and roles of Indonesian physicians are currently eroding. Indonesian physicians, once dominant on the national stage, often play a subordinate role in global health initiatives, as they did during colonial times.

The dreams of Indonesia's nationalist physicians have faded. Despite the central role of physicians and medical students in Indonesia's nationalist movement, medicine did not flourish after independence. On the banner proudly announcing the centennial of Indonesia's national awakening, one of the well-worn clichés of modernity – well-equipped hospitals and surgeons working at operating tables – was glaringly absent. During colonial times, the desire for emancipation and social advancement spurred many Indies physicians to political action; after independence, this desire became somewhat sated – or at least, divorced from nationalist agitation.[45] Most physicians attending the 2008 symposium commenced their medical studies in the late 1950s and early 1960s. Many had vivid memories of the residual nationalist spirit of those days and the pioneering roles physicians played during the first decades after independence. They were perturbed that financial interests appeared to be more important to today's physicians than the idealistic motives that had predominated in the past. The speakers presented the social and political engagement of Indies physicians in colonial times as examples to be emulated by Indonesia's physicians today.[46] By recounting the history of the founding of Boedi Oetomo, they hoped to rekindle a medical awakening, restoring physicians to the leadership roles they once held in the vanguard of the nation. They yearned for the good old days in the late colonial and early national periods, when Indonesian physicians had been, for a few moments, ascendant.

---

[45] See, for example, Benedict R. O'G. Anderson 'Old State, New Society: Indonesia's New Order in Comparative Historical Perspective', *Journal of Asian Studies* 42, no. 3 (1983), 477–96.

[46] The symposium was opened by then vice president Yusuf Kalla. Speakers were: Goenawan Mohamad (novelist and political commentator), Kartono Mohamad (former president of the Indonesian Medical Association), Firman Lubis (Professor of Public Health, University of Indonesia), Max Lane (scholar and translator of Pramoedya Ananta Toer's *Buru Quartet*), Adrian Vickers (Professor of Indonesian Studies, University of Sydney), Herman Keppy (journalist and novelist), R. Z. Leirissa (Professor of History, University of Indonesia), and the author.

1   Abdul Rivai: Medicine and the Enticement of Modernity

As the most educated natives in the Dutch East Indies, Indies physicians were the social group closest to Europeans. Not only were they well educated, but they spoke Dutch, wore European clothing, and lived in or near European neighbourhoods. They hoped to ascend in the colonial social order by conforming to the expectations and standards of the Dutch colonisers, who were situated at the apex of colonial life and embodied worth and social respectability. Indies physicians were encouraged to pursue social advancement at times, by teachers, colonial bureaucrats, and social commentators, but at other times these efforts were ridiculed as the presumption of natives who had forgotten their proper place. In everyday colonial life, the extent of an individual's Europeanness was determined by a complex and shifting set of criteria which included education, occupation, income, cultural refinement, moral character, appearance, ability to speak Dutch, and the location and quality of the family home, as well as other lifestyle factors including dietary preferences and religious practices. Despite their tenacity, Indies physicians found themselves in an ambiguous and, at times, even paradoxical social position. While the pursuit of personal and professional advancement by forging Western identities might be rewarding in specific circumstances, it was as a whole a frustrating endeavour. In response, many developed an almost obsessive concern with their own place and with that of their profession in colonial society.

In this chapter, I analyse the ideas and activities of the first generation of Indies physicians – those who graduated before the end of World War I. I focus on the small group of Indies physicians who pursued advanced medical training in the Netherlands and obtained Dutch medical qualifications. This group influenced the generation as a whole, shaping its professional and political ideas, and leading initiatives to improve the professional status of Indies physicians. Within this group, Abdul Rivai played a pioneering role. Most of these physicians were driven by a profound faith in social evolution and affirmed the vital roles of science, technology, and medicine in bringing progress and prosperity to the Indies. They were convinced that Western-style education and the activities of educated professionals like themselves were essential in furthering social development. Their medical calling, their ideas about the social mission of medicine, and their desire to bring the Indies to a higher plane of civilisation buttressed both their social aspirations and their initiatives to enhance the status of their profession. These same motives led several to take up journalism and to participate in the nationalist movement that was taking shape around them.

Legal Codes and Social Aspirations

The legal code of the Dutch East Indies divided the population into three categories: Europeans, foreign Orientals, and natives.[1] Europeans, the Dutch inhabitants of the Indies and those from other Western countries, were subject to laws similar to those in continental Europe. 'Foreign Orientals' comprised individuals of Chinese and Arab descent, many of whom were traders, businessmen, and shopkeepers. With respect to property and commercial law, they fell under the laws that applied to Europeans; in matters pertaining to individual and family affairs, they followed the traditions of their own ethnic groups. The category of 'natives' consisted of the vast majority of the inhabitants of the archipelago, who were subject to the customary law of their own ethnic groups, generally enforced by village heads and regents. In effect, the Indies system of legal apartheid accorded the various racial and ethnic groups separate spheres characterised by specific legal and administrative expectations. For those in the 'native' category, these were later codified by Dutch legal scholars as various forms of *adat* or customary law. Colonial officials often stated that the Indies legal code protected natives against the intrusion of European legal codes, which were alien to them. Critics argued that it rather enshrined the racialised taxonomies of colonial society in law.

The boundaries between the three legal groups were defined according to race and descent. In practice, however, transitions between them occasionally took place. A small number of privileged foreign Orientals and natives successfully applied to the Governor-General for legal recognition as 'equivalent to European'. Applicants had to demonstrate that they were alienated from their ethnic milieu and, in addition, that they possessed a sufficient number of 'European' sociocultural characteristics including fluency in Dutch, enjoying a certain level of wealth and income, maintaining a European lifestyle, and attaining a certain level of education.[2] In these legal provisions the

[1] Cees Fasseur, 'Cornerstone or Stumbling Block: Racial Classification and the Late Colonial State in Indonesia', in *The Late Colonial State in Indonesia: Political and Economic Foundations of the Netherlands East Indies, 1880–1942*, ed. Robert Cribb (Leiden: KITLV Press, 1994), 31–56; and Robert Cribb, 'Legal Pluralism and Criminal Law in the Dutch Colonial Order', *Indonesia*, no. 90 (2010), 47–66.

[2] Bart Luttikhuis, 'Beyond Race: Constructions of "Europeanness" in Late-Colonial Legal Practice in the Dutch East Indies', *European Review of History* 20, no. 4 (2013), 539–58. See

colonial state defined Europeanness in social, cultural, and economic rather than in ethnic and racial terms, and rewarded applicants who conformed to these standards. Yet natives who were legally 'equivalent to European' were not recognised as such by most colonial Dutchmen. They were definitely not welcome in European social clubs, and Dutchmen derided them as 'Government Gazette Europeans': Europeans in name but not in nature.

From the turn of the twentieth century, Indies physicians became the social group that conformed to the social and cultural expectations of colonial Europeans the most. They were seen as brown Europeans or European-looking natives, occupying contested and often untenable social positions. Their predicament reflected what Ann Laura Stoler has called the 'construction of colonial categories and national identities' and the precarious situation of 'those people who ambiguously straddled, crossed, and threatened these imperial divides'.[3] Individuals inhabiting 'contradictory colonial locations were subject to a frequently shifting set of criteria that allowed them privilege at certain historical moments and pointedly excluded them at others', argues Stoler.[4] European women marrying Indonesian men, poor Europeans living in indigenous neighbourhoods, European men enjoying the company of native concubines, the offspring of such relationships, and Indo-Europeans all occupied ambiguous social positions. Their behaviour, their way of life, their poverty, and the language they spoke – or the peculiar Malay inflection of their Dutch – all had the potential to disqualify them as Europeans.[5] Indies physicians were in a similar situation. Their lifestyle, relatively high incomes, fluency in Dutch, and, for some, legal status as 'equivalent to European', qualified them as Europeans, but their aspirations were perpetually at risk because of their indigenous origins.

Abdul Rivai: Dreams and Aspirations

The first graduate of the Batavia Medical College to receive advanced medical training in the Netherlands was Abdul Rivai, an ambitious and highly

---

also Bart Luttikhuis, 'Negotiating Modernity: Europeanness in Late Colonial Indonesia, 1910–1942' (Dissertation, European University Institute, 2014).

[3] Ann Laura Stoler, *Carnal Knowledge and Imperial Power: Race and the Intimate in Colonial Rule* (Berkeley: University of California Press, 2002), 79.

[4] Stoler, *Carnal Knowledge and Imperial Power*, 40. For a discussion of the role of race, class, and gender in the definition of Europeanness, see Susie Protschky, 'Race, Class, and Gender: Debates over the Character of Social Hierarchies in the Netherlands Indies, circa 1600–1942', *Bijdragen tot de Taal-, Land- en Volkenkunde* 167, no. 4 (2011), 543–56.

[5] For the quandaries facing Indo-Europeans, see Hans Pols, 'Indo-Europeans in the Dutch East Indies: An Indo-European Analysis of a Paradoxical Colonial Category', in *Health and Difference: Rendering Human Variation in Colonial Engagements*, ed. Alexandra Widmer and Veronika Lipphardt (Oxford: Berghahn Books, 2016), 205–23.

articulate young man enamoured with the modern world. It galled him that his local medical qualifications allowed access only to lower-level positions within the colonial medical service that earned less than half the salary of his European colleagues. To Rivai, a European medical degree was a means of professional and social advancement because it allowed him to make the ascent from colonial subject to Dutch citizen. Rivai's ambitions, however, extended beyond improving his personal fortune. He was driven by an unwavering belief in the transformative powers of science, technology, and medicine which would inevitably bring prosperity and progress to the Indies. He was convinced that a highly educated indigenous intellectual elite would be crucial in this transformation, replacing moribund tradition with modern education, and giving the archipelago's inhabitants what was needed to compete in the modern world. Ultimately, Rivai's radical plans for the Indies required the westernisation of its indigenous inhabitants; to enjoy the benefits of modern life, they had to become Dutch.

In March 1895, Rivai graduated from Batavia's Javanese Doctors' School [Dokter Djawa School; the name of the Batavia Medical College from 1851 to 1902]. He immediately confirmed his cosmopolitan aspirations by discarding his traditional Minangkabau outfit in favour of a three-piece suit, black necktie, and Panama hat. 'Dressed as a Dutchman', he visited a portrait studio.[6] Historian Rudolf Mrázek argues that Indonesian dandies like Rivai 'borrowed Dutch clothes to place themselves in the modern colonial society'.[7] Rivai's carefully staged photograph reveals the identity to which he aspired: educated, modern, and cosmopolitan; unfettered by tradition, religious beliefs, or the status of a colonial subject (Figure 1.1). At the same time, his image projects a future nation in which one's social status would be determined by knowledge, skill, and educational accomplishment rather than by race or by one's position in the traditional social hierarchy.[8] Rivai's portrait suggests that for him, emancipation would be achieved only by erasure – by becoming indistinguishable, in the ways that mattered, from Europeans. In his prodigious writings, he aimed to accomplish the same end for all educated natives by redefining what it meant to be a native and a European in colonial life.

[6] Parada Harahap, *Riwajat Dr. A. Rivai* (Medan: Indische Drukkerij, 1939), 5. For early biographical sketches of Rivai, see Hilda Rivai and S. M. Latif, *Dr. A. Rivai Sepintas Laloe* (Np: Np, 1938).

[7] Rudolf Mrázek, 'Indonesian Dandy: The Politics of Clothes in the Late Colonial Period, 1893–1942', in *Outward Appearances: Dressing State and Society in Indonesies*, ed. Henk Schulte Nordholt (Leiden: KITLV Press, 1997), 117–50.

[8] These statements have been inspired by Karen Strassler's analysis of the role of photographic images in the Dutch East Indies. See Karen Strassler, *Refracted Visions: Popular Photography and National Modernity in Java* (Durham, NC: Duke University Press, 2010).

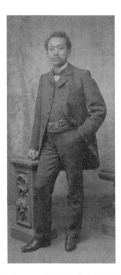

Figure 1.1 Abdul Rivai on New Year's Day, 1902, in Amsterdam. Figure: University of Leiden library, KITLV collection (122953)

In addition to projecting aspirations, photographs have the capacity to negate or reject possible identifications. When Rivai's father received his photograph, he concluded that his son was no longer a Muslim, and dead to him. A number of Minangkabau imams had declared that European dress contradicted the teachings of Islam, that only infidels imitated the dress of *kafirs*. Hats and neckties often received unfavourable mention in imams' religious commentaries – and in a number of fatwas.[9] Wearing European clothing was understood as a declaration that ethnic and religious affiliations were secondary to cultural modernity. For Rivai, Minangkabau outfits represented rigid hierarchies, and stifling ethnic and religious traditions.[10] European dress represented modernity. The cultural dominance of the West was seen as the outcome of the process of global social evolution, which justified conformity

[9] Harahap, *Riwajat Rivai*, 5–6. For the importance of clothing in the Dutch East Indies, see Nico J. G. Kaptein, 'Southeast Asian Debates and Middle East Inspiration: European Dress in Minangkabau at the Beginning of the 20th Century', in *Southeast Asia and the Middle East: Islam, Movement, and the Longue Durée*, ed. Eric Tagliacozzo (Singapore: NUS Press, 2009), 176–95. See also Jean Gelman Taylor, 'Costume and Gender in Colonial Java, 1800–1940', in *Outward Appearances: Dressing State and Society in Indonesies*, ed. Henk Schulte Nordholt (Leiden: KITLV Press, 1997), 85–116; and Kees van Dijk, 'Sarongs, Jubbahs, and Trousers: Appearance as a Means of Distinction and Discrimination', in *Outward Appearances: Dressing State and Society in Indonesies*, ed. Henk Schulte Nordholt (Leiden: KITLV Press, 1997), 39–83.

[10] S. M. Latif, 'Dr. A. Rivai', in *Dr. A. Rivai Sepintas Lalu*, ed. Hilda Rivai and S. M. Latif (Np: Np, 1938), 22.

to European cultural norms and fuelled the broader program of reshaping the Indies according to the Western model.

During his time at the Batavia Medical College, Rivai had repeatedly demonstrated his preference for whatever was Western and modern. He frequently interacted with Europeans and even married a Dutch widow, which was highly unusual at the time (Rivai married three more times, each time to a European woman). He was fluent in Dutch as well as in English, German, and French, and he actively participated in debates on the development of the Indies and the social role of its educated elite. Rivai saw his graduation as only the first step towards participation in the modern world. The Batavia Medical College provided a practical education, and the degrees it conferred were considered inferior to those awarded by European medical schools, which provided a more academic, theoretical course of study. Earning a European medical degree was for Rivai part of an emancipatory strategy that aimed to erase the differences between himself and his European colleagues. In principle, postings and salaries in the colonial medical service were determined by the degree attained, not by one's ethnic background. A Dutch degree would therefore realise his desire for professional advancement and enable him to achieve European social status.

Soon after graduating, Rivai was placed in Medan, the urban centre of the Deli plantation area on the east coast of Sumatra. Within months of their arrival, his young daughter died and Rivai separated from his wife.[11] Because medical students did not have to pay tuition and received modest stipends, they were obliged to work for the colonial medical service for a period of ten years upon completion of their studies. During this time they were permitted to maintain a private practice to compensate for their meagre official incomes. To recruit well-paying private patients, Rivai mingled in wealthy Chinese, Arab, and European circles, demonstrating an uncanny ability to blend in.[12] Nonetheless, he soon had a falling out with the local sultan after naming his dog Sultan. He had an irascible nature, and frequently clashed with his colleagues and superiors in the local medical service who, he thought, failed to appreciate his talents. He tendered his resignation after four years and left for the Netherlands to pursue further study. The leader of Medan's Chinese community gave Rivai a loan of more than forty times his colonial medical service salary to support his studies.

Encouraged by Professor Christiaan Eijkman, past director of the Batavia Medical College and future Nobel Prize winner, and Conrad Theodor van Deventer, Member of Parliament and a fervent adherent of the Ethical Policy,

---

[11] Rivai's first wife returned to Batavia, arriving on 2 September 1895, six months after they had moved to Medan. See 'Passagiers', *Bataviaasch Nieuwsblad*, 28 August 1895, 3.

[12] Latif, 'Dr. A. Rivai', 24.

Rivai began attending classes at the University of Utrecht. Unfortunately, he soon learned that he could not matriculate because he did not have a Dutch high school diploma. After unsuccessfully requesting a waiver from the Minister of Education, he settled in Amsterdam to prepare for the required exams and began working as a journalist. The same year, he founded the biweekly *Pewarta Wolanda* [*Dutch Herald*], which appeared in 1899 and 1900. Although most of its articles were reprinted in the Malay press, the magazine failed to attract paying subscribers, leading to its demise after a mere six months. Not discouraged, Rivai embarked, together with H. C. C. Clockener Brousson, a retired military officer in the colonial army who had previously published a similar newspaper in Batavia, on a more ambitious endeavour: the *Bintang Hindia* [*Star of the Indies*], an illustrated periodical for educated Indonesians.[13] This paper first appeared in 1902. Since the advanced printing technologies needed for an illustrated magazine were not available in the Indies, the *Bintang Hindia* was printed in the Netherlands. By the end of 1904, circulation had reached an astounding 27,000 copies. In 1905, Governor-General van Heutsz, who wholeheartedly supported the ideals of the *Bintang Hindia*, agreed to fund the magazine. Circulation skyrocketed. As Rivai wrote most of the magazine's articles, his views reached an unprecedented number of Indonesian readers.

Sleepless Nights: Articulating a Political Program

Rivai's political program was based on his profound belief in the transformative powers of science and medicine, which had the potential to propel the Indies from its primitive and in some respects barbaric state to civilised modernity. He believed that the lack of mental development that characterised the indigenous population could be rectified by education, which would not only expand knowledge and skills, but inculcate a moral code based on industry, commitment, thrift, and planning. All would be necessary to compete in the modern world. In formulating this program, Rivai combined the enduring interests of his Minangkabau ethnic group in science, education, and progress with his own experiences in the Netherlands. Educated Dutch intellectuals rather than reactionary European colonisers came to embody Rivai's ideals of progress and civilisation. The announcement of the Ethical Policy in 1901, which presented progressive ideals as official colonial policy, reinforced Rivai's convictions. Discussions about progress and development

---

[13] This officer was Henri C. C. Clockener Brousson. On the *Bintang Hindia*, see Ahmat B. Adam, *The Vernacular Press and the Emergence of Modern Indonesian Consciousness* (Ithaca, NY: Southeast Asia Program, Cornell University, 1995), 93–106; and Harry A. Poeze, *In het Land van de Overheerser I: Indonesiërs in Nederland, 1600–1950* (Dordrecht: FORIS, 1986), 26–51; Harry Poeze, 'Early Indonesian Emancipation; Abdul Rivai, Van Heutsz and the Bintang Hindia', *Bijdragen tot de Taal-, Land- en Volkenkunde* 145, no. 1 (1989), 87–106.

among small groups of Indies intellectuals, who were attuned to broader inter-national debates, predated the announcement of the Ethical Policy by more than two decades. Rivai's political program illustrates that an appreciation of science and rational administration were not simply imposed upon the Indies by Europeans, but were rather appropriated by indigenous intellectuals to develop political platforms, plans for the rearrangement of indigenous cultures and traditions, tools for social analysis, and, finally, critiques of colo-nial society.

Rivai was a Minangkabau man. In the nineteenth century, after it became the main stronghold of Islamic modernism in the Indies, the Minangkabau ethnic group valued education highly.[14] Islamic modernists aimed to reconcile Islam with science, rationality, and the demands of progress. They advocated a crit-ical re-examination of the Koran to eliminate extraneous rituals and beliefs that had been added over the course of several centuries. They also hoped that an understanding of science and technology would enable Muslims to halt fur-ther exploitation by Western powers.[15] Starting in the 1880s, Malay-language newspapers circulated in the Indies and regularly featured discussions on pro-gress and development while carrying ample advertisements for modern, mass-produced consumer goods.[16] The readership of these newspapers was limited to the small group of literate men who held clerical positions in businesses, on plantations, or in local administrative offices. Achmad Adam argues that, in the 1880s and 1890s, Indies vernacular newspapers were primarily concerned with searching 'for a way to bring Indonesians to the gates of *kemajuan* or pro-gress'.[17] Papers appearing in the Minangkabau region led the way.

According to historian Rudolf Mrázek, the 'spread of Dutch-style and Dutch-language schools in Minangkabau at the time had no equal anywhere else in the colony'.[18] Almost every day, wrote a colonial official in 1913, the Minangkabau submitted petitions for more Dutch schools. A historian of the area stated: 'The demand to learn Dutch became so great among the

---

[14] For more on the Minangkabau area, see Taufik Abdullah, 'Modernization in the Minangkabau World: West Sumatra in the Early Decades of the Twentieth Century', in *Culture and Politics in Indonesia*, ed. Claire Holt, Benedict R. O'G. Anderson, and James Siegel (Ithaca, NY: Cornell University Press, 1972), 179–245.

[15] See Michael F. Laffan, *The Making of Indonesian Islam: Orientalism and the Narration of a Sufi Past* (Princeton, NJ: Princeton University Press, 2011), 177–89; Michael F. Laffan, *Islamic Nationhood and Colonial Indonesia: The Umma below the Winds* (London: Routledge, 2007).

[16] Henk Schulte Nordholt, 'Modernity and Cultural Citizenship in the Netherlands Indies: An Illustrated Hypothesis', *Journal of Southeast Asian Studies* 42, no. 3 (2011), 435–57; Tom Hoogervorst and Henk Schulte Nordholt, 'Urban Middle Classes in Colonial Java (1900–1942): Images and Language', *Bijdragen tot de Taal-, Land- en Volkenkunde* 173 (2017), 442–74.

[17] Adam, *Vernacular Press*, 80.

[18] Rudolf Mrázek, *Sjahrir: Politics and Exile in Indonesia* (Ithaca, NY: Southeast Asia Program, Cornell University, 1994), 18.

Minangkabau that anyone with the slightest knowledge of the language would establish a backyard school giving crash courses to aspiring civil servants and professionals.'[19] Many young Minangkabau men found employment all over the archipelago in offices, schools, and clinics. Their ability to read, write, and speak Dutch had created new types of employment and previously unimaginable avenues for social advancement. They were also able to read books, magazines, and newspapers, connecting the Indies with the rest of the world. The series of instruction books used for teaching Dutch in the few high schools of the Indies was called, suggestively, *Avenue to the West* [Dutch: *Weg tot het Westen*; Malay: *Djalan ke Barat*].[20] It soon became an axiom among young Minangkabau and, later, among all young Indonesians that one had to master the Dutch language to be modern.

Rivai must have experienced some difficulty when he tried to reconcile his idealistic images of the Netherlands with the generally materialistic, exploitative, and discriminatory behaviour commonly observed among the Dutch in the colonies. Apart from a few inspiring teachers at the Batavia Medical College and a small number of progressive intellectuals, Rivai rarely encountered progressive Dutchmen in the colonies – no educated Indonesian did. This led to a profound subaltern ambivalence. As Francis Gouda has argued, the best qualities of the Dutch, including tolerance, progressiveness, and an appreciation of higher learning, were difficult to find in Dutch colonists.[21] In contrast, after Rivai's arrival in the Netherlands he met several Dutch professors, politicians, and intellectuals who treated him with respect. 'The interests of the natives are discussed more frequently here than in the Indies', he wrote soon after he arrived.[22] Many other Indonesian students found that life in the Netherlands was different from that in the colonies. They interacted freely with fellow students, professors, and intellectuals without experiencing ethnic or racial discrimination.[23] Many fell in love with Dutch women.[24]

---

[19] Elizabeth E. Graves, *The Minangkabau Response to Dutch Colonial Rule in the Nineteenth Century* (Ithaca, NY: Cornell Modern Indonesia Project, 1981), 180; quoted in Mrázek, *Sjahrir*, 20.

[20] About Dutch language education in the Dutch East Indies see Kees Groeneboer, *Gateway to the West: The Dutch Language in Colonial Indonesia 1600–1950, a History of Language Policy* (Amsterdam: Amsterdam University Press, 1998).

[21] Frances Gouda, *Dutch Culture Overseas: Colonial Practice in the Netherlands Indies, 1900–1942* (Amsterdam: Amsterdam University Press, 1995).

[22] Abdul Rivai, 'Demoralisatie van den Javaan', *Oost en West*, 30 Mei 1901, 2.

[23] See, for example, the accounts by Rivai in Bonto van Bijleveld, 'Een Inlandsche Journalist', *Sumatra Post*, 11 June 1901, Section II, 1; and Abdul Rivai, 'Holland, de Inlanders en Nog Iets', *Koloniaal Weekblad* 6, no. 18 (1906), 2.

[24] For details on these amorous affairs, see Poeze, *Land Overheerser*, 35. The Javanese poet Noto Soeroto received ample assistance to extricate himself from an amorous relationship after his partner became pregnant. See René Karels, *Mijn Aardse Leven Vol Moeite en Strijd: Raden Mas Noto Soeroto, Javaan, Dichter, Politicus, 1888–1951* (Leiden: KITLV Press, 2010). The affairs of European students in the Netherlands were similar to those of Filipino students in Spain. See

The Dutch Rivai encountered in the Netherlands provided a stark contrast to colonial Dutchmen. If only the enlightened Dutch in the Netherlands could replace the reactionary, ignorant, and crude Dutch in the colonies, thought Rivai, his vision for the Indies would be within reach. A closer association between the Netherlands and the Dutch East Indies would achieve this. Rivai published the *Pewarta Wolanda* and the *Bintang Hindia* to foster a greater understanding of and affection for the Netherlands and its royal family. Rivai hoped that this would lead them to 'appreciate, even more than they do today, the blessings and benefits brought to them by the Dutch government, which will foster an attachment between the Netherlands and the Indies that will transform the Indies into a Dutch colony in the true sense of the word'.[25] A Dutch journalist who announced the first issue noted that the cover displayed both Queen Emma and Queen Wilhelmina, and contained a poem in high-Malay written by Rivai and dedicated to both queens.[26] Rivai hoped the *Pewarta Wolanda* would make the connection between the Netherlands and the Indies 'stronger and firmer on the higher moral basis of mutual appreciation and respect'.[27] In both papers, Rivai avoided the Dutch colonial presence and drew the attention of his readers towards exemplary Dutch individuals and accomplishments in the Low Countries.

Rivai's journalism also focused on the plight of the archipelago's indigenous population. In a series of articles published just after the turn of the twentieth century, he reported that the Javanese were profoundly demoralised because they were unable to compete with Europeans in the Darwinian struggle for life. Europeans enjoyed the advantage of their education and acquaintance with modern technology.[28] Rivai also characterised Indonesians as primitive and mired in animism and superstition, despite the long presence of Hinduism and Islam. Most were still enchanted by magic incantations [*ilmu*] and amulets, provided by traditional healers [*dukun*], which, they were convinced, could make individuals invincible, extraordinarily powerful, or invisible.[29] These superstitious beliefs were part of a pervasive 'Indo-hypnosis', which, Rivai hoped, psychiatrists would study in the future to counter its pernicious influence.[30] He also recommended that medical students be taught about these

---

Raquel A. G. Reyes, *Love, Passion and Patriotism: Sexuality and the Philippine Propaganda Movement, 1882–1892* (Seattle: University of Washington Press, 2008).

[25] 'Een Maleisch Blad in Nederland', *Sumatra Post*, 25 September 1900, 1.

[26] 'Pewarta Wolanda', *Algemeen Handelsblad*, 9 September 1900, 1. The image portrayed two queens, one of whom was Queen Emma, the wife of King William III, who died in 1890. Because her daughter, the future Queen Wilhelmina, was not yet eighteen, Emma held the throne until 1898. Queen Emma was a very popular member of the Dutch royal family.

[27] Quoted from the prospectus of *Bendera Wolanda*, in 'Maleisch Blad', 1.

[28] Rivai, 'Demoralisatie Javaan', 2.

[29] Abdul Rivai, 'Het Geloof der Inlanders, I', *Algemeen Handelsblad*, 13 August 1901, 7.

[30] Abdul Rivai, 'Het Geloof der Inlanders, II', *Algemeen Handelsblad*, 14 August 1901, 7.

archaic beliefs. Ideally, curing their patients' afflictions would also help eradicate their superstitions.[31] Rivai's portrayal of the Indies' unwashed masses departed dramatically from that of the intellectual elite, which buttressed the latter's exceptional nature.

Rivai attributed the dire condition of the archipelago's indigenous population to the underdevelopment of their minds. In his articles, Rivai made no mention of exploitative labour practices, indentured servitude (as was common in the Deli plantation area), or the brutality of the colonial military forces, exemplified by the butchering of Aceh's population during the previous forty years. Demoralisation was a function instead of cultural backwardness, and both would be cured by modern education. Rivai's diagnosis was acceptable in the Netherlands, as it did not blame Dutch colonialism and allowed Dutch intellectuals a prominent role in ameliorative efforts. Providing educational facilities and, of course, endorsing the Ethical Policy, placed them in a position of exemplary and noble facilitators of progress, rather than ruthless and vicious colonisers. Despite the many parallels between his ideas and those of leading Ethicists, however, Rivai argued that the development of the Indies could be set in motion only by indigenous intellectuals because they were uniquely placed to act as mediators between East and West. While principled Ethicists with technological knowledge and insight into the ethnic cultures of the Indies might provide valuable assistance, they were not able to adopt leadership roles. Only an indigenous intellectual aristocracy could cultivate and disseminate modern forms of thinking, living, and working, because of its proximity to the general population.

Rivai's writings became a manifesto for a small but growing group of educated Indonesians because they laid down an essential and indispensable role for them in modernising the Indies.[32] Rivai named this elite group the young generation [*kaum muda*], which included 'all people of the Indies (young and old) who are no longer willing to follow the obsolete system but are, on the contrary, anxious to achieve self-respect through knowledge and the sciences'.[33] At the time, the designation 'young' referred to individuals who challenged tradition and the status quo by embracing progressive political convictions. Benedict Anderson observed that 'both in Europe and in the colonies "young" and "youth" signified dynamism, progress, self-sacrificing idealism and revolutionary will.'[34] Because of its essential role in firing the engines of progress, Rivai believed that this young generation would soon become the intellectual

---

[31] Abdul Rivai, 'Het Geloof der Inlanders, III', *Algemeen Handelsblad*, 15 August 1901, 7.

[32] For similar developments in India, see Gyan Prakash, *Another Reason: Science and the Imagination of Modern India* (Princeton, NJ: Princeton University Press, 1999).

[33] Quoted in Adam, *Vernacular Press*, 104.

[34] Benedict R. O'G. Anderson, *Imagined Communities: Reflections on the Origin and Spread of Nationalism*, revised and extended edn (London: Verso, 2006 [1983]), 116.

aristocracy [*bangsawan pikiran*], surpassing the traditional one (renamed the old generation [*kaum tua*]), which still exploited the primitive masses (the old-fashioned generation [*kaum kuno*]). Rivai's intellectual aristocracy would elevate the latter through education and guidance. Because of its close similarity to enlightened and educated Europeans, it merited recognition within the highest colonial social tier.

In addition to reactionary Europeans, Rivai's *kaum muda* faced opposition from the traditional aristocracy or *priyayi*, who were not interested in social change. Aristocrats enjoyed a lavish lifestyle by mercilessly exploiting the population, and the colonial administration overlooked it as long as they collected and paid taxes. Aristocrats generally inherited their positions rather than meriting them through education or achievement. They only valued education as far as it was useful to safeguard their children's future: they had no desire for their offspring to pursue useful careers in agriculture, trade, or industry, preferring their sons to become junior government clerks (the 'necessary tools of the colonial government') and work their way up to influential and well-remunerated positions.[35] Rivai wanted the intellectual aristocracy to replace the traditional one, which would assume its rightful place slightly elevated above the masses. Rivai's idealism, then, was elitist: his program was a protest of a recent and growing educated, bourgeois elite against a long-established, traditional one which enjoyed far greater prestige, influence, and economic power. It attacked two fundamental characteristics of colonial society: the stranglehold of the traditional aristocracy, and the fundamental inequality between Europeans and natives, which was most acutely experienced by those natives who had attained an education.

To accelerate the forces of progress, Rivai thought it essential to provide an advanced education to promising Indonesian students. These students would ideally receive part of their education in the Netherlands, where they could acquaint themselves with the latest developments in science, medicine, agriculture, and engineering. They would be able to familiarise themselves with Dutch democratic institutions and be exposed to suitable role models who would display those highly valued Calvinist traits, thrift and diligence.[36] Rivai warned that these students 'should not become Europeanised or pretend to be *blandas* [literally Dutchmen but also a general term for Europeans] who feel too grand to be with their indigenous fellow men'.[37] Upon their return to the Indies, which was required, they had to deliver the fruits of their learning

---

[35] Rivai, 'Demoralisatie Javaan'. Rivai was quoting a phrase Louis Couperus used in *The Silent Force*.

[36] Rivai, 'Demoralisatie Javaan'.

[37] Van Bijleveld, 'Inlandsch Journalist', Section II, 1. This article contained an interview with Abdul Rivai and was reprinted from the *Amsterdamsche Courant*.

by educating the members of their own ethnic group in their native tongue. These bright members of the young generation needed to improve themselves by receiving the best, Western-style education possible without erasing their ties to the Indies.

Like many Indonesian intellectuals at the time, Rivai considered the Dutch language the key to science and learning, even though German, English, and French were more prominent in global science. In the Indies, the ability to speak Dutch had the additional benefit of removing a basic marker of difference between coloniser and colonised.[38] Rivai believed that Malay, Javanese, and the other languages spoken in the archipelago were incapable of expressing scientific concepts and complex ideas. He hoped that the new intellectual aristocracy, in association with the colonial administration, would remedy this defect by stimulating the further development of these languages: 'Malay should be made into a language that is suitable for thinking in order that it can reflect everything that is taking place in the area of progress.'[39] A suitable candidate for a language that could be used throughout the Indies was already present: Malay. It needed only to be updated and modernised.

Establishing an intellectual aristocracy, Rivai thought, would cement the relationship between the Netherlands and the colonies in unprecedented ways. As progress and prosperity reached the Indies, Indonesians would express immense gratitude to the mother country, which would limit the influence of competing alliances:

> When, through the efforts of the colonial government, development has been appropriated by the Javanese people, they will no longer make pilgrimages to Mecca but to the Netherlands; they will no longer face, during their prayers, to the Ka'abah but to The Hague, because they know that the throne of the Dutch Queen is located there, whom they all love, and whose people have brought them happiness and prosperity.[40]

Rivai's ebullient words must have inspired Ethicist van Deventer, who would use nearly identical language several years later to laud Insulinde's awakening upon the founding of Boedi Oetomo.

Although promoting modernity was a regular and important feature of Rivai's writing, perhaps its most significant, and subversive, feat was his subtle rewriting of the fundamental difference between Europeans and Indonesians, coloniser and colonial subject, and white and brown. Rivai redefined this difference as one of mental and moral development or level of civilisation, replacing earlier racial, ethnic, or legal distinctions. Once redefined in this

---

[38] About Dutch ideas on teaching the Dutch language in the Indies see Groeneboer, *Gateway to the West*.

[39] Van Bijleveld, 'Inlandsch Journalist', Section II, 1; see also Rivai, 'Demoralisatie Javaan'.

[40] Rivai, 'Demoralisatie Javaan'.

way, a specific mental quality became the primary indicator of Europeanness, a matter of degree rather than kind. Individuals could become more civilised and climb this hierarchy, or lose the essential characteristics of civilisation by becoming more primitive, and descend. Educated Indonesians might therefore approach, if not reach, the same level as Dutch elite in the Netherlands. Similarly, rude and poorly mannered Europeans in the colonies were on this scale approaching barbarism. Rivai sketched a colonial utopia in which reactionary, materialistic Europeans would be replaced with enlightened and progressive migrants from the Netherlands, which would precipitate a closer association between motherland and colony. Within colonial society too Rivai's intellectual aristocracy would be recognised and accorded due respect, while the traditional aristocracy was relegated to the native realm.

Wahidin Soedirohoesodo, a retired Javanese physician who clamoured for progress, was one of Rivai's early adherents. In 1905, Wahidin used the terms *kaum muda*, *kaum tua*, and *kaum kuno* in a series of articles in his journal *Retnodhoemila*. He urged his readers to embrace modernity, to establish an organisation to promote education among the Javanese, and to publish a Javanese equivalent of the *Bintang Hindia*. He even recommended that his readers contact Abdul Rivai for advice.[41] Wahidin was well informed about Rivai's activities because his son Abdullah was at that time attending art school in the Netherlands, sharing a house with Rivai, and drawing illustrations for the *Bintang Hindia* (Figure 1.2). For several years, Wahidin had attempted to garner support among the Javanese high aristocracy for a scholarship fund. Like Rivai, he favoured teaching Dutch: 'Those who cannot understand Dutch have not yet set foot on the coast of the sea of progress.'[42] He proclaimed:

Let the old-fashioned people stay in the forest and meditate all they want until the end of their lives. However, since the modern age demands progress and the improvement of living conditions, let us take decisive action so that the younger people will not have cause to ridicule those among the young and old who stand in the way of progress.[43]

Wahidin found a receptive audience only when he met Soetomo and several other medical students in 1907. Ironically, the ideas first articulated by an Indies physician studying in the Netherlands were taken up by a retired *Dokter Djawa* in the Indies before they reached the medical students who subsequently founded Boedi Oetomo.

---

[41] Akira Nagazumi, *The Dawn of Indonesian Nationalism: The Early Years of the Budi Utomo, 1908–1918* (Tokyo: Institute of Developing Economies, 1972), 30–31.

[42] Quoted in Nagazumi, *Dawn of Indonesian Nationalism*, 31.

[43] Wahidin Soedirohoesodo, *Retnodhoemila*, May 1905, quoted in Nagazumi, *Dawn of Indonesian Nationalism*, 31.

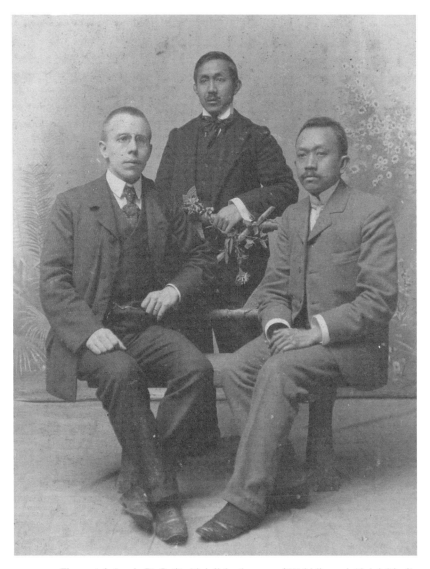

Figure 1.2 Louis D. Petit, Abdullah, the son of Wahidin and Abdul Rivai's housemate, and Abdul Rivai. Abdullah was, at the time, a student at an art school in the Netherlands and illustrated the *Bintang Hindia*. Louis Petit knew many Indies students in the Netherlands and provided various forms of assistance to them. Figure: University of Leiden library, KITLV collection (34440)

A Rude Awakening: Rivai's Return to the Indies

In 1904, Rivai learned that the law regulating admission to Dutch universities had changed: it now exempted graduates of the Batavia Medical College from all preliminary examinations. Rivai soon commenced medical studies at the University of Amsterdam and graduated in June 1908. The following month, he earned a doctorate in medicine from Belgium's University of Ghent. Most European universities required a medical dissertation for a medical doctorate; the University of Ghent required only an oral examination. Rivai subsequently went to England to study eye diseases and married his second wife.[44] He then commenced work at the University of Amsterdam, in the laboratory of Professor Rudolf Hendrik Saltet, one of the most influential professors of public health in the Netherlands. He also visited Paris and attended the Institut Pasteur because he aspired to become the vice director of Batavia's Pasteur Institute.[45]

Rivai's reinvention of himself as a cosmopolitan European professional continued apace. After earning a European medical degree and a doctorate in medicine, speaking Dutch nearly flawlessly, and marrying a European woman, he obtained Dutch citizenship in January 1910. As a consequence, he was a rather unusual native when he returned to the Indies later that year. Legally, he was a European. His European medical degree entitled him to remuneration on the European salary scale, a sabbatical to the Netherlands every seven years, and free repatriation upon retirement. Rivai was soon appointed medical officer in the colonial army, and was stationed at the large army encampment in Cimahi near Bandung. To Rivai, this appointment was an enormous achievement. The military medical service had a higher status and was better resourced than its civilian counterpart, and only Europeans could be appointed as officers. The colonial army was responsible for safeguarding the unity between the Netherlands and the Indies; it had 'pacified' the Indies to prepare it for progress and development. Nonetheless, Rivai frequently argued with his colleagues and superiors because they treated him as a native. Rivai's dreams were shattered:

At school, you think life is rosy. Only later you are disillusioned. You see how you are a physician and also not a physician, how you are closer to the Dutch because of your science but because of that same science you are repelled by them as well. You are not allowed to speak their language but are thrown back on the great pile of uncivilised natives.[46]

---

[44] Her name was Bertha Anne Rautenberg. Unfortunately, nothing is known about her experiences after moving to the Indies with Rivai.

[45] Abdul Rivai, 'Over den Invloed van de Flagellaten op de Zelfreiniging van het Bassinwater', *Geneeskundige Bladen uit Kliniek en Laboratorium voor de Praktijk* 14, no. 9 (1909): 305–44.

[46] Van Bijleveld, 'Inlandsch Journalist', Section II, 1.

The failure of his colleagues to treat him as a European led to great bitterness. Rivai did not, however, disapprove of the colonial social order itself, only of his own position in it and that of other educated natives.

In 1912, Rivai requested a transfer to the colonial medical service in Padang, where he established a private practice on the side. He quickly built an outstanding reputation and was able to earn an impressive income. He was also elected to the city council and bought a new car, delighting in overtaking European colleagues who still travelled by horse and buggy. After disagreements with his superiors in Padang, he decided to leave the life of a civil servant behind and moved to Surabaya, where he established another private practice and was again elected to the city council. Because of his ability to mingle with wealthy Europeans, Chinese merchants, Arab traders, and indigenous aristocrats, his private practice was very successful and profitable. This led his fellow Sumatran Mohamad Amir, a psychiatrist, to call him a merchant rather than a physician.[47]

In 1918, the Dutch colonial administration established the Volksraad, the proto-parliament of the Dutch East Indies which initially had only an advisory function. Twenty-five seats were reserved for Europeans and foreign Orientals; the remaining fifteen seats were for representatives of the indigenous population.[48] The Governor-General appointed half the members to secure an accurate representation of the archipelago's population; the other half was elected by a limited franchise. Rivai's election to the Volksraad highlighted the ambiguities and complexities of legal status, race, and ethnicity. He was elected to a native seat but encountered a legal wrangle because he had become a Dutch citizen and therefore was no longer a native.[49] In the ensuing debates, critics argued about the relative importance of ethnic origin [*landaard*] and legal status. Some argued that a native with Dutch citizenship remained a native; the problem would therefore arise only if Rivai were to apply to become equivalent to European. Others argued that Rivai should resign his seat

---

[47] Mohamad Amir, 'Dr Abdul Rivai', in *Boenga Rampai*, ed. M. Sarqawi (Medan: Centrale Courant en Boekhandel, 1940), 180.

[48] In the first Volksraad, there were fifteen individuals indigenous to the Indies (ten elected, five appointed) and twenty-four Europeans (nine elected, fourteen appointed, and the chairman). See S. L. van der Wal, *De Volksraad en de Staatkundige Ontwikkeling van Nederlands-Indië: Een Bronnenpublicatie*, 2 vols. (Groningen: Wolters, 1964–65), vol. I, 221.

[49] This was the argument presented by the *Bataviaasch Nieuwsblad*, the newspaper generally most sympathetic to the indigenous movement. See, for example, 'Overtrekken!', *Bataviaasch Nieuwsblad*, 18 January 1918, 2; 'Het Lot der Volksraadverkiezing', *Bataviaasch Nieuwsblad*, 19 January 1918, 2; 'Voorlichting', *Bataviaasch Nieuwsblad*, 25 January 1918, 1. Both the *Sumatra Post* and *Nieuws van den Dag voor Nederlandsch-Indië* argued (although not consistently) that naturalisation and ethnic origin ('*landaard*') did not necessarily overlap: 'Dr. Rivai', *Sumatra Post*, 23 January 1918, 10; 'De Verkiezing van Dr. Rivai', *Nieuws van den Dag voor Nederlandsch-Indië*, 30 January 1918, 2. The election of Rivai was covered almost daily for a period of three weeks.

voluntarily and be appointed as a European by the Governor-General. Rivai had been hesitant to join the Volksraad because it would mean giving up his lucrative medical practice, but changed his mind after the vocal protests in the European press against his appointment.[50]

As a member of the Volksraad, Rivai delivered several eloquent and well-researched speeches. The rhetoric of science, development, and enlightened administration was easily appropriated and transformed into a counter-hegemonic discourse critiquing the dire conditions in the colonies and the lack of initiatives by the colonial state. In his maiden speech, for example, Rivai declared that 'the education of the native is the most pressing social issue.'[51] He lamented that 'the level of development of the general population was still low, very low' and severely criticised the educational politics of the colonies, the 'most unsympathetic or antipathic part of colonial politics'.[52] Educational initiatives were implemented only to meet the demands of business and the colonial bureaucracy, he claimed, rather than to advance the indigenous population. Rivai later succeeded in passing a motion to establish a university in the Indies. He also submitted an extensive proposal by the director of the Surabaya Medical College (NIAS) outlining how a university could be established by merging several schools that were already operating. This proposal was supported by the Society of Indies Physicians, which published all relevant material in a special issue of its journal.[53]

Despite Rivai's enthusiasm entering the Volksraad, his next decade was marked by serious illness, disillusionment with colonial politics, and despair. In 1919, he went to Paris to seek treatment for diabetes and tuberculosis. He underwent light and electrotherapy, which he promptly adopted in the private practice he set up in Semarang after his return in 1921. His British wife died the same year, leaving Rivai still more desperate, and unable to work. He married a Dutch apothecary assistant only to leave her two years later.[54] Rivai was again elected to the Volksraad in 1921 but seemed to have lost his passion for politics. He was rarely present when the colonial parliament was in session, earning him the nickname 'Rivai the Silent' after the well-known Dutch monarch William the Silent.[55] In 1926, he left for Switzerland to receive

---

[50] Harahap, *Riwajat Rivai*, citing an article by Rivai in *Bintang Hindia* of 21 August 1929.

[51] Abdul Rivai, 'Algemeene Beschouwingen, 19 Juni 1918', in *Handelingen van den Volksraad, Eerste Gewone Zitting* (Batavia: Volksraad van Nederlandsch-Indië, 1918), 137.

[52] Rivai, 'Algemeene Beschouwingen', 138, 37.

[53] Abdul Rivai, J. T. Terburgh, A. E. Sitsen, and A. de Waart, *Het Hooger Onderwijs Vraagstuk, Speciaal in Veband met het Geneeskundig Onderwijs in Nederlandsch-Indië*, Orgaan van Indische Artsen (Special Issue) (Batavia: VIG, 1919).

[54] Rivai married Dedrika Elisabeth Coerman on 19 July 1922 in Bandung. On 27 August 1924 she moved to the Netherlands where she remarried two years later. The marriage of Rivai and Coerman is not mentioned in the sources on Rivai's life.

[55] See, for example, 'Dr. Abdoel Rivai', *Indische Courant*, 24 November 1926, 1.

further medical treatment. During his convalescence, he met his fourth wife, a German-Swiss woman. He advised Mohamad Hatta, who studied economics in the Netherlands and visited him at his Swiss sanatorium, against political involvement because Sumatrans could expect only marginal success. Rivai subsequently expressed his misgivings about the dominant position of the Javanese in the nationalist movement.[56]

After returning to the Indies in November 1931, Rivai lived only two years, increasingly crippled by physical illness. His patients were shocked because their physician was much sicker than they were.[57] His belief in the Volksraad together with his hope that the Indies might ever resemble a European parliamentary democracy disappeared after he observed that indigenous efforts in the Volksraad had remained without effect. In a series of newspaper articles entitled 'A Colonial Tragedy', he bitterly attacked Indies colonial politics as a farce based on exploiting racial distinctions with the ultimate aim of keeping the indigenous population disenfranchised.[58] He died in Bandung on 16 October 1934. Rivai was one of the most European Indonesians of his time, but at the end of his life saw that all his Europeanness had been a delusion. In the Dutch East Indies, Rivai's Indies origins had proved impossible to overcome.

The First Generation of Indies Physicians with Dutch Medical Degrees

After Rivai discovered that he was unable to enrol at a Dutch medical school, Eijkman, van Deventer, and current STOVIA director H. F. Roll convinced the Minister of Education to change the law, and it was amended in March 1904. European physicians in the Indies were dismayed because this legal change would allow wealthy *Dokters Djawa* to obtain degrees they did not deserve, becoming 'white ravens among our brown intellectuals'.[59] Indies physicians, on the contrary, applauded them, and several immediately made plans to study in the Netherlands.[60] Because Rivai was busy writing for the *Bintang Hindia*, Asmaoen became the first native to receive a Dutch medical degree. He subsequently spent several months at the Institute of Naval and Tropical

[56] Rivai also expressed his misgivings about the dominance of the Javanese in the Indonesian nationalism in a newspaper article: Abdul Rivai, 'Indonesisch of Javaansch Nationalisme', *Het Vaderland*, 25 August 1931, 2.

[57] Latif, 'Dr. A. Rivai', 23.

[58] These essays are reprinted in Harahap, *Riwajat Rivai*, 47–59.

[59] P. Adriani, 'De Toekenning van het Arts-Diploma aan Inlandsche Geneeskundigen', *Soerabaiasch Handelsblad*, 9 May 1904, Section III, 1.

[60] Andrew Goss has captured the idealism and the visions of this first generation well. See Andrew Goss, *The Floracrats: State-Sponsored Science and the Failure of the Enlightenment in Indonesia* (Madison: University of Wisconsin Press, 2011), 96–102.

Medicine in Hamburg. After returning to the Indies, Asmaoen converted to Christianity, obtained Dutch citizenship, married a Dutch woman, and received an appointment as a medical officer in the colonial army. The European press commented:

It is possible to inculcate a lot of knowledge into a Javanese man; one can sprinkle baptismal water on his head; one can dress him in a nice suit with gold stars and braids; one can give him a dignified letter of appointment; one can call him a colleague – but a lot will depend on the man himself … If he demonstrates himself to be … not only a person equal in intellectual, … but also in moral and social respect, he will prevail. Only then will he be considered, primarily, a medical officer and a physician, and, only secondarily, a Javanese.[61]

Several military officers expressed reservations. Would they have to treat this medical officer like a European? Could natives be relied upon to defend the colonial order?[62] Asmaoen's appointment became a source of disappointment and frustration, and he died in 1917, embittered, during leave in the Netherlands.

Mas Boenjamin, who earned his Dutch medical degree in October 1908, was also appointed as a medical officer in the colonial army. Boenjamin was active in Boedi Oetomo and the Association of Indies Physicians. He published a Javanese version of the *Bintang Hindia* named *Magazine for Progressive Javanese* [Javanese: *Oedyånå pårå Prajitnå*], which aimed to provide interesting stories, enrich the Javanese language, and inform readers about the Netherlands. 'The Javanese language needs to be ennobled', he argued; 'it needs to become suitable as a vehicle to render … all thoughts of modern life'.[63] For Boenjamin the first step in this process was adopting the Latin script. Articles in Dutch or Javanese discussed political life in the Netherlands, overpopulation, how to raise Javanese girls, Boedi Oetomo, the Javanese painter Raden Saleh, the social position of Indies physicians, and the new curriculum of the Batavia Medical College (STOVIA). Boenjamin apparently lost interest when he was posted to West Guinea, and the magazine folded after five issues.

The Christian Ambonese brothers Johannes Everhardus and Willem Karel Tehupeiory soon received Dutch medical degrees as well.[64] After graduating from the Batavia Medical College, Johannes established a successful obstetric practice just outside Batavia to finance his and his brother's future

---

[61] 'De Eerste Inlandsche Officier van Gezondheid in Ned.-Indië', *Sumatra Post*, 30 July 1908, Section II, 2.

[62] See, for example, 'Inlandsche Officieren', *Het Nieuws van den Dag voor Nederlandsch-Indië*, 24 June 1910, 1; and 21 July 1910, 1. In both articles, Rivai and Semaoen, the first native officers of health, were mentioned.

[63] [R. Boenjamin], 'Aan Onze Stamgenoten!', *Oedyånå pårå Prajitnå* 1, no. 1 (1909), 2.

[64] For a historical novel containing biographies of the Tehupeiory brothers, see Herman Keppy, *Tussen Ambon en Amsterdam* (Amsterdam: Conserve, 2004).

studies in the Netherlands.[65] In 1903, he joined a scientific expedition through Kalimantan.[66] Johannes wrote for several vernacular newspapers and, while in the Netherlands, wrote articles for Rivai's *Bintang Hindia*.[67] He became a prominent member of the General Dutch Association [Algemeen Nederlands Verbond], which promoted the use of the Dutch language and aimed to unite all Dutch speakers across the globe.[68] Unfortunately, a few days after receiving his medical degree, he died from asphyxiation while sleeping in a hotel room, because of a leaking gas lamp. In 1909, immediately upon his return to the Indies, Willem Karel Tehupeiory established the Ambonese Study Fund for students from Maluku and, with Boenjamin, founded the Association of Indies Physicians. Both organisations were chaired by Maluku Indies physician D. J. Sijahaja.

The hostility of European physicians hindered the careers of their Indies colleagues with Dutch medical degrees. To avoid potential conflict, the Civil Medical Service placed Tehupeiory on the remote island of Bangka, known for its tin mines, where his closest Dutch colleague was hundreds of kilometres away. In 1916, Tehupeiory, his wife, and his two children returned to the Netherlands because they could not adapt to life in the colonies. Tehupeiory's marriage was not successful. While his wife thought that she had attained social respectability and financial security by marrying a physician, Tehupeiory was idealistic and did not care much about money. In 1922, Tehupeiory returned to the Indies because he thought that his professional prospects were better there. He and his wife never saw each other again. Tehupeiory continued to be involved in the Association of Indies Physicians and was nominated for a seat in the Volksraad several times. He died in 1946 in Jakarta, remaining loyal to the Dutch queen and the Netherlands until the end of his life.

The Christian Ambonese physician Hubertus Domingo Jan Apituley was the next Indies physician to receive a Dutch medical degree. Apituley became known for his relentlessly pro-Dutch views in colonial politics. In 1928, he founded, with Tehupeiory, the Maluku Political Union [Moluksch Politiek Verbond], opposing the Ambon Association [Sarekat Ambon], which they

---

[65] J. E. Tehupeiory published a number of interesting case studies in the STOVIA journal: J. E. Tehupeiory, 'Enkele Mededeelingen uit Mijne Verloskundige Praktijk', *Tijdschrift van Inlandsche Geneeskundigen* 11, no. 7, 8, 9, 10 (1903), 97–113.

[66] J. E. Tehupeiory, *Onder de Dajaks in Centraal-Borneo: Een Reisverhaal* (Batavia: Kolff, 1906).

[67] J. E. Tehupeiory wrote a long novel, which appeared in daily instalments in *Bendera Wolanda*. See Johannes Everardus Tehupeiory, 'Raden Adjeng Badaroesmi: Een Nimf uit de Preanger', in *De Njai Moeder van Alle Volken: De Roos uit Tijkembang en Andere Verhalen*, ed. Maya Sutedja-Liem (Leiden: KITLV Press, 2007), 73–174.

[68] J. E. Tehupeiory, *De Inlander Voor en Na de Stichting van het Algemeen Nederlandsch Verbond* (Amsterdam: Boon, 1908). On the Algemeen Nederlandsch Verbond, see Groeneboer, *Gateway to the West*, 240–47; 398–403.

thought had become too radical (Tehupeiory soon relinquished his membership). The new organisation aimed to secure and enhance ties between the Netherlands and the Indies, and was Apituley's mouthpiece when he was a member of the Volksraad from 1922 to 1934. On many occasions, Apituley was the only native member to vote against initiatives of his nationalist colleagues.[69] In 1935, upon retirement, he moved to the Netherlands, where his children attended university. He died there in 1944.

Mas Soewarno, the founding secretary of Boedi Oetomo, received his Dutch medical degree in 1913 and successfully defended a dissertation on trachoma the same year.[70] In 1919, after marrying Dutch physician and novelist Johanna Cornelia van der Kaaden, he returned to the Indies, where the Civil Medical Service employed him to investigate the prevalence of eye disease in eastern Java. He was subsequently appointed lecturer in ophthalmology at the Surabaya Medical College, where he became known for mentoring medical students and encouraging his colleagues to conduct medical research. His wife opened her own private practice in obstetrics and gynaecology in Surabaya.[71] In 1930, they returned with their son to the Netherlands because of Soewarno's tuberculosis, and both opened private practices in The Hague. Johanna wrote three novels with medical themes set in the Indies, revealing a keen insight into the different ethnic groups and their ambivalent feelings towards Western medicine. Her novels were suffused with a strong compassion for suffering individuals but political themes were entirely absent.[72] In late 1945 Soewarno temporarily returned to Indonesia to treat the eye diseases of Europeans who had been interned by the Japanese.[73] He officially became a Dutch citizen in 1956 and replaced his Javanese title 'Mas' with the Dutch first name 'Maarten'.

Several other notable members of the first generation of Indies physicians studied in the Netherlands. Before departing the Indies, Christian Minahasan Philip Laoh had published an elaborate study on beriberi as an infectious disease.[74] After his return to the Indies, he advocated establishing native militias in the Indies to demonstrate loyalty to the Queen. In 1926, Christian Minahasan

---

[69] See Richard Chauvel, *Nationalists, Soldiers and Separatists: The Ambonese Islands from Colonialism to Revolt, 1880–1950* (Leiden: KITLV Press, 2008), 142.

[70] Mas Soewarno, *Over Eenige Vormen van Irisdepigmentatie* (Amsterdam: De Bussy, 1919).

[71] L. Kaiser, 'In Memoriam Mevr. Dr. J. C. Soewarno-van der Kaaden', *Nederlands Tijdschrift voor Geneeskunde* 109, no. 5 (1965), 243–44.

[72] Johanna Cornelia Soewarno-van der Kaaden, *Nonna Dokter* (Bussum: Van Dishoek, 1936); *De Weg naar Pelantoegan* (Leiden: Stafleu, 1936); *De Bonte Slendang* (Bussum: Van Dishoek, 1942).

[73] M. Soewarno, 'Iets over Kampogen', *Nederlands Tijdschrift voor Geneeskunde* 90 (14 January 1946), 213–16.

[74] Ph. Laoh, *Iets over de Aetiologie, Prophylaxis en Therapie der Beri-Beri: Bijdragen tot de Kennis der Infectie-Ziekten* (Batavia: Kolff, 1903).

surgeon, gynaecologist, and X-ray specialist Heinig Frederik Lumentut announced that he had convincing evidence that cancer was caused by radioactive substances, which, he claimed, could also cure it. He left the Indies to conduct further research on his theory at the Institut de Radium in Paris, where he was a colleague of Pierre and Marie Curie. He became sick soon after and died in 1936. After he received his Dutch medical degree, Javanese physician Mas Radjiman became the court physician at Solo's sultanate, serving Sunan Pakubuwono X. He always had a strong interest in philosophy and ardently promoted Javanese culture throughout his life. In 1945, he rose to national prominence when he joined Sukarno and Hatta on a mission to discuss independence with the Japanese.

The twenty physicians from the Indies who obtained medical degrees in the Netherlands before World War I exerted a profound influence on the Indies medical profession. Despite marked differences in ethnicity, religious affiliation, type of medical practice, and the extent of their political involvement, there were striking similarities. They were united in their belief in modern medicine and in their loyalty to the medical profession. They were enthralled by the world of science and medicine, and advocated education for the indigenous population. They all supported increasing the quality of medical education in the Indies and improving the working conditions of Indies physicians. They also embraced Rivai's idealistic visions of a future society in which education and professional accomplishment erased the impediments of colour and descent. Their professional identity as physicians inspired some of them to engage in a range of social, cultural, and political activities. Many were members of the General Dutch Association [Algemeen Nederlands Verbond] and several were active as journalists, members of city councils, and ethnic associations. Two became members of the Volksraad and used their positions to pursue the issues which animated their cohort: increases in the remuneration of Indies physicians, the enhancement of the medical curriculum, increases in funding for the public health service, and improvements in sanitary conditions in the Indies.

Conclusion

From the 1880s, the Indies vernacular press tirelessly promoted progress, development, and the importance of education in transforming the Indies from a traditional into a modern society. It attributed European hegemony in the colonies to education and technological advancement, and assumed that the deep chasm separating Europeans from natives could be bridged through the efforts of a new, intellectual elite – and considered themselves its pioneering members. Rivai and his cohort were committed to pursuing individual social advancement. They expected that conforming to European social and cultural standards, holding European academic qualifications, and obtaining European legal status would allow entry into the European social sphere. Most soon realised that these hopes were unrealistic. Instead, they found themselves occupying ambiguous, even paradoxical social positions in colonial life. Some grew frustrated or fell into despair. Others sought to understand their predicament through an almost obsessive analysis of colonial life. Still others became involved with the Association of Indies Physicians, which worked to improve the social position of their profession.

It would be easy to dismiss Rivai's fanatical emulation of European appearances, qualifications, and related characteristics as colonial mimicry. Several European physicians did indeed criticise their would-be Indies colleagues as mere imitators lacking moral and intellectual substance. Rivai's political program was similarly dismissed as little more than advocating a derivative makeover of the Indies in a European fashion. This type of critique was levelled against Rivai in the late 1920s and 1930s by Indies intellectuals, of whom psychiatrist, Theosophist, and fellow Sumatran Mohamad Amir was the most outspoken. Amir disparaged the disciples of the gospel of progress in strong language: 'At that time, when we had just woken up from our sleep, we became counterfeiters, mere parrots, while looking at the West as the Himalaya; the voice of the West was more valuable than the Gospel or the Koran.'[75] Rivai had always been 'intoxicated by new things, fashionable things', he wrote, 'and thought that everything that embodied "progress" deserved praise'.[76] Amir claimed that Rivai had given up the archipelago's rich cultural heritage for Western science: 'a Malay soul hypnotised by the West' attempting to be 'more Western than the West'.[77] Amir disdained the profound elitism of this small group of educated Indonesians, who declared everybody else to be old-fashioned, outdated, primitive, and stupid. He thought that the Indies should chart its own course in the process of modernisation, assisted by Western science, technology, and medicine, but not guided by it.[78]

Indies intellectuals did not long consider the Netherlands the prime model of modernity. After the industrialised slaughter of World War I became known, Western modernity lost its lustre, and many Indonesian intellectuals turned to a highly idealised image of indigenous cultures of the Indies to bolster Indonesian nationalism. To them, the traditional village, once an emblem of

---

[75] Mohamad Amir, 'Kemadjuan', in *Boenga Rampai*, ed. M. Sarqawi (Medan: Centrale Courant en Boekhandel, 1940), 107–08.
[76] Amir, 'Kemadjuan', 107.
[77] Amir, 'Rivai', 185, 184.
[78] Amir, 'Kemadjuan', 108.

backwardness soon to be overtaken by modern life, was now transformed into the main reservoir of traditional culture, social cohesion, and a deeply communitarian spirit. Consequently, the damage done to these traditional villages became a potent argument against colonialism while the revitalisation of their unique spirit indicated the pathway of the future country's alternate form of modernity.

2   The Enchantment of Cosmopolitan Science: Student Life at the Dutch East Indies Medical Colleges

In 1851, a modest initiative to teach medicine to indigenous young men commenced at Batavia's military hospital. Students arrived from all over Java to enrol in a two-year course. As the medical curriculum was updated and expanded, students came from the whole archipelago. In 1902, when the school moved to new, purpose-built quarters and was renamed the School for the Education of Native Physicians [School tot Opleiding van Inlandsche Artsen] (STOVIA), it offered a nine-year training program. The Dutch government had inaugurated the Ethical Policy the previous year, strengthening the indigenous voices that had advocated development and modernity for more than two decades. In the final years of the nineteenth century, student life at the Batavia Medical College became distinctly European. Students spoke Dutch with each other, were instructed in the latest findings of Western medical science, and spent their spare time in a metropolitan city. They had busy extracurricular lives playing sports, participating in student associations, reading newspapers, and partying. In conduct, dress, language, aesthetic preference, and ideals, they appeared 'modern'. They believed intensely in the power of medical science, which they saw as quintessentially rational and scientific, and were filled with pride in their school and in their future profession. Simultaneously, pupils came to regard the indigenous world of the Indies as diseased and primitive, and in need of the remedies of Western medicine. Medicine entailed for them a mission to bring hygienic modernity to the Indies.[1]

With the announcement of the Ethical Policy, the strengthening of the medical curriculum, and its move to the new premises, the symbolic significance of the Batavia Medical College increased markedly. It continued to be the only place in the colony where natives could receive training in scientific and experimental methods. Until the 1920s, when an engineering and a law school were established, it offered the most advanced form of education in the Indies. A second medical college was established in Surabaya in 1913. Here and in Batavia, instructors sought to awaken rational and moral sensibilities in what

---

[1] The phrase 'hygienic modernity' is derived from Ruth Rogaski, *Hygienic Modernity: Meanings of Health and Disease in Treaty-Port China* (Berkeley: University of California Press, 2004).

they viewed as young, native, and therefore still primitive minds to produce mature, modern, and moral ones respecting evidence and desiring truth, as well as being dedicated to the welfare of humanity. The medical colleges were unusual colonial laboratories which blurred the boundaries between native and European, brown and white. During their education, students transgressed the distinctions which constituted colonial society.[2] Graduates emerged with hybrid identities and found it difficult to find their places in colonial society. As well as producing physicians willing to work in the budding Indies planta-tion economy at lower salaries than Europeans, the medical colleges came to epitomise the promises (or, as critics would later argue, the mistakes) of the Ethical Policy.

Medical Education in the Dutch East Indies

Medical education in the Dutch East Indies began inauspiciously. After surveying the devastating effects of a typhoid epidemic in Central Java in 1847, Willem Bosch, then director of the colonial medical service, recommended that young Javanese men of good standing receive instruction in medicine.[3] The first medical college in the Indies was the Javanese Doctors' School [Dokter Djawa School], established in 1851. It consisted of a few rooms set aside in Batavia's military hospital and offered a two-year training course, taught in Malay, for assistant physicians and vaccinators.[4] Graduates received the title 'Javanese Physician' [*Dokter Djawa*], even after the school began admitting students from all ethnic groups. In the following decades, the medical cur-riculum was progressively expanded.[5] Dutch was introduced as the language of instruction in 1875 and laboratory work became increasingly important in the 1890s. By the turn of the twentieth century it had become a fully-fledged medical college.

During the first fifteen years of operation (1851–66), it was not unusual for young Javanese aristocrats to enrol.[6] When it became clear that *Dokters Djawa*

---

[2] Suman Seth, 'Colonial History and Postcolonial Science Studies', *Radical History Review*, no. 127 (2017), 67; for parallel developments in India, see Gyan Prakash, *Another Reason: Science and the Imagination of Modern India* (Princeton, NJ: Princeton University Press, 1999).

[3] Liesbeth Hesselink, *Healers on the Colonial Market: Native Doctors and Midwives in the Dutch East Indies* (Leiden: KITLV Press, 2011), 60–72.

[4] Hesselink, *Healers on the Colonial Market*, 60–81. For other overviews of the history of the Batavia Medical School, see Gabrielle Lauw, 'De Dokter Djawa School te Batavia (1850–1875)', *Spiegel Historiael: Maandblad voor Geschiedenis en Archeologie* 23, no. 2 (1988), 75–79; A. de Waart, ed. *Ontwikkeling van het Geneeskundig Onderwijs te Weltevreden, 1851–1926* (Weltevreden: Kolff, 1926); Cornelis Leonard van der Burg, 'Schets eener Geschiedenis der School voor Inlandsche Geneeskundigen (Dokter Djawa) te Batavia', *Indische Gids* 18 (1896), 1862–76.

[5] Hesselink, *Healers on the Colonial Market*, 93–99.

[6] Hesselink, *Healers on the Colonial Market*, 85.

received a remuneration equivalent to that of lower government clerks and less than indigenous teachers, they lost interest. The colonial administration also failed to create a symbolic position for the school's graduates within the traditional aristocratic hierarchy: *Dokters Djawa* were not allowed to carry parasols [*pajung*] or other aristocratic regalia.[7] Regents and other members of the upper layer of the indigenous aristocracy generally relied on their wealth and connections to secure the futures of their sons. In 1872, the colonial administration established three modest schools to train students for high administrative positions [*Hoofdenschool* or *Sekolah Raja*]. Because the tuition fees were exorbitant, these schools were only available to wealthy aristocratic families eager to secure well-remunerated jobs for their sons.

Members of the lower ranks of the indigenous aristocracy were aware that the careers of their sons depended on the education they received, since they had no means of securing their future careers in other ways. The medical colleges were attractive because medical training was free. Not surprisingly, these colleges acquired a reputation as schools for the impecunious. In 1927, C. D. de Langen, instructor in internal medicine at the STOVIA, referred to the medical college as the school for the poor [*sekolah miskin*].[8] An Indies physician agreed: 'The STOVIA is frequented mostly by children from the *lower* aristocratic circles.'[9] In exchange for free education and a modest allowance to buy food and basic necessities, students were obliged to work for the colonial administration for a period of ten years upon graduation. The graduates of the Indies medical colleges, in turn, felt a deep-seated rancour towards the higher aristocracy, which, they claimed, comprised lazy, overpaid, and vain individuals very different from educated, moral, and hard-working individuals like themselves. From the turn of the twentieth century, the traditional and intellectual aristocracies were persistently at loggerheads.

In the 1870s the use of Malay, the archipelago's lingua franca, as the language of instruction became one of the most significant obstacles to medical education. The instructors barely spoke it and it was the second language for most students. Moreover, teachers found it difficult to find suitable Malay equivalents for scientific terms, and translation was time-consuming. A former teacher described how, as a consequence, an unusual language developed at

---

[7] Hesselink, *Healers on the Colonial Market*, 117; Liesbeth Hesselink, 'The Unbearable Absence of Parasols: The Formidable Weight of a Colonial Java Status Symbol', *IIAS Newsletter*, no. 45 (2007), 26.

[8] C. D. de Langen, 'Beroepsbelangen', *Orgaan der Vereeniging van Indische Geneeskundigen* 16, no. 1 (1927), 13.

[9] Mohamad Amir, 'Rondom een Indisch Jeugdcongres', *Opbouw* 10, no. 2 (1927), 74; my emphasis. See also Margono Djojohadikusumo, *Herinneringen uit 3 Tijdperken: Een Geschreven Familie-Overlevering* (Jakarta: Indira, 1970), 43.

the school, 'a mixture of Malay, Dutch, and Latin'.[10] Because of this linguistic handicap, most teachers opted to avoid prescribed subjects such as anatomy, chemistry, and physics, and focused instead on instilling practical skills, hoping to produce 'useful assistants instead of useless physicians'.[11] After years of unsatisfactory experiences, instructors concluded that Malay was suitable for bartering and trade, but not for scientific instruction and rational thought. In 1875, Dutch became the language of instruction and a two-year preparatory course was added to the five-year medical course. Students initially had difficulty mastering Dutch because they did not use it in everyday conversation. This changed after the student body became more ethnically diverse and more students had received some Dutch language instruction before matriculating. In the 1880s, Dutch became the primary language for all students at the medical colleges.

In 1888, when future Nobel Laureate Christiaan Eijkman was appointed director, the Dokter Djawa School became a prestigious educational institute. Eijkman made his laboratory, established to investigate beriberi, available for teaching purposes. Believing that beriberi was an infectious disease, he had brought the latest bacteriological equipment from the Netherlands.[12] After 1890, students served rotations and internships at the polyclinics of the military hospital where Batavia's inhabitants received free surgical, ophthalmological, and general medical care. In 1896, Eijkman's successor, Hermanus Frederik Roll, suggested extending medical training to six years. The following year, three wealthy Deli planters who had successfully introduced health programs for the indentured labourers on their plantations – decreasing labour turnover and increasing profits – funded a new building. Roll's ambitious plans were implemented in 1902 and the college was renamed the School for the Education of Native Physicians [School tot Opleiding van Inlandsche Artsen] (STOVIA), granting the title of 'Native Physician' [*Inlandsch Arts*]. The new quarters comprised several teaching spaces, rooms for dissection and laboratory experiments, and dormitories. An entrance examination was introduced. Around twenty students enrolled in the preparatory course and twelve in the medical course annually.

In 1913, the curriculum was expanded again and a new name, the School for the Education of Indies Physicians [School tot Opleiding van Indische Artsen]

---

[10] J. Alken, 'De School voor Doctor Djawa', *Indisch Genootschap*, 28 February 1882, 2. For the discussions around the 1875 reform, see Hesselink, *Healers on the Colonial Market*, 100–01, 111–13.

[11] Van den Burg, 'Schets eener Geschiedenis', 1968.

[12] Eijkman's research demonstrated that the cause of beriberi was a nutritional deficiency, and stimulated later research on vitamins and other essential nutrients. On Eijkman see Kenneth J. Carpenter, *Beriberi, White Rice, and Vitamin B: A Disease, a Cause, and a Cure* (Berkeley: University of California Press, 2000).

(the acronym remained STOVIA), was adopted. The college now conveyed the degree of 'Indies Physician' [*Indisch Arts*]. The preparatory course was extended to three years and the medical course to seven – ten years in total. The Batavia Medical College now accepted all inhabitants of the Indies and, for the first time, women, although they were not allowed to stay in the dormitories and their numbers remained low. Even though European, Arab, and Chinese students could enrol for medical training, their number remained negligible. The same year, a second medical college opened in Surabaya: the Netherlands Indies Physicians School [Nederlandsch-Indische Artsen School] (NIAS), which also awarded the degree of 'Indies Physician'. The Surabaya Medical College, like the school in Batavia, had an unpromising start. The preparatory department was housed in a large but poorly equipped residential house.[13] During World War I, books and teaching material were difficult to obtain and the arrival of teachers was delayed. Only seven microscopes were available for all the students, and 'only one skeleton and one anatomical atlas'.[14] Almost all classes were taught by the college's director, A. E. Sitsen. In 1923, the NIAS buildings were completed (Figure 2.1; they are part of the Faculty of Medicine at Airlangga University today), the first three Indies physicians graduated, and Soetomo, who had completed his advanced medical training in the Netherlands, was appointed as instructor in dermatology. In the following years, the Surabaya Medical College hired several Indies physicians as instructors after they had received advanced medical training in Europe. In 1928, the School for the Education of Indies Dentists [School ter Opleiding van Indische Tandheelkundigen] (STOVIT) opened next to the NIAS.

In Batavia, engineers finished a new and much larger building in July 1920 which would house the medical college (these buildings are now part of the Faculty of Medicine at the University of Indonesia). This was the outcome of an ambitious plan to arrange medical research, medical care, and medical education in close proximity. The school was located next to the recently inaugurated Central Civil Hospital [Centrale Burgerlijke Ziekeninrichting] (CBZ) and a new medical laboratory, informally named the Eijkman Institute. During the years prior to 1920, the STOVIA building had become increasingly cramped and a number of dormitory halls had been converted to laboratory space. From

---

[13] For histories of the NIAS, see 'De Nederlandsch-Indische Artsenschool (NIAS) te Soerabaja', in *NIAS Jaarboek 1932* (Surabaya: Kolff, 1932), 53–58; R. J. F. Zeben, 'Rede', in *NIAS-STOVIT Lustrum Almanak 1938* (Soerabaja: Kolff, 1938), 9–20; Widohariadi and Bambang Permono, *Peringatan 70 Tahun Pendidikan Dokter di Surabaya* (Surabaya: Gideon, 1983); Widohariadi and Bambang Permono, *Peringatan 90 Tahun Pendidikan Dokter di Surabaya* (Surabaya: Fakultas Kedoktoran Universitas Airlingga, 2003); Sandiantoro, *Jejak Jiwa, di Listasan Zaman (1913– 2013): Mengenang yang Silam, Meretas Masa Depan* (Surabaya: Peringatan 1 Abad Pendidikan Dokter di Surabaya, 2013).

[14] Soetopo, 'Bij de Viering van het Derde Lustrum van de NIAS te Soerabaia', *NIAS Orgaan* 3, no. 1 (1928), 53.

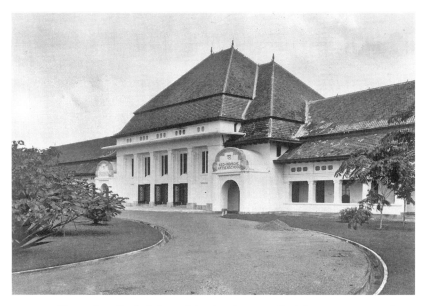

Figure 2.1 The building of the Surabaya Medical College (NIAS). Figure courtesy of the Dutch National Museum of Ethnology, Leiden (TM10002343)

1918, classes were transferred to the still incomplete new buildings and all rooms of the old building became dormitories. To mark the opening of the new buildings and to create a favourable impression abroad, the fourth Congress of the Far-Eastern Association of Tropical Medicine was held there in August 1921.[15] In 1927, the Batavia Medical School [Geneeskundige Hoogeschool], which awarded degrees equivalent to European university-affiliated medical schools, was established. From that moment, the STOVIA no longer accepted new students and its buildings were transferred to the new medical school.

Student Life

Sociologists investigating post-war medical education in Europe and North America agree that attending medical school was (and continues to be) a transformative experience.[16] Studying medicine not only involves acquiring

---

[15] L. S. A. M. von Römer, *Historical Sketches: An Introduction to the Fourth Congress of the Far Eastern Association of Tropical Medicine, to Be Held at Batavia from 6th to 13th August 1921* (Batavia: Javasche Boekhandel en Drukkerij, 1921).

[16] For some classical studies, see, for example, Robert K. Merton, George G. Reader, and Patricia L. Kendall, *The Student-Physician: Introductory Studies in the Sociology of Medical Education* (Cambridge, MA: Harvard University Press for the Commonwealth Fund, 1957); Howard S. Becker, Blanche Geer, Everett C. Hughes, and Anselm M. Strauss, *Boys in White: Student Culture in Medical School* (Chicago: University of Chicago Press, 1961); Renée

vast amounts of knowledge and attaining large numbers of skills but also profoundly changes a student's disposition, cognitive orientation, emotional style, and behaviour. Medical students, in particular, become emotionally detached after dissecting human cadavers and interacting with despairing patients during rotations and internships. They also tend to develop physiological and reductionist perspectives on disease, their patients, and the human body which displace social, political, cultural, and spiritual factors. Students form strong bonds with each other and identify with their future profession; at the same time, ties to friends and family weaken. During the later years of their training, they increasingly conform to implicit but pervasive professional standards in their speech, actions, reactions, and emotions. These findings are particularly pertinent to medical students in the Dutch East Indies, because students enrolled at a younger age, were more isolated from their families, and lived in school environments entirely unlike their childhood surroundings. By the same measure, the Indies medical schools were ideal colonial laboratories for the transformation of young native teenagers into educated, modern, and cosmopolitan men.

Batavia and Surabaya were large metropolitan centres in the Dutch East Indies. The many impressive buildings and the various possibilities for entertainment gave colour to student life. 'Apart from becoming a Stovian', said one student, 'you become a Batavian!'[17] Another spoke of his deep love for the people of Batavia, their sense of humour, tolerance, and the many ethnic groups which together created a unique 'Betawi' blend of life.[18] An NIAS student remembered his arrival in Surabaya 'with its busy traffic, not in any way less than that in Batavia, with its beautiful harbour and its shopping palaces'.[19] For many students, attending medical school meant leaving the slow and stagnant life of small rural villages for the energetic, sometimes frenetic life of the metropolis. The medical schools opened a gateway not only to science but to the modern world.

The STOVIA was located next to the military hospital in the modern centre of Batavia and was surrounded by high walls – a separation from the outside world which was both real and symbolic. Naturally, these walls inspired countless efforts to scale them, typically at night.[20] The school buildings

---

C. Fox, *Experiment Perilous: Physicians and Patients Facing the Unknown* (New Brunswick, NJ: Transaction, 1998); Renée C. Fox, *Essays in Medical Sociology: Journeys into the Field* (New Brunswick, NJ: Transaction, 1988).

[17] A., 'STOVIA Schetsen, 1913–1923', in *STOVIA Almanak 1924* (Weltevreden: Kolff, 1924), 170.

[18] 'Betawi' was the common name for Batavia among the indigenous population; it also refers to the group who originally lived in the area before the Dutch conquered their city. Johnny, 'Bekentenissen', in *STOVIA Almanak 1925* (Weltevreden: Kolff, 1925), 155–58.

[19] Noeroe'l Soem, 'Moeder!: Lief en Leed van een NIASser', in *NIAS-STOVIT Lustrum Almanak 1938* (Soerabaja: Kolff, 1938), 107.

[20] One of the student essays written for a lesson in the Dutch language which was part of the preparatory course at the STOVIA deals with the various methods students had designed to

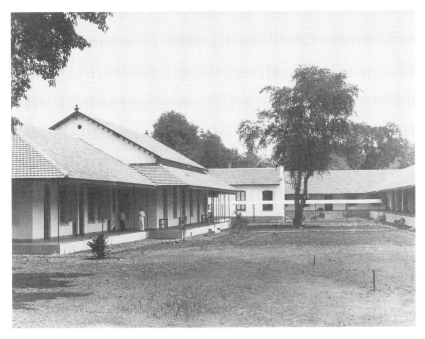

Figure 2.2 Courtyard of the Batavia Medical College (STOVIA) in 1902.
Figure: University of Leiden library, KITLV collection (35819)

enclosed a pleasant courtyard with large and shady trees. In the centre was a recreation hall with two billiard tables, comfortable chairs, and a large table with newspapers and periodicals. Buildings with shared bedrooms for the older students and an athletics hall (Figure 2.2) were also placed in the court-yard. The buildings at the back were taken up by four large dormitories for the younger students (Figure 2.3). Student life was highly structured. 'In those days', commented one graduate, 'we were treated as … soldiers. Everything went by the clock'.[21] Students woke at six, showered, and dressed. Classes ran from seven to one. During the afternoon, students rested, played music, studied, or had lunch outside the school. Javanese and Sumatran students organised canteens for lunch. From seven in the evening, students toiled, under super-vision, in the study halls. At ten, a roll call was held in the central courtyard.

escape the STOVIA at night. See Aboe Bakar, 'Het leven van den STOVIAAN', written in 1916. Collection Nederlandstalige opstellen J. Toot, KITLV Archival Collections DH 1274.

[21] Jacob Samallo, 'Herinneringen uit het Leven van de Élèves der STOVIA 25 Jaar Geleden', in *Ontwikkeling van het Geneeskundig Onderwijs te Weltevreden, 1851–1926*, ed. A. de Waart (Weltevreden: Kolff, 1926), 290.

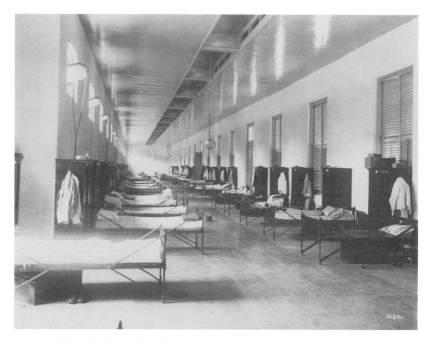

Figure 2.3 Dormitory for the younger students at the Batavia Medical College (STOVIA). Figure: University of Leiden library, KITLV collection (35818)

At ten, eleven, or twelve, depending on their age, students were sent to their dormitories and the lights were switched off.[22] Two attendants, both veterans of the colonial army, supervised all students. Transgressing the rules led to punishment or even expulsion. Students were permitted to leave the school buildings on Saturday evenings and on Sundays during the day.

As there was no dormitory at the Surabaya Medical College, students were housed in more than 100 households. The advanced students took their classes in the hospital, which was a good distance away. As a consequence, students were dispersed across the city. In 1916, the *NIAS Magazine* commenced publication, informing students of events at the school and increasing a sense of community. The following year, the NIAS Association was established to organise the celebration of the fifth anniversary of the school's founding. It sought to provide parties, cultural evenings, lectures, and sports events.[23] In the following years, students established clubs for chess, fencing, sports, music, and debating, as well as a Javanese cultural group. In 1930, students founded the NIAS Cooperative Society, which allowed them to buy clothing, books,

[22] Derde-jaars, 'Roemloos Einde', in *STOVIA Almanak 1924* (Weltevreden: Kolff, 1924), 188–94.
[23] 'De NIAS Vereeniging', in *NIAS Jaarboek 1932* (Surabaya: Kolff, 1932), 93–111.

and bicycles with discounts and on instalment plans. A clubhouse opened the following year. It had two billiard tables and became the social hub for student life.[24]

During their formative years, students at both medical colleges faced the challenge of navigating between indigenous and Western cultures. Like most teenagers, they devoted significant amounts of time to constructing, rehearsing, and performing their personal and professional identities. In conversations, newsletters, magazines, and yearbooks, they discussed life events, philosophical musings, and the unique nature of student life. They elaborated on their exhaustion from too much studying, the cruelty of professors setting difficult exams, the thrills of city life, infatuations, their pride in their school, and the fear of failure and expulsion. They also shared highlights, including sports, parties, and special events.[25] They articulated hybrid and consciously modern identities while they were socialised as physicians, and their behaviour, mannerisms, ways of talking, and appearance converged.

Matriculation was a rite of passage. During the first month, new students were 'greens' and subject to mild abuse by older students who taught them the school's ways.[26] Newly arrived medical students identified role models amongst the older cohorts and the college's instructors. They admired the senior students doing internships in local hospitals, dressed in impressive long, white coats. Older pupils became substitute parents, since all of them were, in a way, orphans.[27] At the NIAS, new students were told that they should find themselves 'a father in spirit' among the older students.[28] Close bonds developed between students to replace family ties. As one commented: 'For five years he had been living together with them, five years of his *Sturm und Drang* period. They were brothers to him, his class-mates.'[29] These bonds formed the basis

---

[24] 'Ons Clubhuis', in *NIAS Jaarboek 1932* (Surabaya: Kolff, 1932), 112–24.

[25] About love see, for example, 'Herderszangen', in *STOVIA Almanak 1923* (Weltevreden: Kolff, 1923), 165–66; Job, 'Bij de Uitdragers', in *STOVIA Almanak 1925* (Weltevreden: Kolff, 1925), 165–69; about partying, drinking, and hangovers see, for example, 'Fantasy', in *STOVIA Almanak 1925* (Weltevreden: Kolff, 1925), 150–52; about studying, the strain caused by exams, and the fear of failure and expulsion, see, for example, A. R., 'Wanneer Pluizer zijn Slag Slaat', in *STOVIA Almanak 1923* (Weltevreden: Kolff, 1923), 197–200; A. H., 'Zorgen', in *STOVIA Almanak 1925* (Weltevreden: Kolff, 1925), 159–61; Pirngadi Gonggopoetro, 'Ontslagen', in *STOVIA Almanak 1923* (Weltevreden: Kolff, 1923); J. L., 'Fragment uit 't Schoolleven', in *STOVIA Almanak 1926* (Weltevreden: Kolff, 1926), 253–58; and Samallo, 'Herinneringen STOVIA', 293.

[26] Samallo, 'Herinningen STOVIA', 189; Mohamad Roem, 'Tradisi Berpolitik', in *45 Tahun Sumpah Pemuda*, ed. Yayasan Gedung-Gedung Bersejarah Jakarta (Jakarta: Gunung Agung, 1974), 246–47; Mams, 'De Eerste Ontgroeningsavond', in *NIAS Lustrum Almanak 1933–1934* (Surabaya: NIAS, 1934), 249–42; Een Oude, 'Ontgroenen!', in *NIAS Lustrum Almanak 1933–1934* (Surabaya: NIAS, 1934), 266–68.

[27] 'Geestelijk Leven op de NIAS', *NIAS Orgaan* 11, no. 1-2-3 (1938), 19.

[28] 'Mijlpalen', *NIAS Orgaan* 11, no. 1-2-3 (1938), 24.

[29] Gonggopoetro, 'Ontslagen', 190.

for the personal and professional ties between Indies physicians. They became, in turn, a model for the new nation of Indonesia, in which regional and ethnic ties were also superseded by those joining citizens to each other and to the nation state.

In 1912, several STOVIA students lobbied successfully for the rescindment of the regulation requiring them to dress in ethnic attire, which was unusual in Batavia, and marked them as natives.[30] Western outfits, they argued, would elicit the respect rightly accorded to Indies physicians. By 1925, students dressed in silk socks, silk tie, jacket, trousers, and shirts: the best Western clothing they could afford.[31] Leading physician Hanafiah remembered that the day he enrolled at the STOVIA wearing his Minangkabau outfit, an older student took him to the tailor where all students had their clothes made to measure.[32]

For almost all students, medical college provided the first entrance into the world of science. One pupil recalled his sense of wonder as he took his first steps into the field of medicine:

How unforgettable the impressions were! Entering the dissecting room and viewing the anatomical preparations for the first time; this became the cause of many a terrible dream. Then the physiological experiments on animals, which caused my wounded heart to protest in silence. And now this investigation of traitorous micro-organisms, the sworn enemies of man.[33]

These musings occurred to this student while he was viewing microbes through the lens of a microscope (Figure 2.4). He had lost track of time and was alone in the laboratory; everyone else had left for the day, but he was unperturbed. He experienced an epiphany: he 'heard the voice of a sublime calling' and became aware that 'the study of nature would deepen my knowledge and widen the horizons of my ideas'.[34] Another student praised the impressive powers of the microscope:

The microscope has given us the power to study the previously invisible world of life, a world the size of which is impossible to estimate. How beautiful is the image that opens itself up before our eyes when we pay attention to the countless micro-organisms, the diversity of which most likely exceeds the number of grains of sand in the Sahara desert … Isn't it incredibly wonderful how a stethoscope and a test tube can unveil the most intricate secrets of human suffering.[35]

---

[30] Hesselink, *Healers on the Colonial Market*, 169–70, 200–01; Hans van Miert, *Een Koel Hoofd en een Warm Hart: Nationalisme, Javanisme en Jeugdbeweging in Nederlands-Indië, 1918–1930* (Amsterdam: Bataafsche Leeuw, 1995), 44.

[31] 'Trilbeelden', in *STOVIA Almanak 1926* (Weltevreden: Kolff, 1926), 240–45.

[32] Mohamad Ali Hanafiah, *77 Tahun Riwayat Hidup* (Jakarta: Author, 1977), 24.

[33] B. D. [Bahder Djohan], 'A Student's Idyls', in *STOVIA Almanak 1923* (Weltevreden: Kolff, 1923), 187. The original is in English.

[34] B. D., 'Student's Idyls', 188.

[35] M., 'De Medische Wetenschap', in *STOVIA Almanak 1923* (Weltevreden: Kolff, 1923), 180–81.

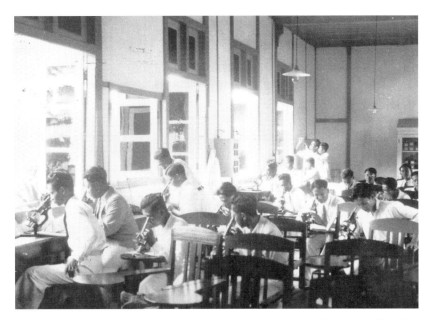

Figure 2.4 Students at the Surabaya Medical College (NIAS) using microscopes. Figure courtesy of the NIAS Museum, Faculty of Medicine, Airlangga University

Science provided the means to see what had been hidden. It could explain the happenings in the surface world; indeed, it could make them seem dull. The limitless potential of science was a recurring theme in student writings.

Like medical students everywhere, students at the Indies colleges came to apply a medical and physiological perspective to everyday situations. Latin phrases and seemingly scientific language featured in descriptions of everyday events and emphasised the students' other-worldliness. One student admired a painting of Adam and Eve while noticing how Adam's bronzed, bent-over body clearly showed the *inscriptiones tendineae* of his moderately tensed *rectus abdominis*.[36] Another saw 'in his sweetheart's lovely and delicate face only a mass of tiny muscles'.[37] A third wrote a series of medical and physiological descriptions of his fellow students, claiming that he relied on his clinical gaze for reliable diagnoses.[38] He commented favourably on the *glutaei* [the large muscles in the buttocks] of a European student, who always wore a straw hat

---

[36] Job, 'Bij de Uitdragers', 167.
[37] Marco B., 'Brief van een Derdejaars NIASser aan zijn Meisje', *NIAS Orgaan* 11, no. 1-2-3 (1938), 21.
[38] 'Tjoh', 'NIAS Zoologie', *NIAS Orgaan* 1, no. 2 (1926), 30.

to shelter the site of 'a couple of ganglion cells'.[39] The author apologised for the 'dissection style' of his writing; he was taking anatomy classes.[40] Students acquired a physiological and pathological gaze, a gaze they would later turn upon the colonial social body to analyse its workings.

While some students found time to write light-hearted pieces for college magazines and yearbooks, a great deal of time was spent studying, which was often tedious and exhausting. During the evenings, an eerie silence filled the study halls: 'They are sitting, bent over thick books, and study until they are no longer able to, until they are tired, mentally tired and blunted, and go to bed … Only the scribbling of pens over lecture notes and, every once in a while, the turning of a page can be heard.'[41] Students worked very hard. 'In bathrooms, in the garden, on the beds, while eating, everywhere the élèves [pupils] walked carrying or reading books.'[42] Instructors scheduled exams every three months to check progress, which significantly affected the students' moods in the weeks leading up to them.[43] For one student, exams were 'that mysterious enemy … and the great suffering of the Stovian', which forced him to forgo excursions, parties, and other pastimes.[44] Another compared exams to a battle-field, where one had to fight for victory; when he thought he had failed, he had recurring nightmares.[45] When one NIAS student died, his obituary suggested that one factor in his demise was exhaustion from endless studying.[46] Students frequently diagnosed themselves with neurasthenia, then a well-known neuro-logical condition characterised by extreme fatigue, listlessness, irritability, and insomnia.

At times, however, students allowed romance to interfere with their studies. Infatuations were frequent and engrossing: 'Stormy, full of passion, crazy, and illogical is love.'[47] One student met a young woman during a trip to Sumatra and became besotted with her.[48] Another was overcome with shyness when he fell for a shop attendant.[49] One pupil found life empty and without purpose while he longed for the day he would meet his beloved again.[50] Another student

[39] 'Tjoh', 'NIAS Zoologie', 30.
[40] 'Tjoh', 'NIAS Zoologie, II', *NIAS Orgaan* 1, no. 3 (1926), 59.
[41] A. R., 'Pluizer', 197, 198.
[42] M. A. Hanafiah, 'Sepuluh Tahun dalam Asrama STOVIA', in *125 Tahun Pendidikan Dokter di Indonesia 1851–1976*, ed. M. A. Hanafiah, Bahder Djohan, and Surono (Jakarta: FKUI, 1976), 103.
[43] Bahder Djohan, 'Algemeen Verslag over het Jaar 1925', in *STOVIA Almanak 1926* (Weltevreden: Kolff, 1926), 88.
[44] A., 'STOVIA Schetsen', 171.
[45] A. H., 'Zorgen', 159.
[46] A. Manap, 'In Memoriam R. Soetedjo', *NIAS Orgaan* 11–12, no. 4-1-2 (1938), 49.
[47] A., 'STOVIA Schetsen', 176.
[48] Sursum Corda, 'De Vreemdeling', in *STOVIA Almanak 1924* (Weltevreden: Kolff, 1924), 201–04.
[49] Job, 'Bij de Uitdragers', 164–69.
[50] Z., 'Zoeken', in *STOVIA Almanak 1924* (Weltevreden: Kolff, 1924), 199–200.

reviewed his romantic attachments in recent years and the emotional turmoil they had caused him, and decided he needed to focus on his studies and not indulge such silly thoughts.[51]

Partying too was inseparable from student life. STOVIA students especially liked the festivities marking the end of exams at the Batavia Botanical and Zoological Gardens. Attended by the mayor, members of the city council, officers of the public health service, teachers, and other dignitaries, they featured sports demonstrations, dance and theatre performances, and live music. Students would dance afterwards into the early hours. In 1923, more than 3,000 people took part in these festivities.[52] In 1930, the NIAS Association organised a large celebration marking the opening of the new school buildings seven years earlier, simply because it had excess funds. The anniversaries of the various student clubs were also celebrated. Some pupils spent too much time at the NIAS clubhouse; several were known to sleep on the billiard tables. Following parties, students often used sickness as an excuse for not attending early morning lectures.[53] The prohibition against drinking alcohol common among Muslims was not strictly observed at the colleges, and it was not uncommon for students to drink too much at student parties.

In an essay entitled 'The Standard Work', an anonymous student provided a humorous description of a mad scientist who had made a special study of *Homo Sapiens Bataviensis, variety STOVIA*. This species 'lives together in a colony, Hospital Road 32. Has its own manners and customs. Its own language … Very easy to differentiate from *Homo Sapiens Bataviensis Vulgaris* or the common people'. The fifth section of the essay concerned psychology and mental life: 'love and heart-neuroses … the frequency of neurasthenia in relation to exams … wallet-asthenia … *guna-guna* [black magic] and the magical mysticism of Java … the over-stimulation of the political centre [of the brain, and] the admissibility of [newspapers] as daily reading material'.[54] The students' interest in politics was also noted. This new type of human, the mad scientist found, displayed a fascinating blend of traditional traits and modern ideals. A new, hybrid colonial subject was in the making.

Teachers and Role Models

Students held their instructors in high esteem. They were particularly fond of teachers who advocated the further expansion of the medical curriculum

---

[51] Ja-Ben, 'Van Groen naar Rood', in *NIAS Lustrum Almanak 1933–1934* (Surabaya: NIAS, 1934), 243–47.

[52] See, for example, 'STOVIA aan het Feesten', *Bataviaasch Nieuwsblad*, 11 May 1917, 2; 'De STOVIA Fuif', *Het Nieuws van de Dag voor Nederlandsch-Indië*, 2 May 1922, 5.

[53] 'Aether-Trillingen', in *NIAS Lustrum Almanak 1933–1934* (Surabaya: NIAS, 1934), 219.

[54] Orion, 'Het Standaardwerk', in *STOVIA-Almanak 1923* (Weltevreden: Kolff, 1923), 172, 175.

and supported the cause of Indies physicians. They revered Dr Roll, generally referred to as Father Roll, 'a name he deserved with honour'.[55] Roll had been involved in removing bureaucratic obstacles for Indies physicians wishing to pursue advanced medical training in the Netherlands. In 1908, when most teachers wanted to expel Soetomo because of his involvement with Boedi Oetomo, Roll defended him. The following year, when a committee on the organisation of medical education recommended lowering standards to increase the number of graduates, Roll made his opposition known.[56] 'This school needs to graduate *full*, not *half* physicians', he often stated.[57] Roll conducted an informal survey among Dutch medical professors that showed the high esteem in which they held Indies physicians.[58] 'For the fact that medical study at the STOVIA has taken such a high flight', wrote an Indies physician in 1927, 'we inhabitants of the Indies primarily have to thank Dr Roll'.[59]

Instructors organised extracurricular activities to help shape their students after European ideals. There were several student associations, modelled on their Dutch counterparts. 'The student associations have a very important place in our student society', wrote Minangkabau medical student Bahder Djohan, editor of the STOVIA yearbooks (and future president of the University of Indonesia).[60] There was a gymnastics and fencing club, a soccer club (which had a strong local reputation), a music society, a club devoted to Javanese music, song, and dance, a chess club, a Sumatran *pencak silat* (martial arts) club, a tennis club, and a Hawaiian Band club, which won several prizes at citywide competitions. Roll was especially proud of the large recreation hall, which 'met a real need to keep students out of the *kampong*'.[61] The only significant gap in the medical students' hermetic world was the lack of cooking facilities. As a former teacher related, students who spent time in the *kampong* to have lunch were exposed to European drifters, inferior kinds of Indo-Europeans, criminal natives who had fled their villages, and the lower classes generally. Placing pupils with respectable European families would have a more salubrious and civilising effect.[62]

[55] Samallo, 'Herinneringen STOVIA', 290.
[56] H. F. Roll, *Is Reorganisatie van de School tot Opleiding van Inlandsche Artsen te Weltevreden Nogmaals Nodig?* (Dordrecht: Morks & Geuze, 1909).
[57] Samallo, 'Herinneringen STOVIA', 291.
[58] Roll, *Reorganisatie STOVIA Nodig?*, 15–16. Indies physicians frequently quoted this survey.
[59] Samallo, 'Herinneringen STOVIA', 291.
[60] Bahder Djohan, 'School tot Opleiding van Indische Artsen: Verslag over 1923', in *STOVIA Almanak 1924* (Weltevreden: Kolff, 1924), 79.
[61] H. F. Roll, *Jaarlijksch Verslag der School tot Opleiding van Inl. Artsen te Weltevreden over den Cursus 1902/1903* (Batavia: Landsdrukkerij, 1903), 13.
[62] A. J. H. Scherp, 'De Inrichting der Gouvernements-Internaten voor Inlandsche Jonglieden in Nederlands-Indië in Verband met de Zedelijke Vorming der Leerlingen', *Indisch Genootschap*, 26 Maart 1907, 219–41. Scherp had been an instructor at the STOVIA for six years. Scherp's

Others recommended that the STOVIA provide meals, but this never eventuated.[63]

Some instructors encouraged their students to conduct research and to publish their findings. In 1893, the Dokter Djawa School initiated the *Journal for Native Physicians* [*Tijdschrift voor Inlandsche Geneeskundigen*], which was distributed to all students and graduates. The first issues featured articles on tropical anaemia, the use of mercury as a laxative, phlebotomy, indigenous and Chinese medications, and 'climate therapy' for malaria. Students and recent graduates wrote several articles and instructors wrote the rest. During the first decade of the twentieth century, topics such as X-rays, diet and beri-beri, plague, and new theories on malaria received attention. In the 1910s there were articles on hookworm disease, tuberculosis, syphilis, dysentery, the use of microscopes, and the role of rats in spreading the bubonic plague. In 1915, C. D. de vowed to increase the number of submissions from Indies physicians and advanced students. He hoped that the journal would eventually contain only articles written by Indies physicians.[64] By the early 1920s, the journal's editorial board consisted almost entirely of Indies physicians and was soon viewed as the indigenous counterpart of the *Medical Journal of the Dutch Indies* [*Geneeskundig Tijdschrift voor Nederlandsch-Indië*], the leading medical journal in the colonies.[65]

In 1923, de Langen encouraged senior STOVIA students to establish a medical discussion group, where students could present their research and discuss recent publications. To mark the occasion, he brought cigarettes, cigars, and a case of cold beer to the first meeting.[66] He also made his library and collection of medical journals available.[67] Students viewed de Langen as a genuinely supportive and charismatic leader. When he left Batavia for the Netherlands in 1926, the Association of Indies Physicians organised a banquet in his honour. Several members made laudatory speeches, praising him as someone who had encouraged 'Indies physicians to become men of science, who inspired them to become energetic minds, able to conduct scientific research'.[68] They presented him with souvenirs from across the Dutch East Indies and two paintings by

critique on schools in the Indies was vague and unspecific; Abendanon added a postscript indicating that the critique expressed in the piece was *not* applicable to the STOVIA.

[63] Willem Karel Tehupeiory, 'Iets over de Inlandsche Geneeskundigen', *Indisch Genootschap*, 28 January 1908, 101–34.

[64] C. D. de Langen, 'Aan de Lezers!', *Tijdschrift voor Inlandsche Geneeskundigen* 23, no. 1 (1915), 1–4.

[65] Raden Seno, 'Ons Tijdschrift', *Tijdschrift voor Indische Geneeskundigen* 27, no. 2 (1919), 1–6.

[66] Pirngadi, 'Medisch Dispuut Gezelschap', in *STOVIA Almanak 1924* (Weltevreden: Kolff, 1924), 147.

[67] F. L. Tobing, 'Medisch Dispuut Gezelschap', in *STOVIA Almanak 1925* (Weltevreden: Kolff, 1925), 136–37.

[68] 'Het Vertrek van C.D. de Langen', *Orgaan der Vereeniging van Indische Geneeskundigen* 15, no. 1 (1926), 65.

well-known indigenous artists.[69] De Langen returned only a few years later to become a professor at the Batavia Medical School.

When Indies physicians were appointed as assistant instructors at the STOVIA and as instructors at the NIAS, they provided support to students beyond their academic tuition. When Soewarno, instructor in ophthalmology at the Surabaya Medical College and co-founder of Boedi Oetomo, moved to Europe for health reasons, he was praised as a 'fatherly friend of all NIAS students and Indies physicians'.[70] Special note was made of the group he had organised for recent graduates to discuss their research in progress.[71] His colleague Soerjatin had similarly become an 'unforgettable figure' for all his efforts for the 'parentless' students at the NIAS.[72] Upon his death in 1938, Soetomo – 'Father Tom' – was praised for his mildness and fatherly attitude, as well as for his many contributions to medical science in the Indies and to student life at the Surabaya Medical College: 'Every NIASser can be proud to call himself a student of Dr. Soetomo.'[73] Isolated from their families, students looked for surrogate fathers and found 'siblings' in older students. They saw in these men their futures, and watched with interest as the stature of their profession rose with them.

Esprit de corps

Because of their many shared experiences, their shared exhaustion and anxiety, and their shared ideals, a strong *esprit de corps* developed among medical students. 'Friendship, rooted in STOVIAN soil [and] solidified by many years of student agony, is lasting', reflected one.[74] Pupils were proud of their school and their status as medical students. Officially, students at the Batavia Medical College were called *élèves* [pupils]; informally, they called themselves Stovians [*Stoviaanen*] or *klèpèks*, a Malay bastardisation of either *élèves* or Asclepius, or both. Djohan commented that students were 'happy to be called a Klepek, because this name is so closely associated with the STOVIA dormitory at the Kampong Ketapang [just outside the school] and well known to everyone in Batavia'.[75] Students at the NIAS were just as proud of their school. In the 1930s many of them were gratified that political activity at the Surabaya

---

[69] 'Vertrek de Langen', 66.

[70] 'Bij het Vertrek van Dr. Soewarno', *NIAS Orgaan* 4, no. 3 (1930), 6.

[71] 'Assistentenavond', *NIAS Orgaan* 3, no. 2 (1930), 16.

[72] 'Dokter Soerjatin Hoofd-Indisch-Arts', *NIAS Orgaan* 4, no. 3 (1930), 7.

[73] Soewarno, 'Dr. R. Soetomo + (1888–1938)', *NIAS Orgaan* 11, 12, no. 4-1-2 (1938), 44.

[74] J. S. Warouw, 'In Memoriam: Sam Nendu', in *STOVIA Almanak 1924* (Weltevreden: Kolff, 1924), 163.

[75] Djohan, 'Algemeen Verslag 1925', 97.

Medical College continued while it had diminished in Batavia with its elite medical school.[76]

Students often contemplated the great responsibilities that awaited them after graduation. They were guided by 'ineradicable inspirations for country and people [and by] national expectations'.[77] As physicians, they would be responsible for treating the sick and educating the population in the principles of health and hygiene.[78] Medical students thought a physician was more useful than a lawyer, soldier, or bureaucrat; 'more significant for his country and his people than a bureaucratic machine that continuously eats paper and drinks ink, only to become old and yellow like the papers of his department'.[79] Medicine was the ultimately modern profession in that it was responsible for drawing out the ill effects of traditional society. Students viewed traditional mores as 'a brake on our progress'.[80] One expressed his aversion to the traditional aristocracy as follows: 'He is not of noble birth, but he will demonstrate that he can put something in front of his name; instead of an "R. M." [Raden Mas; Javanese noble title] it would be the "Dr" title [a doctorate in medicine].'[81]

The students' aspirations to be cosmopolitan professionals could offend both Europeans and indigenous intellectuals. A commentator in the radical journal *Hindia Poetra* argued that the 1923 STOVIA yearbook was 'a pure copy of the Dutch ones', while criticising it for its lack of attention to the indigenous youth movements and for the absence of articles in the indigenous languages of the archipelago.[82] Sumatran physician Mohamad Amir lamented that the Almanac had 'slavishly followed' European equivalents – medical students 'had lost contact with their Indonesian cultural heritage'.[83] The editors of the 1925 yearbook took issue with those statements:

We intended, in issuing our yearbook, first of all, to highlight issues specific for the STOVIA. The existing political associations within our institution, which focus on politico-nationalistic and socio-economic issues, are too broad and fall outside the

---

[76] See, for example, Suhario 'Kecik' Padmodiwiryo, *Student Soldiers: A Memoir of the Battle that Sparked Indonesia's National Revolution* (Jakarta: Yayasan Pustaka Obor Indonesia, 2015).

[77] A., 'STOVIA Schetsen', 179.

[78] S., 'Toen Hij Nog NIASser Was', in *NIAS Jaarboek 1932* (Surabaya: Kolff, 1932), 211.

[79] Gandiwan D. I., 'Bij een Mijlpaal', in *STOVIA Almanak 1923* (Weltevreden: Kolff, 1923), 208.

[80] Datoe Hitam, 'Iets over Adat en Traditie in Verband met de Jongeren', *NIAS Orgaan* 1, no. 2 (1926), 31–33.

[81] Gonggopoetro, 'Ontslagen', 192.

[82] 'Twee Lezenswaardige Geschriften', *Hindia Poetra: Orgaan van de Indonesische Vereeniging* 1 (1923), 47.

[83] Mohamad Amir, quoted in Koloniaal Onderwijscongres, *Stenografisch Verslag van het Verhandelde op het Derde Koloniaal Onderwijscongres* (Groningen: Wolters, 1924), 165. Also see his critique on student life at the STOVIA: Mohamad Amir, 'De Medische Hoogeschool te Batavia', *Opbouw* 8 (1926), 932–45.

scope of our STOVIA society ... The material in the yearbook is what makes the heart of us medical students tick.[84]

The head of the editorial team, Bahder Djohan, was no stranger to student politics and probably had strategic reasons to remain silent about the political activities of medical students. Publications by medical students were generally silent about broader political issues but became almost fanatical when their school's pride or the status of Indies physicians were at stake.[85]

Because of the many years they spent together, their shared identity as medical students and aspiring medical professionals came to surpass their ethnic identity. In the words of Djohan: 'Arriving from different parts of the archipelago, often from different social environments, these young men are suddenly placed in the middle of a group of people who, although they aspire to achieve the same goal, are entirely foreign to them, both in their essence and their character.'[86] In their ten years at the STOVIA, students developed strong bonds and a common identity. The NIAS fostered similar sentiments: 'For us the NIAS is a mirror of the unity of the Indies archipelago, because here we see representatives of maybe not all, but surely of many population groups which originate on its many islands.'[87] The shared identity of medical students was academic, modern, and Western. Dutch was their first language. Once they were allowed to wear European clothing, they did. The strong and enduring professional bond between these aspiring physicians superseded their ethnic affiliations.

Medical Politics and Nationalist Sentiment

In student writings, discussions on the reputation of the medical colleges, the status of Indies physicians, and the latter's social responsibilities abounded. Medical students were particularly sensitive when they perceived that they, their institution, or their future profession were not sufficiently appreciated. They saw themselves as combatants in the 'bitter struggle fought by Indies physicians to receive the deference and respect that is due to them in the greater society'.[88] Most students favoured transforming the medical colleges into medical schools equivalent to those in Europe; students from the Indies would then be able to gain full medical degrees without undertaking the expensive

---

[84] 'Voorwoord', in STOVIA Almanak 1925 (Weltevreden: Kolff, 1925), 3.
[85] See, for example, Sardjito, 'De Toelating van Indische Geneeskundigen, Abituriënten van de STOVIA en de NIAS tot de Universiteit en Hoogeschool', NIAS Orgaan 11, no. 1-2-3 (1938), 6–18.
[86] Djohan, 'STOVIA Verslag 1923', 83.
[87] 'Toespraak van de Vertegenwoordiger der NIASsers tot den Directeur van de Jubileerende Scholen', in NIAS-STOVIT Lustrum Almanak 1938 (Soerabaja: Kolff, 1938), 25.
[88] 'Sport- en Kunstvereeniging', in STOVIA Almanak 1925 (Weltevreden: Kolff, 1925), 110.

journey to the Netherlands. This would also end the two-tier medical system and remedy the constant discrimination suffered by Indies physicians. They regularly argued that the education provided at the Batavia Medical College was already sophisticated, and needed little expansion – it was merely a matter of 'a name change'.[89] Students felt that old-fashioned colonial administrators and hostile European physicians had a vested interest in this mostly artificial classification.

Students observed the conditions under which the greater part of the indigenous population lived as part of their training. Rotations in the *kampong* exposed them to abject poverty and unhygienic conditions and demonstrated the need for public health programs.[90] Students observed that many young children died unnecessarily.[91] Yearbooks included such aphorisms as 'exaggerated interest in so-called tropical diseases obscures the gynaecological suffering that takes place in the intimacy of *kampong* houses', and 'on Java, at least three times more mothers and new-born children died than there were plague victims.'[92] For many students, these *kampong* visits sharpened their political sensitivities and their sense of responsibility. They saw that the population urgently needed more health facilities, new hygienic measures, and better public health education. A recent graduate noted that unhygienic habits were common among the poorly educated native population. People washed clothing and food, bathed, and defecated in the streams, which were also the main source of drinking water.[93] Such anecdotes reinforced the social responsibility of graduates: 'It is a high task of the Indies physician to educate the population and to treat their ailments.'[94] They therefore advocated extensive public health education campaigns and more generous appropriations for medical care.

According to Bahder Djohan, it was the duty of future physicians to 'infiltrate the great, wide society'.[95] He advised medical students to participate in the many youth organisations of the Indies: 'Because of their study and position, many [medical students] are destined to stand in the first lines in the middle of their people and it is advisable that, before they enter the big society, they are aware of the factors which determine social life in this young

[89] 'Aphorism', in *STOVIA-Almanak 1925* (Weltevreden: Kolff, 1925), 174.
[90] Aboe Bakar, 'Herinneringen en Overpeinzingen', in *Ontwikkeling van het Geneeskundig Onderwijs te Weltevreden, 1851–1926*, ed. A. de Waart (Weltevreden: Kolff, 1926), 330, 332. See also 'Zijn Eerste Nacht', in *NIAS Jaarboek 1932* (Surabaya: Kolff, 1932), 197–201.
[91] Remboelan, 'Treurig', *NIAS Orgaan* 1, no. 3 (1926), 48.
[92] 'Aphorism 77 and 78', in *STOVIA Almanak 1925*, 172.
[93] Sh., 'Bij 't Portret van Dr. Th. G. van Vogelpoel', in *STOVIA Almanak 1926* (Weltevreden: Kolff, 1926), 151–56; Tabib, 'Vacantie-Indrukken: De Stads-Hygiëne van Semarang', *NIAS Orgaan* 4, no. 2 (1929), 11–14.
[94] Otede, 'Geneeskunde en de Inlandsche Bevolking', *NIAS Orgaan* 1, no. 2 (1926), 34–46.
[95] Bahder Djohan, 'Algemeen Verslag over het Jaar 1924', in *STOVIA Almanak 1925* (Weltevreden: Kolff, 1925), 84–85.

country which only recently has been opened up.'[96] The majority of youth associations were founded by medical students, and their most active members originally came from the STOVIA. This was because 'the *klèpèk* is occupied with social questions', explained Djohan, 'and because many weighty problems are discussed within the walls of the dormitory'.[97] He held that such participation contributed to the social development of students and prepared them for their later responsibilities. Attending medical college fostered their intellectual development; student associations helped expose them to broader social, cultural, and political issues. 'A physician standing in the middle of social life and his people is naturally appointed as their representative', wrote a student. 'He naturally is exceptionally well suited to be the spiritual father of his people.'[98]

Some nationalist sentiment was present in the yearbooks and student magazines, but it was muted. One student, for example, wrote how he was saddened by the deplorable condition of the elephants [*gadjah*] locked up in Solo's zoo and mused how Gadjah Mada [the immensely powerful and legendary general of Java's Majapahit Empire] would pity them – if only they could become kings of the forest again.[99] Another student gave an affectionate account of a meeting with his uncle who had been a teacher at a Dutch high school but now lived a secluded life high in the mountains. His uncle was a 'real worker for building the father-land' and it was rumoured he was in 'close contact with the most prominent leaders of the indigenous movement'.[100] He was revered by the local population as a spiritual leader and was the puppeteer of local *wayang kulit* shows. This uncle advised his nephew to remain true to his ideals as a physician and to continue his work for the independence of the nation. Because he aspired to foster a people healthy in body and spirit, he needed to maintain a pure body and an exalted spirit by avoiding everything that could potentially cause disease. After all, 'someone who goes to the STOVIA is the ongoing focus of public attention.'[101] The figure of an older spiritual leader living in a remote area was a familiar one, as was the emphasis on spiritual purity. In this short essay, Javanese spirituality, the wisdom of the elders, and medicine were connected with the nationalist movement.

---

[96] Djohan, 'Algemeen Verslag 1925', 98.
[97] Djohan, 'Algemeen Verslag 1925', 97.
[98] S., 'The Positie van de Medische Scholen in Indonesië', in *NIAS Lustrum Almanak 1933–1934* (Batavia: Kolff, 1934), 24. The article is signed only with 'S.'. It portrays a maturity of vision that would be unusual among medical students. It could have been written by Soetomo, who was a teacher at the medical school.
[99] M., 'Bij de Olifanten van Soerakarta', in *STOVIA Almanac 1923* (Batavia: Kolff, 1923), 183–84.
[100] D. I., 'Mijlpaal', 210.
[101] D. I., 'Mijlpaal', 215.

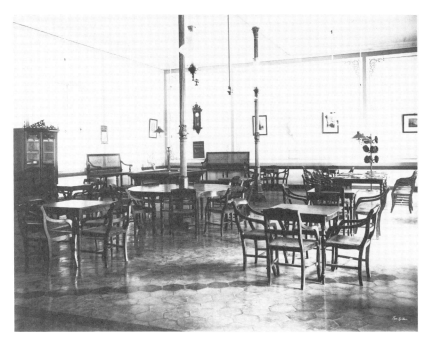

Figure 2.5 The recreation room at the Batavia Medical College (STOVIA) in 1902. Figure: University of Leiden library, KITLV collection (35817)

The founding of Boedi Oetomo was the outcome of the vibrant intellectual life at the Batavia Medical College. Ten years after it was established, Goenawan Mangoenkoesoemo fondly recalled how his friend 'Soetomo and other class-mates brought pleasant and less pleasant newspaper articles with them from the newspaper table which we discussed during the evening study hours.'[102] Soetomo actively supported the interests of the Javanese people, 'arguing with his whole body'.[103] These were treasured times; 'these cosy gatherings, often disturbed by the noisy, scratchy voice of the dormitory supervisor, were the cradle of *Boedi Oetomo*.'[104] Discussions at the STOVIA continued during the following two decades. Mohamad Roem recalled the reading table in the recreation room (Figure 2.5) with affection because the discussions around it had stimulated his political awareness. Rather than

[102] Goenawan Mangoenkoesoemo, 'De Geboorte van Boedi-Oetomo', in *Soembangsih: Gedenkboek Boedi-Oetomo 1908 – 20 Mei – 1918* (Amsterdam: Nederlandsch-Indië Oud en Nieuw, 1918), 9.
[103] Mangoenkoesoemo, 'Geboorte Boedi Oetomo', 9.
[104] Mangoenkoesoemo, 'Geboorte Boedi Oetomo', 9.

reading newspapers and magazines himself, Roem preferred to listen to the conversations of the older students.[105] Pirngadi related how, one evening, Satiman, the founder of the student association Young Java, announced that he had made the ten-minute walk to the Concordia Military Club to demand a greater say in colonial affairs for the indigenous population. It was a daring feat and led to an official reprimand. This impressed Pirngadi so much that he started to think about politics.[106]

The interest and encouragement of a small number of Europeans also played an important role in this political awakening. Henri Clockener Brousson, who later founded the *Bintang Hindia* with Abdul Rivai, maintained cordial relationships with medical students around the turn of the twentieth century. With medical student J. E. Tehupeiory, he edited the *Soldiers' Newspaper* [*Soerat Chabar Soldadoe*] for indigenous soldiers in the colonial army, which appeared in 1900–01, and *Dutch Flag* [*Bandera Wolanda*] for soldiers and students, which appeared in 1901–03. Indo-European journalist E. F. E. Douwes Dekker remembered how both Soetomo and Goenawan Mangoenkoesoemo came to his house to consult his extensive library and to discuss political issues.[107] Also welcoming to Indonesian students was one of the most influential Theosophists in the Indies, D. van Hinloopen Labberton.[108] Theosophists believed in the spiritual harmony of all humankind, reincarnation, and the essential unity of all religions, which they believed found their source in deep spiritual impulses. They opposed the materialism and individualism they thought had run rampant in the West and advocated for the equality of all human beings, and had faith in the irresistible power of evolution and progress. Several medical students, including Soetomo, Tjipto Mangoenkoesoemo, and Mohamad Amir, were deeply influenced by theosophical ideas.[109] According to van Hinloopen Labberton, the task of the colonial administration was to provide education to

---

[105] Roem, 'Tradisi Berpolitik', 249. For Roem, see George McTurnan Kahin, 'In Memoriam: Mohamad Roem (1908–1983)', *Indonesia*, no. 37 (1984), 134–38.

[106] Pirngadi, 'Afscheid', *Jong Java* 11, no. 19–20 (1–15 October 1926), 3.

[107] E. F. E. Douwes Dekker, 'Mijn Ontmoeting met Soetomo', *Kritiek en Opbouw* (1, 16 October 1938), 246–48, 264–65. Douwes Dekker often overstated his importance, but other sources confirm his contacts with medical students. See D. M. G. Koch, *Verantwoording: Een Halve Eeuw in Indonesië* (The Hague/Bandung: Van Hoeve, 1956), 44. See also Akira Nagazumi, *The Dawn of Indonesian Nationalism: The Early Years of the Budi Utomo, 1908–1918* (Tokyo: Institute of Developing Economies, 1972), 35.

[108] Laurie J. Sears, 'Intellectuals, Theosophy and Failed Narratives of the Nation in Late Colonial Java', in *A Companion to Postcolonial Studies*, ed. Henry Schwarz and Sangeeta Ray (London: Blackwell, 2004), 333–59; Iskandar P. Nugraha, *Teosofi, Nasionalisme and Elite Modern Indonesia* (Jakarta: Kommunitas Bambu, 2011); H. A. O. Tollenaere, *The Politics of Divine Wisdom: Theosophy and Labour, National, and Women's Movements in Indonesia and South Asia, 1875–1947* (Nijmegen: Katholieke Universiteit Nijmegen, 1996).

[109] D. van Hinloopen Labberton, *Theosofie in Verband met Boedi-Oetomo/Theosophie oentoek Boedi-Oetomo* (Batavia: Boekhandel & Drukkerij Kho Tjeng Bie, 1909). The connections between spiritualism and abolitionism because of the belief in the equality of humankind has

the indigenous population to further the development of the Indies, and those indigenous individuals who had received advanced education were to play a leading role. In 1918, he became a member of the Volksraad and consistently supported moderate indigenous initiatives.

Conclusion

As well as creating a strong professional identity and an intense belief in the power of medicine, the experience of attending medical school created strong bonds between students. Student life was full of exhilarating experiences such as identifying the cause of a disease while investigating samples under a microscope, the excitement of acquiring new knowledge, organising and attending parties, running student associations, watching and participating in sports, engaging in mischief, and evading dormitory supervisors. In combination with the nausea experienced when first dissecting a human body, the gloomy and tense weeks before exams, the anxiety of being subjugated to the whims of instructors, the nagging fear of expulsion, and romantic disappointment, they shared unique experiences that fostered life-long friendships and a strong collective identity. As Benedict Anderson has argued, schools and other educational institutions played an important role in the creation of the idea of the Indies nation because they created 'a self-contained, coherent universe of experience' superimposed neatly upon the geography of the Indies.[110] It was the strong and enduring professional bonds between these aspiring physicians that superseded the earlier familial and ethnic affiliation upon which the nation of Indonesia was modelled.

Schools, colleges, and universities with their associated dormitories have always been important sites for young men and women to articulate, rehearse, and perform their identities. Students have often been motivated by the vision of impending change, convinced that they are in many ways superior to their forebears. Medical students in the Dutch East Indies were no exception. They defined their identities in contrast with archaic older generations and in terms of their future profession, which, they were convinced, had the tools for improving the lives of all inhabitants of the archipelago. Always appearing self-assured, these students were quick to appoint themselves heralds of modernity and harbingers of the future. They remembered their early childhood with fondness and a tinge of nostalgia but nevertheless relegated it to a distant, less enlightened past, while articulating their identity as young intellectuals

been highlighted by Ann Deborah Braude, *Radical Spirits: Spiritualism and Women's Rights in Nineteenth-Century America* (Boston, MA: Beacon Press, 1989).

[110] Benedict R. O'G. Anderson, *Imagined Communities: Reflections on the Origin and Spread of Nationalism*, rev. and extended edn (London: Verso, 2006 [1983]), 123.

destined to bring the blessings of modern medicine to the people and to change society for the better. The medical colleges of the Indies, as two unusual colonial laboratories, transformed native subjects by fostering modern, rational, and moral identities. During their student years, these identities could be endlessly performed and celebrated. Only after graduation did they have to face the unforgiving realities of colonial life.

3   The Indies Youth Movements: Progress, Westernisation, and Cultural Pride

Employing the intellectual tools they had acquired during their medical training, Indies physicians and medical students became diagnosticians of colonial society. They analysed the process of social evolution and identified factors that might impede or accelerate it, and diagnosed threats to the health of the colonial social body while thinking of ways to neutralise them. Yet despite their apparent consensus about their social role, they presented divergent and at times incompatible views on the ills of colonial society, the direction of the nationalist movement, and the future of the archipelago. A number of physician-intellectuals urged the archipelago's inhabitants to embrace modernity, relinquish outdated traditions, and aspire to westernisation. Others exhorted them to embrace their various ethnic traditions, enrich artistic expression, and revitalise their cultures with modern tools. Still others hoped to unite all ethnic groups in the Indies into an all-encompassing Indonesian identity that could be mobilised for the nationalist struggle, accomplished through westernisation, creating shared cultural traditions, merging existing ethnic traditions, or adherence to Islam.[1] To add even more variation to these options, a number preferred enlisting elites while others pursued more egalitarian approaches. During the first congress of Boedi Oetomo, held in October 1908, these differing visions came to the fore and caused considerable friction among speakers and participants.

Diversity in political opinions increased still further after the congress. When Indies physician Tjipto Mangoenkoesoemo and former medical student Soewardi Soerjaningrat joined the Indies Party [Indische Partij] and started to advocate independence, they were promptly exiled and their party was outlawed. After his return from exile, Soewardi and (then) Dr Radjiman Wediodipoero urged their fellow Javanese to celebrate their own culture because they viewed it as the principal source of social cohesion, solidarity,

---

[1] For an elaboration of these views, see R. E. Elson, 'Constructing the Nation: Ethnicity, Race, Modernity and Citizenship in Early Indonesian Thought', *Asian Ethnicity* 6, no. 3 (2005), 145–60; R. E. Elson, *The Idea of Indonesia: A History* (Cambridge: Cambridge University Press, 2008).

and political engagement. Students at the medical colleges established associations for younger students at high schools and professional schools. Ethnic affiliation was the basis of these associations, which, following Rivai, were given names like Young Java [Jong Java] and Young Sumatra [Jong Sumatra]. Lectures, outings, sports competitions, and scouting events were their regular activities. These associations increased students' awareness of cultural, social, and political issues, and, for some, they provided a springboard for later political activity.

The First Year of Boedi Oetomo

When Boedi Oetomo was founded on 20 May 1908, Soetomo and the group of medical students around him decided to recruit members, develop a program, and establish contacts with progressive regents [*bupati*] before launching the organisation publicly.[2] The launch event would be a conference in October 1908, to be held in Yogyakarta, and its organisation took considerable time, energy, and money. They 'gave up their watches, sarongs, head-clothes, and even their allowances for the fasting month' to fund the gathering.[3] Goenawan Mangoenkoesoemo recalled that students locked themselves 'in the chemistry laboratory and used agar poured on slates to hectograph announcements which were distributed later to our members as flying newsletters'.[4] Soetomo and his fellow students frequently met with Wahidin and Douwes Dekker to discuss organisational matters. They published a manifesto advocating increasing educational opportunities, and stimulating trade and industry among the Javanese. The regents issued a more limited program proposing scholarships for students from respectable (that is, aristocratic) homes. Even before the first congress was held, it was clear that the medical students envisaged a different course for the organisation than the regents, but this hardly dampened recruitment efforts. When the congress began, the association had 1,200 members.

The first congress, held at Yogyakarta's teachers' college, was attended by 300 individuals, including several progressive regents and a few princes of Yogyakarta's two sultanates. Journalist Douwes Dekker called the congress a 'turning point in Indies history' because the voice of the Javanese was heard publicly for the first time.[5] Wahidin, the president, related that

---

[2] Goenawan Mangoenkoesoemo, 'De Geboorte van Boedi-Oetomo', in *Soembangsih: Gedenkboek Boedi-Oetomo 1908 – 20 Mei – 1918* (Amsterdam: Nederlandsch-Indië Oud en Nieuw, 1918), 13; see also Akira Nagazumi, *The Dawn of Indonesian Nationalism: The Early Years of the Budi Utomo, 1908–1918* (Tokyo: Institute of Developing Economies, 1972), 38–44.

[3] R. Soetomo, *Towards a Glorious Indonesia* (Athens: Ohio University Center for International Studies, 1987), 76.

[4] G. Mangoenkoesoemo, 'Geboorte Boedi Oetomo', 14.

[5] 'Het Eerste Nationaal Javaansche Congress te Djokja, I', *Bataviaasch Nieuwsblad*, 5 October 1908, Section II, 2. E. F. E. Douwes Dekker was the reporter present at the congress. His reporting was hardly neutral: it is clear that his sympathies were with the medical students.

hc had inoculated new ideas for years and was now witnessing the fruits of his labours.[6] One reporter was pleasantly surprised that 'the intellectuals of a people that had been mentally subjugated for centuries now preach the gospel of development.'[7] For another, 'it was more a western than an eastern congress … because Young Java battled for western civilisation.'[8] The congress, in his judgement, was not revolutionary in nature, since it propagated Dutch ideas, in particular those of the Ethical Policy.[9]

In his opening speech, Wahidin related, in Malay, how the struggle for existence had become increasingly difficult for the Javanese. Education could remedy this, but the Javanese should not, warned Wahidin, become 'imitation Westerners [and] descend into an inadequate imitation of western customs and traditions'.[10] They should instead be creative and selective: 'What we should adopt from the European is his knowledge, his science, his concepts of hygiene, mental development, and social improvement.'[11] This would enable Javanese individuals to discard mistaken and outdated elements of their *adat*. Javanese intellectuals could play leading roles only if they did not lose their roots in traditional culture. Soetomo also noted the widespread thirst for progress and development among the Javanese. He hoped that more educational facilities might be established, since education was 'the key to all locks, provide[d] access to all the sciences, and [was] the source of everything good'.[12] Education in trade, industry, and the arts would fuel the development of a viable Javanese middle class, he argued – something that had been absent thus far. Several other speakers reinforced the need for education, progress, and development.

The address of the Indies physician Radjiman Wediopoero, Wahidin's adopted son, struck a decidedly different chord.[13] Radjiman made an obeisance [*sembah*] to the aristocrats in the audience before arguing, in high Javanese, that the Javanese did not need 'Dutch or western science as they are not amenable to western civilisation and development'.[14] Using elaborate philosophical, biological, and medical arguments, he reasoned that culture and civilisation

 [6] 'Eerste Javaansch Congres, I', Section II, 2.
 [7] 'Boedi Oetomo', *Sumatra Post*, 7 October 1908, 1.
 [8] 'Het Eerste Javaansche Congres, I', *Jong Indië* 1, no. 15 (10 October 1908), 129.
 [9] 'Het Eerste Javaansche Congres, II', *Jong Indië* 1, no. 16 (17 October 1908), 142.
 [10] 'Het Eerste Nationaal Javaansche Congress te Djokja, II', *Bataviaasch Nieuwsblad*, 6 October 1908, Section II, 1; 'Het Eerste Nationaal Javaansche Congres I', *Bataviaasch Nieuwsblad*, 5 October 1908, 1. For the congress, see also Nagazumi, *Dawn of Indonesian Nationalism*, 44–47.
 [11] Soetomo, quoted in 'Eerste Javaansch Congres, II', Section II, 1.
 [12] Soetomo, quoted in 'Eerste Javaansche Congres, II', Section II, 2. Soetomo's speech was written by Goenawan Mangoenkoesoemo; see Soetomo, *Towards a Glorious Indonesia*, 78.
 [13] For a biography, see Soebaryo Mangunwidodo, *Dr. K. R. T. Radjiman Wediodiningrat: Perjalanan Seorang Putra Bangsa 1879–1952* (Jakarta: Yayasan Dr. K. R. T. Radjiman Wediodiningrat, 1994).
 [14] Radjiman, quoted in 'Het Eerste Nationaal Javaansche Congress te Djokja, III', *Bataviaasch Nieuwsblad*, 7 October 1908, Section II, 1.

depended on the mental and emotional development of ethnic groups, and was therefore the result of the unique interactions of these groups with specific natural environments over the course of centuries. As a consequence, Javanese students could acquire only a superficial understanding of Dutch culture and could never fully understand complex Western ideas. Radjiman continued by praising Java's rich cultural heritage and concluded that the Javanese did not need to pursue Western civilisation. Their own impressive culture provided everything they needed. The attending princes and regents clapped enthusiastically; the rest of the audience was stunned and whistled in disapproval.

Tjipto Mangoenkoesomo, visibly upset by Radjiman's speech, declared, in Dutch, that the Javanese arts and culture praised by Radjiman were luxuries for wealthy aristocrats, and irrelevant to the common people. Over the past three centuries, argued Tjipto, Western nations had been able to increase prosperity through industrialisation, and this had given the greatest benefit to the lower classes. On Java, Western-style development had the capacity to ensure that the average Javanese has 'his daily plate of rice'.[15] Tjipto rejected the idea that Western-style education robbed the Javanese of their cultural identity; it would rather prepare them for the modern world. He received a deafening applause; the audience, including the lower aristocrats, yelled and cheered loudly. The princes and regents sat silently, stone-faced. One Dutch commentator thought that Tjipto's had been a courageous act, 'upholding the right of the lower Javanese classes to exist' in one of the strongholds of the Javanese aristocracy.[16] In the closing address, Goenawan Mangoenkoesoemo, Tjipto's younger brother, Soetomo's closest friend and co-founder of Boedi Oetomo, proclaimed that the organisation's work was 'in the *desa* [villages]' because it was there that 'millions and millions still walk around in the deepest darkness of ignorance; it is there that light has to be ignited'.[17]

Soetomo's views and those of his fellow medical students carried the day at the congress, but met resistance beyond it. They had hoped to limit the role of Java's traditional aristocracy, both within the organisation and in Javanese society, and to expand the influence of educated individuals. Soon after the congress, the students lost their leading role in Boedi Oetomo. Colonial bureaucrats were manoeuvring behind the scenes to alter the course of the new organisation. Soetomo wrote drily: 'the glorious leadership of *Boedi Oetomo* was transferred to more mature people' – such as the high aristocrats who had applauded Radjiman's speech.[18]

---

[15] 'Eerste Javaansch Congres, III', Section II, 2.
[16] A. J. H. van Eyken, *Voordracht over de Jong Javaansche Beweging* (The Hague: Korthuis, 1909), 28.
[17] 'Het Eerste Nationaal Javaansche Congress te Djokja, V', *Bataviaasch Nieuwsblad*, 10 October 1908, Section II, 1.
[18] Soetomo, *Towards a Glorious Indonesia*, 85.

Tjipto Mangoenkoesoemo, the Unification of the Indies, and the Call for Independence

Tjipto Mangoenkoesoemo was the eldest son in a lesser aristocratic family (he consistently demurred to use the Javanese title *Mas*).[19] His father had an unusually successful career. He began as a Malay teacher at a provincial indigenous primary school, was promoted to the position of headmaster at a primary school in Semarang, and then became an administrative assistant to the Semarang municipal council. Tjipto's ten siblings included three physicians, an engineer, and a lawyer, and his sisters played significant roles in the nationalist women's movement. Tjipto was scrupulously honest, highly principled, uncompromising, and fiercely egalitarian.[20] During his days at the Batavia Medical College, he publicly identified with the common people by wearing a simple Javanese outfit normally worn by the lower classes, and by smoking clove [*kretek*] cigarettes. Tjipto opposed the exploitative hierarchies in both Javanese and European social spheres, and advocated for the expansion of educational opportunities for the whole indigenous population. He severed ties with Boedi Oetomo after the first congress because he found it too elitist and conservative.[21]

Because of his uncompromising nature, Tjipto often attracted controversy. In 1908, for example, the colonial health service transferred him to Demak, where he annoyed the local regent by ostentatiously keeping a carriage with two horses for his medical duties. According to the local *adat*, this privilege was restricted to regents and their immediate families. To make matters worse, Tjipto refused to rein in his horses and move his carriage to the side of the road when the regent drove by. He also had disagreements with European colleagues. When a malaria epidemic broke out, European medical officer J. T. Terburgh appointed ten assistants [*mantris*] to distribute quinine among the population. Because these *mantris* viewed Tjipto as their immediate superior, they complained to him about their insufficient salaries. Tjipto immediately informed a local European official, which antagonised Terburgh, who claimed that all Javanese refused to work unless they were paid above their station and that humanitarian motives were alien to them. Tjipto warned that if Terburgh did not approve the proposed salary increases, he would resign, and then did so when Terburgh refused. His superiors informed him that he had been too

---

[19] For biographical information on Tjipto, see Savitri Prastiti Scherer, 'Harmony and Dissonance: Early Nationalist Thought on Java' (MA thesis, Cornell University, 1975), 102–81; Takashi Shiraishi, *An Age in Motion: Popular Radicalism in Java, 1912–1926* (Ithaca, NY: Cornell University Press, 1990), 88–96, 117–27,165–93, 209–16.

[20] D. M. G. Koch, 'Dr. Tjipto Mangoenkoesoemo', in *Batig Slot: Figuren uit het Oude Indië* (Amsterdam: De Brug/Djambatan, 1960), 149.

[21] Tjipto Mangoenkoesoemo, 'The Volgende Fase in de Javaansche Beweging'. Quoted in 'Beweging in de Inlandsche Wereld', *Sumatra Post*, 25 September 1912, 1.

sensitive. 'Clearly', Tjipto later commented, 'that medical officer's social status was so far elevated above mine, that for anyone to point out that he was wrong would signify a revolution in existing relationships'.[22]

The following year, Tjipto established a private practice in Solo where he broke etiquette again, riding his horse in the main town square as only the *Sunan* was permitted to do.[23] When plague broke out in East Java in 1911, he immediately volunteered his services and was placed near Malang. By an unfortunate twist of fate, Terburgh once again became his superior, and immediately inquired why Tjipto's stipend was higher than that of his colleagues. Tjipto's salary was delayed by three months while it was reviewed. When he borrowed money from an indigenous official to make ends meet, a European official, seeing a chance to get even with this troublemaker, charged him with embezzlement.[24] To resolve matters, Tjipto was transferred, even though his superiors knew the charges were false. In July 1912, he was knighted in the Order of Orange Nassau for his selfless efforts in the plague eradication campaign.[25] The clarity of his political views and his devotion to fighting the plague earned him a stellar reputation among the indigenous population. His knighthood gave him the freedom to pursue his political ideals.

Tjipto was critical of attempts to stimulate Javanese culture; these were 'petrifying spells' turning the Javanese into 'mental fossils'; they would hardly benefit from 'hauling antiquities from our cluttered attic'.[26] Javanese culture was 'beautiful', certainly, but it did 'not meet the demands of life in these times'.[27] It might be retained as a 'private hobby'.[28] He argued that Java's cultural heritage had been irrevocably tainted by the caste system, and that this was perpetuated by the Javanese language, which assigned each social class a separate linguistic repertoire. 'The psyche of the Javanese people needs to be changed', declared Tjipto, 'to such an extent that a change of language, or more cynically a killing of a language becomes urgent'.[29] Attempts to keep the Javanese 'unspoiled' by limiting or excluding Western influence interfered

[22] Tjipto Mangoenkoesoemo, 'Ervaringen uit het Leven: Kracht Boven Recht', *De Expres*, 30 September 1912, 1.

[23] M. Balfas, *Dr. Tjipto Mangoenkoesoemo: Demokrat Sedjati* (Djakarta: Djambatan, 1952), 36; Scherer, 'Harmony and Dissonance', 118–19.

[24] T. Mangoenkoesoemo, 'Ervaringen Leven', 1.

[25] 'Koninklijke Onderscheidingen', *Het Nieuws van den Dag voor Nederlandsch-Indië*, 13 July 1912, 2.

[26] Tjipto Mangoenkoesoemo, 'Geestelijke Immobiliteit Ge-Eischt', *Het Tijdschrift*, 1 September 1912, 18; Tjipto Mangoenkoesoemo, 'Iets over Javaansche Cultuurontwikkeling: Prae-Advies', in *Congres voor Javaansche Cultuur-Ontwikkeling* (Semarang: Misset, 1918), 21.

[27] Tjipto Mangoenkoesoemo, 'Het Indisch Nationalisme en zijn Rechtvaardiging', in *Javaansch of Indisch Nationalisme: Pro en Contra* (Semarang: Benjamins, 1918), 27.

[28] T. Mangoenkoesoemo, 'Javaansche Cultuurontwikkeling', 34.

[29] Tjipto Mangoenkoesomo, cited in R. M. Soewardi Soerjaningrat, 'Welke Plaats Behooren bij het Onderwijs in te Nemen, Eensdeels de Inheemsche Talen (Ook het Chineesch en Arabisch),

with the natural process of social evolution, which led inevitably to decline and possible extinction. Learning Dutch was essential: 'To deprive us of the Dutch language', he argued, 'equals shutting down our evolution'.[30] For Tjipto, celebrating the cultural traditions of the Indies impeded the unification of all people from the archipelago – a plethora of peoples already unified in their subjection to the Dutch crown.

By 1910, Douwes Dekker was looking for ways to reach a large audience for his increasingly radical political ideas – he was the first intellectual to advocate independence for the Indies.[31] He was a great-nephew of Eduard Douwes Dekker who, in 1860, published *Max Havelaar* under the pen name Multatuli. It was a sustained critique of Dutch colonialism and is now widely seen as the most influential Dutch novel ever written. In his newspaper and magazine, the younger Douwes Dekker covered the exploitation of the indigenous population by avaricious aristocrats, ruthless businessmen, and corrupt colonial officials. He also laid out his plans to organise a political party uniting all individuals who considered the Indies their homeland, irrespective of whether they were natives, foreign Orientals, Indo-Europeans, or Europeans. In 1911, Douwes Dekker established the Indies Party [Indische Partij] and embarked on a hugely successful recruitment campaign in September 1912. Travelling all over Java by train, he was met by hundreds of supporters at every station.[32] When he visited Serang (West Java), local regent and host Achmad Djajadiningrat noted the excitement and reported how a solicitor and a lower Javanese official spoke with each other in an informal manner. Later an indigenous clerk and the wife of a European assistant shattered colonial conventions by dancing together.[33]

In 1912, Douwes Dekker convinced Tjipto to become the vice chair of the Indies Party and the associate editor of its newspaper, *The Express [De Expres]*, which significantly strengthened its appeal among the indigenous population. Tjipto agreed only reluctantly, since he shared Douwes Dekker's political

---

Anderdeels het Nederlandsch?: Prae-Advies', in *Prae-Adviezen van het Eerste Koloniaal Onderwijscongres* (The Hague: Korthals, 1916), 55.

[30] T. Mangoenkoesoemo, 'Javaansche Cultuurontwikkeling', 16.

[31] For biographies of Ernest François Eugène Dekker, see Paul W. van der Veur, *The Lion and the Gadfly: Dutch Colonialism and the Spirit of E. F. E. Douwes Dekker* (Leiden: KITLV Press, 2006); Frans Glissenaar, *D. D.: Het Leven van E. F. E. Douwes Dekker* (Hilversum: Verloren, 1999). E. F. E. Douwes Dekker also published an autobiographical account: E. F. E. Douwes Dekker and Harumi Wanasita, *70 Jaar Konsekwent* (Bandoeng: A. C. Nix, 1949). In particular Robert Elson has emphasised the revolutionary character of Douwes Dekker's ideas. See Elson, *The Idea of Indonesia*.

[32] For a report of this tour, see E. F. E. Douwes Dekker, 'De Indische Partij: Verslag der Progaganda-Deputatie', *Het Tijdschrift* 2, no. 4 (15 October 1912), 97–146.

[33] P. A. Achmad Djajadiningrat, *Herinneringen van Pangeran Aria Achmad Djajadiningrat* (Batavia: Kolff, 1936), 283.

ideals but had doubts about his populist methods.[34] In his idealistic writings for *De Expres*, Tjipto superimposed metaphors derived from Darwin's evolutionary theory on idealist philosophies detailing the inexorable progress of mental and spiritual development. He argued, in accordance with Theosophist principles, that the process of evolution would eventually result in a brotherhood encompassing all humankind: 'Evolution, unfolding, development – comprised in all these concepts is growth, from the singular to the composite, from the primitive to the complicated, in the same way as the thousand-fold composite organism grows out of the original cell.'[35]

R. M. Soewardi Soerjaningrat, an aristocrat who left the STOVIA without graduating, joined the Indies Party soon after Tjipto. During the first months of 1913, the colonial administration began planning celebrations to mark the centennial of the liberation of the Netherlands from Napoleon's grasp, and requested donations and active participation from Europeans and natives alike. Tjipto and Soewardi formed a committee to protest the absurdity of these requests. Their committee published a highly ironic political pamphlet, now considered the most famous one in the history of the Indies: 'If I ever were a Dutchman [*Als ik eens Nederlander was*]'. If he ever were a Dutchman, wrote Soewardi, he would never request the oppressed population of the Indies to contribute to any liberation ceremony until that population had itself been liberated.[36] The pamphlet hit a nerve and the authorities acted swiftly. Tjipto, Soewardi, and several others were arrested during a raid involving more than 1,500 police officers. Weeks later, the Governor-General exiled Tjipto, Soewardi, and Douwes Dekker to separate remote areas (all others were released within days of their arrest). The three requested and were permitted to be exiled to the Netherlands instead. They left the Indies on separate ships in September 1913.[37]

Because of his severe asthma and increasing weakness and fatigue, Tjipto was allowed to return to the Indies in August 1914. He re-established his private practice in Solo and took an active part in organising labourers on local plantations. He was appointed a member of the Volksraad in 1918 and used this

---

[34] Tjipto Mangoenkoesoemo, *Open Brief aan Mijne Landgenoten* (Kepandjen: Author, 1912). This letter was reprinted, in full, in *De Expres*, 27 November 1913, 1.

[35] Tjipto Mangoenkoesoemo, 'Eenheid', *Het Tijdschrift* 1, no. 12 (15 February 1912), 402.

[36] *Als Ik Eens Nederlander Was* (Bandoeng: Inlandsch Comité tot Herdenking van Neêrlands Honderdjarige Vrijheid, 1913). For a fascinating interpretation of this pamphlet, see James T. Siegel, *Fetish, Recognition, Revolution* (Princeton, NJ: Princeton University Press, 1997), 26–37.

[37] All material related to their exile was published as: E. F. E. Douwes Dekker, Tjipto Mangoenkoesoemo, and R. M. Soewardi Soerjaningrat, *Onze Verbanning* (Schiedam: De Indiër, 1913).

platform to broadcast his radical ideas. He openly doubted the effectiveness of
the new colonial parliament because only a few of its members had received
medical training:

The powers of the national body are destroyed by a cancerous tumour. Medical science
currently does not know any better means to fight cancer than the knife. I used to be
naïve and assumed that the *Volksraad* would act like a surgeon to stop further growth
of this cancer. I was very naïve! Experience has taught me that, in reality, the *Volksraad*
is a quack who cannot be trusted with a knife. It is not responsible toward the patient
because it never completed a full medical education.[38]

According to Tjipto, only physicians were able to counteract conditions as
severe as these. In 1920, he was banned from the Principalities (the area around
Solo and Yogyakarta) after being charged with instigating political unrest.[39] He
moved to Bandung, where he frequently met his former associates Douwes
Dekker and Soewardi, also returned from exile.

Tjipto's influence on the young Sukarno was his most significant legacy.
Sukarno, who would become the most influential leader of the nationalist
movement and Indonesia's first president, was a student at the Bandung
Technical School in 1925. There he established a study club in which Tjipto
and Douwes Dekker participated. Two years later he called Tjipto his 'chief'.[40]
Tjipto was involved in the founding of Sukarno's Indonesian National Party
[Partai Nasional Indonesia] (PNI) in 1927. In an interview conducted in 1959,
Sukarno, without any hesitation, identified Tjipto as the person who had
influenced him most.[41] Tjipto was again exiled in 1927 for his continuing pol-
itical activities. He was sent this time to Banda, a tiny island in the eastern part
of the archipelago which had been of great interest to the United Dutch East
Indies Company as the only place where nutmeg trees grew. Seven years later,
Indonesia's future vice president Mohammad Hatta and nationalist leaders
Iwa Koesoema Soemantri and Sutan Sjahrir were sent to join him.[42] Tjipto's
health steadily deteriorated on Banda. He was transferred to Makassar in 1941,
released three months later, and died in 1943.

---

[38] Tjipto Mangoenkoesoemo, 'Algemeene Beschouwingen, 14 Nov 1918', in *Handelingen van den
      Volksraad, Tweede Gewone Zitting* (Batavia: Volksraad van Nederlandsch-Indië, 1918), 168.
[39] Shiraishi, *Age in Motion*, 211.
[40] Bob Heering, *Soekarno: Founding Father of Indonesia, 1901–1945* (Leiden: KITLV Press,
      2002), 109.
[41] Scherer, 'Harmony and Dissonance', 149.
[42] See Des Alwi, *Friends and Exiles: A Memoir of the Nutmeg Isles and the Indonesian Nationalist
      Movement* (Ithaca, NY: Southeast Asia Program, Cornell University, 2008); Des Alwi, *Bersama
      Hatta, Syahrir, Dr. Tjipto & Iwa K. Soemantri di Banda Naira* (Jakarta: Dian Rakyat, 2002);
      Rudolf Mrázek, *Sjahrir: Politics and Exile in Indonesia* (Ithaca, NY: Southeast Asia Program,
      Cornell University, 1994), 154–208.

Western Civilisation and Its Discontents

Physicians Abdul Rivai and Tjipto Mangoenkoesoemo viewed cultural traditions as impediments to progress. After World War I, a new culturalist approach gained adherents among Indonesian nationalists, who came to criticise their predecessors for internalising European contempt for the archipelago's cultural heritage. These cultures, they argued, could serve as the foundation for viable alternatives to Western modernity. Their ideas garnered support during World War I, which demonstrated to many that modern science and technology simply augmented warfare, causing millions of deaths. In 1919 Goenawan Mangoenkoesoemo proclaimed: 'Today's Europe is sick, sick because of large ideas, propagated by large predecessors.'[43] He was critical of Javanese men who thought that by wearing 'hat and trousers [they] had also taken over Dutch virtues'.[44] By persistently imitating Europeans in dress and appearance, they ran the risk of 'forgetting to maintain their own culture'.[45] Nationalist intellectuals must instead 'show the people that their own civilisation is suitable to them and requires its full care and maintenance'.[46] They should work 'neither to kill nor to preserve her, but to keep her sufficiently alive, elastic, and powerful to deal with the vicissitudes of everyday life'.[47] As long as everyone remained dazzled by the West and continued to despise their own culture, he argued, they could never see themselves as equal to Europeans and would be, at best, slavish imitators.

Soewardi later described his growing disenchantment with European culture; his earlier adulation of what was Western and modern struck him as sadly misguided:

We [Indonesians] had a feeling of satisfaction or mild delight every time we had the opportunity to be among Europeans, speak Dutch even to our own countrymen, appear in western clothing, and arrange our houses in a western style. We even went further in our imitation: a small party at home would be too pedestrian and banal without western food, a jazz band, a glass of Dutch gin from Schiedam, which were necessary to 'modern' sociability and 'European' freedom usually on display on such occasions … We may certainly sigh together with Rabindranath Tagore: 'Our life is a quotation from that of the westerner, our voice an echo of that of Europe, instead of intellectuals we are nothing but bags full of information, there exists such an emptiness in our mind that we are not in a position to absorb what is beautiful and worthy.'[48]

---

[43] Goenawan Mangoenkoesoemo, 'What Heeft Indonesië Noodig? II', *Hindia Poetra* 1, no. 9 (1919), 194.

[44] Goenawan Mangoenkoesoemo, 'What Heeft Indonesië Noodig? III', *Hindia Poetra* 1, no. 10 (1919): 210.

[45] G. Mangoenkoesoemo, 'What Heeft Indonesië Noodig? III', 210.

[46] G. Mangoenkoesoemo, 'What Heeft Indonesië Noodig? III', 211.

[47] G. Mangoenkoesoemo, 'What Heeft Indonesië Noodig? III', 211.

[48] Ki Hadjar Dewantara, 'Some Aspects of National Education and the Taman Siswa Insitute of Jogjakarta', *Indonesia*, no. 5 (1967), 150–68.

In 1922, Soewardi renamed himself Ki Hadjar Dewantara and dropped the aristocratic titles *Raden Mas*. That same year, he established the first Garden of Pupils [*Taman Siswa*] school in Yogyakarta with a curriculum based on Javanese culture.[49] Over the next two decades, many *Taman Siswa* schools were established in the archipelago. These schools operated outside the orbit of the colonial administration, which labelled them 'wild schools' and sought to curb their activities.

The interest in traditional culture and ethnic traditions could easily be mistaken for nostalgia, celebrating the innocence of childhood, or for conservatism, reaffirming tradition, reasserting the authority of traditional heads, or warding off the corrosive effects of modernisation. Ernest Gellner, one of the most influential scholars of nationalism, has proposed an alternative explanation in which interest in traditional culture is a symptom of the transition of an agrarian society into an industrial one.[50] The idealisation of tradition, he argues, is a product of the imagination of metropolitan intellectuals, appropriating Orientalist notions to bolster their nationalist ideals. When Indies physicians and other nationalists extolled the vitality of traditional communities or viewed them as living and breathing organisms, they emphasised their modern surgical skills rather than the abilities of traditional healers to guide the further growth of these communities. Instead of affirming tradition, then, they sought to reshape it and put it to political ends.

Intellectuals who valorised the archipelago's ethnic cultures were joined by European and American Theosophists, and intellectuals associated with the Java Institute, founded in Solo in 1919. Theosophists promoted the deep spirituality, affinity with nature, and communitarian attitudes of the Javanese against Western materialism, egoism, and alienation.[51] In some instances they located Javanese spirituality in the distant past, long before the Dutch came to the Indies; in others it was relegated to a distant future when the original Eastern spirituality had been reawakened. Indonesian nationalists started to emphasise the vitality of *adat*, the vibrancy of artistic crafts, oral traditions, religious and tribal rituals, and the communitarian social organisation of organic traditional communities. Many nationalists grew increasingly convinced that an orientation towards Eastern, or Asian, principles and values would provide new energy to their movement. Indigenous cultures could be the bases for

---

[49] Kenji Tsuchiya, *Democracy and Leadership: The Rise of the Taman Siswa Movement in Indonesia* (Honolulu: University of Hawaii Press, 1987).

[50] Ernest Gellner, *Nations and Nationalism*, 2nd edn (Malden, MA: Blackwell, 2006), 38–51, 52–57.

[51] H. A. O Tollenaere, *The Politics of Divine Wisdom: Theosophy and Labour, National, and Women's Movements in Indonesia and South Asia, 1875–1947* (Nijmegen: Katholieke Universiteit Nijmegen, 1996) and Ethan Mark, '"Asia's" Transwar Lineage: Nationalism, Marxism, and "Greater Asia" in an Indonesian Inflection', *Journal of Asian Studies* 65, no. 3 (2006), 461–93.

solidarity, pride, and resistance, and indeed, the archipelago's cultural heritage offered the foundations for a unique local modernity in place of a derivative Western one. Accordingly, the corrosion of traditional culture and communities became a powerful critique against Dutch colonialism, and an argument for greater self-determination and, later, independence.

The Indies Youth Associations

During the second decade of the twentieth century, medical students became interested in their own ethnic groups, cultures, languages, histories, *adat*, and religious practices. They were hardly nostalgic; they did not advocate return to the past but looked for ways to revitalise and adapt traditional culture for the future. Their interest was intellectual in nature. They consulted the latest academic studies by Dutch scholars rather than meeting the elders of their ethnic groups; they fashioned alternative telic narratives that buttressed their broader social, cultural, and political interests. Most rhetoric on traditional culture came not from cultural heartlands but from the schools and colleges of the cities.

The medical students who founded Boedi Oetomo advocated the expansion of educational opportunities to improve the fate of the Javanese. They had aimed to unite Javanese high school students, particularly those attending elite, Dutch-speaking high schools, and students at the handful of institutions offering advanced education. After Boedi Oetomo became a regents' organisation, students at both medical colleges again took the lead and established a number of youth associations based on ethnic affiliation. They established Young Java [Jong Java] in 1915, the Young Sumatra Union [Jong Sumatranen Bond] and the Minahasa Student Association [Minahassa Studeerenden Vereeniging] in 1917, Young Ambon [Jong Ambon] in 1919, and Young Batak [Jong Batak] in 1926. Medical students did not play a leading role in the Young Muslim Association [Jong Islamieten Bond], which was established in 1925. Although they were discouraged from engaging in political activity, participation in these movements nonetheless provided a springboard for many members' activities in the nationalist movement. Members of these youth associations discussed the various political programs advocated by Indies physicians and other nationalists, which ranged from complete westernisation to revitalising traditional cultures, from realising independence to building closer ties with the Netherlands, and from building new elites to empowering the masses.

The youth associations organised lectures, social and cultural events, discussion groups, outings, scouting groups, and sports competitions. Their aim was to build unity among students. Except for Young Java, these groups played minor roles in the larger ethnic groups they aimed to represent. At times, students who were active in these associations caused considerable friction when they returned home to spend the holidays with their parents, who were not pleased with their appearance (Western-style clothing) and alien ideas.[52] As Sumatran Mohamad Amir observed:

Great is the influence of students when they return to their respective islands during the holidays. They no longer feel *senang* [happy, at ease] in their environment, they see unjust situations, they have far-reaching ideals and have many conflicts with their family in particular with respect to marriage. Yet they bring to the countryside a new civilisation from the west, new manners, new family ideals, objects, books, stories, and knowledge.[53]

There was a specific rupture between the students' new ideas about romantic love and partner choice, and the traditional ideas of their families. Students spoke with disdain of arranged marriages, the practice of marrying very young women, and polygamy. The home front rarely appreciated such innovations.

Young Java

In 1915, several Javanese medical students established Three Lofty Goals [Tri Koro Dharmo], which aimed to create a bond between all indigenous students, encourage personal development, and promote the study of indigenous languages, traditions, and arts.[54] Despite its archipelago-wide ambitions, Tri Koro Dharmo focused on unifying Javanese students and fostering appreciation of their language and culture. In 1918, the organisation had six branches and more than 700 members. Four years later it had eighteen branches and some 3,000 members. In 1918, its members decided to rename themselves as Jong Java and published a magazine with the same name (Figure 3.1).[55] The association's Dutch name and Dutch-language periodical emphasised the westernisation of its members, but still it searched for a redemptive understanding of Javanese culture.

One of the founders of Tri Koro Dharmo was medical student Satiman, who was known as outspoken and sometimes tactless. He often scolded his fellow students for imitating Europeans – speaking Dutch exclusively, wearing

---

[52] Mohamad Amir, 'Familieplichten', *Jong Sumatra* 1 (1918), 136–40.

[53] Mohamad Amir, 'Rondom een Indisch Jeugdcongres', *Opbouw* 10, no. 2 (1927), 75.

[54] Koentjoro Poerbapranato, 'Het Offer van Jong-Java aan het Altaar van het Vaderland', in *Gedenkboek Jong Java 1915 – 7 Maart – 1930: Kitab Peringatan Jong-Java* (Jakatera: Pedoman Besar Jong-Java, 1930), 43.

[55] For an excellent overview of Jong Java, see Hans van Miert, *Een Koel Hoofd en een Warm Hart: Nationalisme, Javanisme en Jeugdbeweging in Nederlands-Indië, 1918–1930* (Amsterdam: Bataafsche Leeuw, 1995), 44–64. See also Leo Suryadinata, 'Indonesian Nationalism and the Pre-War Youth Movement: A Reexamination', *Journal of Southeast Asian Studies* 9, no. 1 (1978), 99–114; Mr, 'Jong-Java, 1915–1922', in *Jong-Java's Jaarboekje, 1923* (Weltevreden: Kolff, 1923), 115–29.

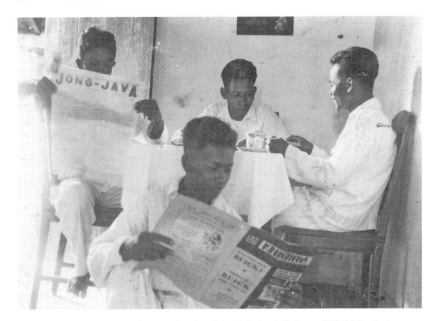

Figure 3.1 Students at the Surabaya Medical College (NIAS) in their spare time. Figure courtesy of the NIAS Museum, Faculty of Medicine, Airlangga University

European clothing, and appreciating everything modern and Western. Satiman was convinced that nationalist activity must be based on a common cultural heritage rather than mere accidents of geography or a shared status as colonial subjects. Tri Koro Dharmo aimed to prepare its members for future leadership roles. It sought to provide a cultural education for its members to avoid their transformation into 'entirely different beings, who, after spending years of isolation in schools, descend onto earth with extra-terrestrial wisdom'.[56] Satiman advocated academic methods to achieve this, including the study of ancient scriptures and Dutch archaeology. He also appealed to a sense of nostalgia: 'Don't you see the leaves of the *klapperboom* [palm tree] waving, don't you feel the coolness of the *waringin* [banyan tree], don't you smell the *melati* [jasmine] flowers, don't you hear the cooing of the *perkoetoets* [turtledoves] and the chirping of the *glatiks* [weaverbirds] swimming on the green *sawahs* [rice fields]?'[57]

---

[56] Satiman, 'Onze Vereeniging Tri Koro Dharmo', in *Maju Setapak*, ed. Pitut Soeharto and A. Zainoel Ihsan (Jakarta: Aksara Jayasakti, 1981 [1916]), 6.
[57] Satiman, 'Onze Vereeniging', 9.

Popular among members of Jong Java were discussions of Java's glorious past as embodied in the vast Majapahit Empire, which at its apex in the fourteenth century encompassed all Indonesia, Malaysia, southern Thailand, and part of the Philippines. Only a small number of Javanese court officials knew about this empire at the beginning of the century, but it became widely known after Dutch scholars unearthed several key manuscripts and an accessible history appeared.[58] Javanese intellectuals quickly developed an appealing narrative: Dutch colonialism had destroyed this powerful kingdom but it would rise again, with even greater strength, in the near future. Javanese history showed, for Jong Java leaders, that the 'Easterner is, in not a single respect, inferior to the Westerner.'[59] Medical student Soekiman, Satiman's brother and later president of Jong Java, put it eloquently: 'In deep admiration we kneel for our ancestors, who created temples such as the Borobudur and the Prambanan … besides this feeling of reverence, we sense in our minds the emanation of a growing force, a force that makes us strong in our attempts to rise from our state of our current impotence, our inability to act.'[60] With ingenuity and creativity, Soekiman and others mobilised Java's past to foment cultural pride for nationalist purposes. In 1918, Soekiman issued a more radical call for the unification of the archipelago's ethnic groups and for economic and political independence.[61]

Jong Java and all other student associations were forced to abandon political activities to achieve legal status in 1923.[62] From this point they organised sports competitions during their events and annual meetings, which helped to foster *esprit-de-corps* and ethnic pride. Attendance rose dramatically.[63] Within Jong Java, medical student Moewardi took the lead in organising boy scout and girl guide clubs to foster physical, mental, and spiritual development, and the other associations followed suit. In the 1920s, as the political climate in the Indies became increasingly repressive, leaders of the youth movements advocated preparation for the future instead of political activity.[64] Moewardi's colleague

---

[58] Willemine Fruin-Mees, *Geschiedenis van Java: Het Hindoetijdperk* (Weltevreden: Commissie voor de Volkslectuur, 1919).

[59] Soekiman, 'De Beteekenis van het Javaansche Cultuur Congres', *Jong Java* 3, no. 11 (1918), 160.

[60] Soekiman, 'Beteekenis', 160.

[61] Soekiman, 'Rede Uitgesproken ten Tweeden Jong-Java Congresse', *Jong-Java* (1918), 223–27.

[62] Mochtar Atmosoeprodjo, 'Jong-Java en de Politiek', in *Gedenkboek Jong Java 1915 – 7 Maart – 1930: Kitab Peringatan Jong-Java* (Jakatera: Pedoman Besar Jong-Java, 1930), 67–73.

[63] Soewandi, 'Jong-Java en Sport', in *Gedenkboek Jong Java 1915 – 7 Maart – 1930: Kitab Peringatan Jong-Java* (Jakatera: Pedoman Besar Jong-Java, 1930), 118–21. See also the report of the seventh conference, held in 1927, which devotes a great number of its pages to sports: *Jong-Java: Congresnummer 7e Jong-Java Congres* (Weltevreden: Indonesische Drukkerij, 1925).

[64] For Moewardi's ideas on scouting in Jong Java, see Moewardi, 'Kepandoean dalam Jong-Java', in *Gedenkboek Jong Java 1915 – 7 Maart – 1930: Kitab Peringatan Jong-Java* (Jakatera: Pedoman Besar Jong-Java, 1930), 141–80.

Pirngadi admonished students that being truly Javanese entailed much more than performing traditional dances and being mesmerised by *gamelan* music. Pirngadi also advised against participating in politics and encouraged students to join the boy scouts and girl guides instead because they would learn cooperation, courage, and self-sacrifice.[65] During the 1920s, scouting became very popular in the Indies and scouting clubs emerged throughout the archipelago.[66] Physical education, sports, scouting, and debating clubs were part of the effort to prepare for the future.[67]

Young Sumatra

In 1917, a number of medical students from Sumatra established the Young Sumatra Union [Jong Sumatranen Bond]. The founding meeting, at the Batavia Medical College, was attended by some 150 students.[68] Its aims closely mirrored those of Tri Koro Dharmo: to explore the history of Sumatra and its inhabitants; to investigate its cultures and languages; to strengthen the bonds between Sumatran students; and to prepare members for their future roles as leaders and educators.[69] It looked to stimulate further development in Sumatra by using Western knowledge to discard, enrich, or transform Sumatran cultural traditions.[70] In 1918 the association established a journal with the name *Jong Sumatra*, which was the key means of uniting its membership. The first president was medical student Tengkoe [Prince] Mansoer, son of the Sultan of Asahan; one of the two secretaries was his fellow medical student Mohamad Amir, the main ideologist and president of the association from 1920 to 1922.

The members of the Jong Sumatranen Bond faced an interesting and perhaps insurmountable challenge in that the inhabitants of their island did not view themselves as Sumatrans. They belonged to several ethnic groups, were geographically dispersed, and spoke many different languages. There was no common Sumatran culture, language, or identity.[71] Amir nonetheless argued that Sumatra's unity was perceptible at a psychological level since all

---

[65] Pirngadi, 'Afscheid', *Jong Java* 11, no. 19–20 (1–15 October 1926), 4.
[66] 'De Inlandsche Beweging: Een Overzicht', *Sumatra Post*, 10 January 1927, 1.
[67] For the fund that provided scholarships to Javanese students, see Sarwono Prawirohardjo, 'Nasib Studiefonds Kita Dikemoedian Hari', in *Gedenkboek Jong Java 1915 – 7 Maart – 1930: Kitab Peringatan Jong-Java* (Jakatera: Pedoman Besar Jong-Java, 1930), 182–205.
[68] For an overview of the history of the Jong Sumatranen Bond, see Hans van Miert, 'The "Land of the Future": The Jong Sumatranen Bond (1917–1930) and Its Image of the Nation', *Modern Asian Studies* 30, no. 3 (1996), 591–616; Miert, *Koel Hoofd Warm Hart*, 65–91.
[69] Abdoel Rachman, 'Jong Sumatra, Heil U!', *Wederopbouw* 1, no. 1 (1918), 11.
[70] See, for example, 'Fauna', 'Kemadjuan', *Jong Sumatra* 1 (1918), 221–24.
[71] Anthony Reid, 'The Identity of "Sumatra" in History', in *Cultures and Societies of North Sumatra*, ed. R. Carle (Berlin/Hamburg: Dietrich Reimer, 1987), 25–42.

Sumatrans had lived, for thousands of years, in the same natural environment. Skull measurements were of limited significance, argued Amir; only an appreciation of the vast island's 'cosmic rhythm' revealed its inner unity.[72] The ideal of uniting Sumatra came from Sumatrans residing elsewhere, such as students attending school on Java.[73] Despite organising several activities (of which a soccer competition in the Deli area was the most successful), the association remained without a following in its own heartland.

The members of Jong Sumatra hoped that exploring Sumatran history and culture would assist its various ethnic groups to transcend rivalries. Reading Dutch archaeology, members learned that the cities of Palembang and Jambi had been capitals of the once powerful Sriwidjaja Empire. Amir often conveyed the latest results of Dutch archaeological research in his articles.[74] The articles about *adat*, however, were more interesting. Time and again, Amir railed against stultifying traditions that inhibited personal development. 'The East is the land of the caste system', he proclaimed; 'of fossilised principles, of rigid, age-old institutions, in one word of *bondage* ... as a consequence of the fatal overgrowth of the authority of the *adat* and the family'.[75] He particularly criticised the position of women, who were seen as 'procreators and work machines ... akin to prisoners or slaves'.[76] Amir criticised arranged marriages, polygamy, the marrying of young girls, the lack of education among young women, and the complete lack of basic hygienic principles. He strongly supported the budding women's movement in Sumatra because it could correct many of these injustices. On *adat*, however, Amir was ambivalent. He expressed his admiration, but rarely elaborated on its virtues and often criticised its limitations.

According to Amir and other members of Jong Sumatra, nations were defined by a shared culture. 'An ethnic group [*volk*] without culture is no ethnic group at all', wrote Amir, 'even less a nation; such an ethnic group does not have a soul and will die out. A group which neglects its own culture (art, religion, *adat*, philosophy) and kneels for someone else's culture is a degenerated and lost group'.[77] It was imperative for Sumatran students to avoid becoming imitation Europeans, argued Amir, or individuals with a full understanding of

[72] Mohamad Amir, 'Sumatra's Eenheid: Bijdrage tot een Dynamisch-Psychologische Her-Stelling van het Probleem', in *Gedenknummer van Jong Sumatra, 1917–1922* (Weltevreden: Jong Sumatranen Bond, 1923), 19.

[73] 'Jong Sumatranenbond', *Sumatra Post*, 17 January 1918, Section III, 3.

[74] See, for example, Mohamad Amir, 'De Hindoe's op Sumatra', *Jong Sumatra* 1, no. 4 (1918), 57–60; Amir, 'Iets over de Sumatranen als Zeevarend Volk', 36–43. See also, for example, Bahder Djohan, 'De Strijd der Padries', in *Gedenk-Nummer van Jong Sumatra, 1917–1922* (Weltevreden: Jong Sumatranen Bond, 1923), 58–63.

[75] Mohamad Amir, 'De Vrouwenbeweging ter Sumatra's Westkust', *Jong Sumatra* 2, no. 1 (1919), 3.

[76] Amir, 'Vrouwenbeweging', 7.

[77] A. [Mohamad Amir], 'Op den Uitkijk', *Jong Sumatra* 4 (1921), 153.

Europe's intellectual accomplishments but only a partial grasp of European culture. They needed to become true Sumatrans, although they had to avoid adulating Sumatran culture, which some thought far superior to the materialism and individualism of the West. Only a meaningful integration of East and West, opined Amir, could revitalise the indigenous cultures of the Indies. It was a lofty ideal, and Amir offered little practical advice on how to achieve it except that, as a devout Theosophist, he recommended a deepening of religious sentiment because of its unifying force.[78]

Jong Sumatra supported the use of Malay, a language originally spoken on the east coast of Sumatra and the Malay Peninsula. A coarse form of Malay had become the lingua franca of the archipelago and was soon adopted by both the nationalist movement and the colonial administration as a common language for all inhabitants of the archipelago. At the first annual congress of Jong Sumatra, held in July 1919 in Padang, Bahder Djohan, president of the association from 1923 to 1926, argued that language created a powerful bond between people.[79] Instead of abandoning Malay as an outdated language, he urged his audience to usher it to a higher level: 'A Malay literature, our literature, understood and comprehended by us, has to be born to save our people, no, to save *youth*, those *who have strayed*.'[80] He hoped that a Malay literary association would soon be established; the magazine *Jong Sumatra* served as an important forum for Malay literature in the meantime.

The unity the Jong Sumatranen Bond hoped to establish suffered a blow of sorts when medical student Djabangoen Harahap established the Young Batak Union [Jong Bataks Bond] in 1925 to investigate, discuss, and modernise its own unique culture.[81] The various Batak groups, living in the Sumatra highlands, were perceived as backward; it was rumoured that cannibalism had been common a few generations ago. Most educated Bataks who found employment away from the Batak heartland did not disclose their ethnic background. The Batak association failed, however, to unite all Batak groups. Only the Toba Bataks came to refer to themselves as Batak; the Karo, Simulungun, Pakpak-Dairi, Ankola-Mandailing groups refused to do so. Even the name Jong Batak was therefore contested from the beginning.[82] Only groups living

---

[78] Mohamad Amir, 'Godsdienst en Spes-Patria', *Jong Sumatra* 1 (1918), 161–65.
[79] For Djohan's recollections of the Jong Sumatranen Bond, see Bahder Djohan, 'Gerakan Pemuda Membawa Perobahan Mental', in *45 Tahun Sumpah Pemuda* (Jakarta: Gunung Agung, 1974), 171–75.
[80] Bahder Djohan, 'De Maleische Taal en Hare Toekomst', *Jong Sumatra* 1 (1918), 167; see also Mohamad Amir, 'Letterkundige Verpoozingen', *Jong Sumatra* 2 (1919), 133–34.
[81] Aminoeddin Pohan, 'Een Reorganisatie van den Jong Sumatranenbond', *Jong Batak* 1, no. 2 (1926), 30–33; Sanoesi Pane, 'JSB-JBB', *Jong Batak* 1, no. 3 (1926), 58–60; Gindo Siregar, 'Het Bestaansrecht van een Jong Bataks Bond', *Jong Batak* 1, no. 1 (1926), 3–6.
[82] The name was discussed by Aminoeddin Pohan, 'Rede op de Oprichtingsvergadering', *Jong Batak* 1, no. 1 (1926), 7–11; and Sanoesi Pane, 'Nationalisme', *Jong Batak* 1, no. 1 (1926),

in close proximity could understand each other through their linguistic differences. Religious differences caused problems as well: several students were prepared to join a Christian group; others saw this as a betrayal of their culture.[83] The most successful activities of Jong Batak appeared to be soccer matches, chess games, and nature outings, organised by the few Bataks attending institutions of higher learning in the large urban centres of Sumatra and Java.[84] The short history of Jong Batak and Jong Sumatra illustrates the significant hurdles in attempts to base nationalist activity on shared cultural traditions.

Minahasa Student Association

The inhabitants of the Minahasa area in northern Sulawesi, together with the Christians of the Moluccan islands, have always held an anomalous position in the Dutch East Indies. Both groups converted to Christianity early, and enjoyed access to education provided by missionary groups and the colonial administration.[85] Many educated Minahasans moved to other parts of the archipelago, taking up positions in the colonial army and the lower ranks of the government bureaucracy. Because of their religion, their close cultural affinity with the Dutch, and their role within the colonies, most Minahasans saw themselves as a privileged group, and indeed their association with the colonial administration had resulted in economic prosperity, ample educational opportunities, and better career prospects. Minahasans proudly called their area the twelfth province of the Netherlands, after the eleven in Europe, and were acutely aware that the colonial administrations had always relied on them (and the Ambonese or Moluccans), for soldiers, policemen, and clerical workers. Not surprisingly, the social and political leaders among them were unwilling to jeopardise their privileged position in the colonies and had strong reservations

16. It was also discussed during the first meetings: 'Verslag van de Oprichtingsvergardering', *Jong Batak* 1, no. 1 (1926), 20–22; 'Verslag van de Voorvergardering van de JBB', *Jong Batak* 1, no. 1 (1926), 22–23. For a history of the Batak area, see Leonard Y. Andaya, 'The Trans-Sumatra Trade and the Ethnicization of the "Batak"', *Bijdragen tot de Taal-, Land- en Volkenkunde* 158, no. 3 (2002), 367–409; Anthony Reid, 'Sumatran Bataks: From Statelessness to Indonesian Diaspora', in *Imperial Alchemy: Nationalism and Political Identity in Southeast Asia* (Cambridge: Cambridge University Press, 2009), 145–86.

[83] 'Etna Lambda', 'De JBB en de Godsdiensten', *Jong Batak* 1, no. 4/5 (1926), 88–89.

[84] Sanoesi Pane, 'Onze Werkwijze', *Jong Batak* 1, no. 4/5 (1926), 76–79.

[85] For incisive analyses of the social and political position of the Minahasa region in the Dutch East Indies, see David Henley, 'Nationalism and Regionalism in Colonial Indonesia: The Case of Minahasa', *Indonesia*, no. 55 (1993), 91–112; and David Henley, *Nationalism and Regionalism in a Colonial Context: Minahasa in the Dutch East Indies* (Leiden: KITLV Press, 1996). Christian minorities in the Indies were generally ambivalent about the Indies nationalist movement. For an analysis of the ideas of Christian leaders in the Indies, see Gerry van Klinken, *Minorities, Modernity and the Emerging Nation: Christians in Indonesia, a Biographical Approach* (Leiden: KITLV Press, 2003), in particular the chapter of G. S. S. J. Ratulangi.

about the activities of the Indies nationalist movement. The Minahasa Student Association was therefore very different.

In early 1918, medical student Tom Kandou established the Minahasa Student Association [Studeerenden-Vereeniging Minahassa] at a meeting at the Batavia Medical College, 'surrounded by mysterious bottles and medical instruments'.[86] Thirty-four students attended. Minahasan ideas and interests deserved wider attention, Kandou declared. Despite their undisputed allegiance to the Dutch crown, the colonial administration rarely consulted Minahasans and Minahasans rarely spoke out. Kandou highlighted the desire for education and further development among Minahasans and argued that their ties with the Netherlands should be strengthened.[87] Dutch, not Malay, should be the primary language in Minahasa – 'Dutch is a perfect language … the key to the temple of knowledge and the arts … able to bring us to our goal of the highest level of development.'[88] One month later, the first issue of the association's periodical appeared, printed on bright orange paper, the colour of the Dutch royal family.

The Minahasa student association provided opportunities for students to socialise, deepen their understanding of Minahasan history and culture, and prepare them for leadership positions after graduation.[89] In its periodical, there was little discussion of the unique nature of Minahasan culture and how it could be preserved or updated. Instead, authors reflected that the easy access to Dutch schools enjoyed by Minahasans had caused an exodus of educated young people, leaving the area in disarray.[90] Residents of the most advanced area on the island of Sulawesi, Minahasans, Kandou believed, were responsible for fostering the further development of the whole island.[91] Instead of supporting Rivai's aristocracy of learning, Kandou advocated leadership roles for the most advanced ethnic groups – Minahasans and Christian

[86] T. A. Kandou, 'Rede ter Opening van de Eerste Jaarvergadering der Studeerenden-Vereeniging Minahassa', *Orgaan van de Studeerenden Vereeniging Minahassa* 1, no. 9 (March 1919), 135; R. C. L. Senduk, '1918–1928', *Jong Celebes* 4, no. 3–4 (1928), 2; reprinted in Pitut Soeharto and A. Zainoel Ihsan, eds., *Maju Setapak*, vol. 3, *Capita Selecta* (Jakarta: Aksara Jayasakti, 1981), 145–46.

[87] T. A. Kandou, 'De Evolutie bij de Minahassers', *Orgaan van de Studeerenden Vereeniging Minahassa* 1, no. 1 (1918), 9–16. See also Ms [A. Maramis], 'De Geestelijke Opleving in de Minahassa', *Orgaan van de Studeerenden Vereeniging Minahassa* 1, no. 1 (1918), 19–21.

[88] T. A. Kandou, 'De Minahassers en 't Nederlands', *Orgaan van de Studeerenden-vereeniging Minahassa* 1, no. 2 (15 March 1918), 28.

[89] Kandou, 'Evolutie Minahassers', 14.

[90] A. H. M., 'Quo Vadis', *Orgaan der Vereeniging van Indische Geneeskundigen* 1, no. 2 (1918), 22–3; Ms [A. Maramis], 'De Exodus van Minahassers', *Orgaan van de Studeerenden Vereeniging Minahassa* 1, no. 3 (1918), 33–38.

[91] T. A. Kandou, 'De Civilisatie van Celebes door Minahassers', *Orgaan van de Studeerenden Vereeniging Minahassa* 1, no. 3 (1918), 40–43; T. A. Kandou, 'Minahassa's Studeerende Jongelingschap en Haar Toekomstige Taak', *Orgaan van de Studeerenden Vereeniging Minahassa* 1, no. 8 (February 1919), 113–17; S. J. Warouw, 'Nationalisme', *Orgaan van de Studeerenden Vereeniging Minahassa* 2, no. 2 (May 1922), 36–42.

Moluccans. Not surprisingly, these ideas met a cold reception elsewhere on Sulawesi.

In 1931, Kandou divorced his Minahasan wife and moved to the Netherlands for specialist training in psychiatry. He died there in 1940.[92] The next chair of the Minahasa Student Association was medical student Sam Warouw, who was more pessimistic about the role of education and more sceptical about the benefits of speaking Dutch. In his at times impenetrable prose, full of citations of Western philosophers and sociologists, he argued that Western education and Western language had only encouraged young people to pursue careers outside Minahasa, forsaking their duty to their region. He sketched an image of ambitious students 'getting dizzy because of excessive modernisation and confused by all that abominable and pointless Dutch activity', while the Minahasan nation lay bereft of farmers and craftsman.[93] During the Indonesian revolution, Warouw advocated passionately for the establishment of a federal Indonesian state with strong ties to the Netherlands and, later, independence for Minahasa. He was the minister of health and, briefly, the president of the State of East Indonesia, which the Dutch established in December 1946 to counter the influence of the Republic. After independence, Warouw returned to his medical career.

Conclusion

Medical students founded almost all of the Indies student associations and occupied key leadership roles in them. Their opinions and those of other participants reflected broader changes in the nationalist movement as a whole. Unlike the advocates of progress and development, Indies intellectuals increasingly emphasised the importance of modernising traditional culture and finding a balance between European modernity and the plurality of ethnic cultures in the Indies. They began to counter views of the indigenous population as primitive and backward, and praised the vitality of traditional culture, citing its glorious past and its possible futures. Many political, academic, and social leaders began their careers as members of these associations, which provided their first contact with the nationalist movement and introduced them to broader social and political ideas.

Several members of Jong Java played significant roles in the Indonesian nationalist movement and the Republic of Indonesia. In 1918, Satiman

---

[92] During his time in the Netherlands, he co-wrote a book on psychoses with leading Dutch psychiatrist Eugène A. D. E. Carp. See E. A. D. E. Carp, Anthonius Henri Fortanier, and T. A. Kandou, *Psychosen op Exogenen Grondslag en Geestelijke Defecttoestanden* (Amsterdam: Scheltema & Holkema, 1937).

[93] Warouw, 'Nationalisme', 14.

co-founded the journal *Reconstruction* [*Wederopbouw*], published by the Committee for Javanese Nationalism and the Association of Javanese Intellectuals. In the 1930s, he was involved in various Islamic political associations. He received a Dutch medical degree in 1929 and established a private practice in Solo, where he participated in the founding of an Islamic Institute of Higher Learning. Soekiman studied in the Netherlands from 1923 to 1925 and was president of the Indonesian Association at a time when it was becoming increasingly radical. After his return, he participated actively in various Islamic political associations, and was, in time, the seventh prime minister of the Republic of Indonesia.[94] Members of Jong Sumatra included Bahder Djohan, Indonesia's founding vice president, Mohammad Hatta, lawyer Mohammad Jamin, and physician/politician Mohamad Amir. Jong Batak counted brothers Sanoesi and Armijn Pane as members; both became popular novelists and literary commentators. Nationalist G. S. S. J. Ratulangi wrote several essays for Jong Celebes, which replaced Jong Minahasa. Boedi Oetomo continued as a moderate political party, and merged in 1935 with Soetomo's moderate Greater Indonesia Party (Perindra) in 1935. Jong Ambon was founded by Johannes Leimena, who was Indonesia's minister of health for most of the 1950s and early 1960s.

Apart from presenting programs of social and political change for specific ethnic groups and areas, the Indies youth movements also held discussions on the future of the Indies as a whole. In particular, their leaders began coordinating their activities more closely and came to view amalgamation positively. On 28 October 1928, at a joint meeting, members from all Indonesian youth movements took the now famous youth oath [*sumpah pemuda*] and pledged allegiance to one motherland, one nation, and one language [*satu bangsa, satu Negara, satu bahasa*], sang *Indonesia Raya* [*Great Indonesia*], the future national anthem, for the first time, and voted to merge all youth movements into one: Young Indonesia [*Indonesia Moeda*].[95]

---

[94] For a biography, see Amir Hamzah Wiryosukarto, *Wawasan Politik Seorang Muslim Patriot: Kumpulan Karangan* (Jakarta: YP2LPM, 1984).
[95] See Elson, *The Idea of Indonesia*, 64–72.

4 Professional Aspirations and Colonial Ambivalence: The Association of Indies Physicians

Medical students at the Indies medical colleges cherished their cosmopolitan identity and yearned to join the ranks of the educated elite. Upon graduation, however, they were confronted with the harsh realities of colonial life and the realisation that the social position of Indies physicians was ambiguous and contested. Dutchmen resisted their attempts to penetrate the European social sphere and treated them as they treated other natives: with disdain. European physicians were hostile and frequently questioned the qualifications, character, and morality of their native colleagues. They portrayed them as rootless and dangerously over-educated imitation Europeans who had forgotten their proper place in colonial society. The colonial administration reinforced this disdain by remunerating Indies physicians poorly, placing them at the lower end of the traditional hierarchy. Higher aristocrats took their cue from the administration and did not treat Indies physicians very well. Denied entry into the European social sphere and snubbed by the upper layers of the traditional aristocracy, Indies physicians occupied an unenviable social position. The idealism and optimism that had characterised them as medical students were replaced by disappointment and frustration. It would spur some of them into organised protest and political activism.

It was one of the most absurd features of colonial life that the individuals with the highest educational accomplishments were forced to occupy the fringes of both European and indigenous social circles. As early as 1898, renowned Islamist scholar Christiaan Snouck Hurgronje, one of the most influential advocates of the Ethical Policy and advisor for native affairs to the colonial administration, described the position of *Dokters Djawa* as 'fully unsatisfactory and not in agreement with the education they have enjoyed'.[1] Despite standing 'far above the majority of indigenous civil servants' their rank remained 'one of the lowest' and their income was insufficient to meet 'demands related to engagement in the *priyayi* world'.[2] Pursuing emancipation

---

[1] Christiaan Snouck Hurgronje, *Ambtelijke Adviezen van C. Snouck Hurgronje 1889–1936*, vol. 2 (The Hague: Nijhoff, 1959), 1040. This advice was dated 21 March 1898.
[2] Snouck Hurgronje, *Ambtelijke Adviezen*, 2, 1040.

and equality with Europeans, they acted in 1909, founding the Association of Indies Physicians so that they would have a public voice. The Association provided mutual support, represented their interests, and lobbied for better remuneration and improved working conditions. Above all, it attempted, through organised activity, to enhance their social status. Their emancipatory efforts culminated in 1918, when three Indies physicians became members of the first Volksraad. Debates in the Dutch colonial press about Indies physicians were unusually intense. Conservative commentators considered the physicians' emancipatory program premature, even ill conceived; progressives occasionally praised their courage. Debates on the social position of Indies physicians reflected and informed broader disagreements about the nature, desirability, and potential pitfalls of the Ethical Policy and the future of the Dutch colonial project as a whole.

A Medical Perspective on the Indigenous Population

Even before the Ethical Policy was officially inaugurated in 1901, it attracted widespread critique from plantation owners, policy makers, and social commentators as unduly expensive, overly idealistic, and inappropriate for the Dutch East Indies. Critics were particularly concerned by the Policy's program of Western-style education which aimed to train a sufficient number of lower colonial functionaries to support its implementation. In 1907, physician Jacob Herman Friedrich Kohlbrugge published *Glances into the Soul of the Javanese*, the first scholarly critique of the Ethical Policy, arguing that anything beyond the most basic form of education unhinged native minds and corroded indigenous communities. Primitive and animistic beliefs, argued Kohlbrugge, held the Javanese mind in a resolute grip, obstructing all attempts at education and improvement (Figure 4.1).[3] Providing a Western-style education to such minds, Kohlbrugge warned, was not only misguided but also dangerous, since it created a rootless group of urban quasi-intellectuals alienated from their culture and ethnic group. These corrupted natives, he argued, threatened to rupture the colonial social order.

As an alternative to the Ethical Policy, Kohlbrugge presented a psychological colonial policy, based on insights into 'the mental life of the people, which one acquires through … psychology'.[4] This alternative, he argued,

---

[3] J. H. F. Kohlbrugge, *Blikken in het Zieleleven van den Javaan en Zijner Overheerschers* (Leiden: Brill, 1907).

[4] J. H. F. Kohlbrugge, 'Psychologische Koloniale Politiek', *Vereeniging Moederland en Koloniën* 8, no. 2 (1907), 37. For his practical suggestions, see Kohlbrugge, *Blikken*; 'Psychologische Koloniale Politiek', and 'Zielkunde als Grondslag van Koloniaal Beleid', *Militaire Gids* 27 (1908), 229–51.

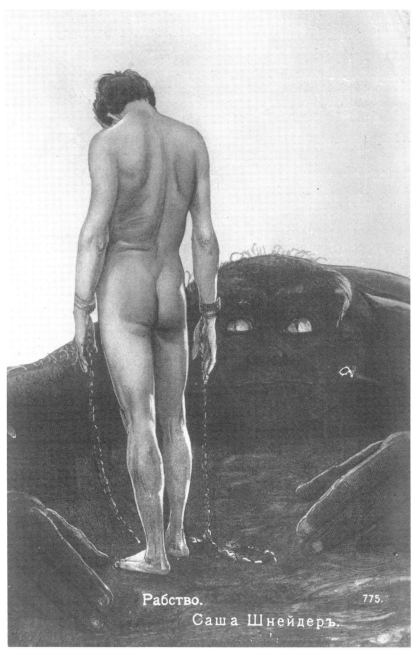

Рабство.

Саша Шнейдеръ.

775.

Figure 4.1 Sascha Schneider: A feeling of dependence. This figure graced the cover of Kohlbrugge's *Glances into the Soul of the Javanese and Their Rulers* and represents the force of animism. Antique postcard, author's collection

would not disregard the 'peculiar nature of the character of the Javanese'.[5] By emphasising the differences between Eastern and Western minds, Kohlbrugge disputed the view that the Javanese were merely lagging behind and would eventually catch up, with Dutch assistance. He argued that Western-style education would erode traditional culture and the communitarian spirit of traditional village life. Keeping Europeans and natives in separate spheres through a policy of association would, he continued, allow each group to develop according to its own inner dynamic.[6] This approach would respect indigenous customs, religious beliefs, and traditions by interfering as little as possible in indigenous affairs.

Kohlbrugge used psychological and anthropological arguments to mark the essential difference between natives and Europeans. Biological research on racial difference and medical theories of cerebral development had served the same purpose in other contexts. Kohlbrugge instead highlighted the impact of specific and enduring cultural factors. Animism, the belief that the natural and human worlds are suffused with a spiritual reality, provided 'the key to the secret' of the Javanese soul.[7] Quoting Abdul Rivai's views on the primitive nature of native minds approvingly, Kohlbrugge asserted that Javanese minds were highly suggestible, emotional, erratic, superstitious, and childlike.[8] Their lack of individualism, inability to plan ahead, irrationality, pervasive laziness, and deeply emotional nature meant that Javanese society could develop only very slowly, if at all. The tropical climate also stifled mental activity.[9] Compelling Javanese people to develop their higher mental faculties would inevitably result in neurasthenia, insanity, and suicide. Western-style education, Kohlbrugge warned, would only create a band of discontented intellectuals or a 'scientific proletariat' likely to foment strife and insurrection: 'Such half-baked scholars are an impatient and dangerous race, in particular when they originate from and live in the middle of the completely uneducated, unthinking, and suggestible masses.'[10]

While Kohlbrugge did not explicitly discuss Indies physicians, he singled out Roll as the main culprit in instilling a harmful desire for higher education in natives. This desire, he asserted, had been foisted upon the Javanese by misguided Ethicists, but 'perhaps the greatest influence could be ascribed to Roll.'[11]

---

[5] Kohlbrugge, 'Zielkunde', 236.
[6] For similar considerations in the French empire, see Martin Deming Lewis, 'One Hundred Million Frenchmen: The "Assimilation" Theory in French Colonial Policy', *Comparative Studies in Society and History* 4, no. 2 (1962), 129–53.
[7] Kohlbrugge, *Blikken*, 99.
[8] Kohlbrugge quoted Abdul Rivai, 'Het Geloof der Inlanders, I', *Algemeen Handelsblad*, 13 August 1901, 7 and from four further instalments.
[9] Kohlbrugge, *Blikken*, 93.
[10] Kohlbrugge, *Blikken*, 66, 95–96.
[11] J. H. F. Kohlbrugge, 'Welken Weg Moeten Wij Volgen om den Javaan te Ontwikkelen?', *Vereeniging Moederland en Koloniën* 8, no. 7 (1908), 37.

Kohlbrugge's appraisal of the Ethical Policy received little attention at the time.[12] Only Snouck Hurgronje wrote a rebuttal, calling Kohlbrugge's booklet undisciplined, anecdotal, and far too selective in its use of scholarship.[13] Indies physicians did not pay much attention either: Kohlbrugge was seen as a cantankerous and petulant loner who had an uncanny ability to antagonise virtually everyone. When, a few years later, similar arguments started to appear in the colonial press, it became clear that reactionary colonial backroom chatter had become public discourse. With increasing frequency, politicians, social commentators, and European physicians deployed similar arguments. As a consequence, the social aspirations of Indies physicians took centre stage in the broader debate about the Ethical Policy. Indies physicians and other intellectuals could no longer avoid addressing the political uses of medical and biological theories by conservative colonial commentators.

The Report on the Reorganisation of the Colonial Medical Service

Before the turn of the twentieth century, the Indies medical service primarily served the needs of soldiers, military officers, and high administrators. The afflictions of the European inhabitants of the colonies received treatment only if medical personnel were not otherwise occupied and sufficient resources were available. During the previous century, several critics had advocated separating the military and civil medical services.[14] After the inauguration of the Ethical Policy, commentators advocated the expansion of medical care to the indigenous population. In 1906, the colonial administration appointed a committee to study these issues consisting of several military medical officers and J. Schülein, chairman of the Union of (European) Physicians in the Dutch Indies [Bond van Geneesheeren in Nederlandsch-Indië]. Two years later, the committee's long-awaited report appeared. It detailed the deplorable state of the health facilities for the indigenous population (which, at the time, only

[12] One exception was Boeka [P. C. C. Hansen], 'Naar Aanleiding van het Belangrijke Boek van Dr. Kohlbrugge', *Indische Gids* 30 (1908), 480–87. Boeka disagreed with Kohlbrugge's conclusions and discussed a great number of topics in his review, none of which was mentioned in Kohlbrugge's book.

[13] Kohlbrugge drew extensively on the work of C. Poensen, a protestant missionary. See Christiaan Snouck Hurgronje, 'Blikken in het Zieleleven van den Javaan?', *De Gids* 71, no. 3 (1908), 423–47.

[14] For two early proposals, see Een Geneesheer in Indië [Cornelis Swaving], *Twee Voorstellen in het Belang van de Nederlandsche Bezittingen in Oost-Indië* (Groningen: Wolters, 1850); C. Swaving, 'Voorstel tot Verbetering van den Burgerlijken Geneeskundigen Dienst in Nederlandsch-Indië', *Nederlands Tijdschrift voor Geneeskunde* 17 (1873), 549–53; see also 'Historisch Overzicht van de Voorstellen tot Reorganisatie van den Burgerlijken Geneeskundigen Dienst', in *Rapport der Commissie tot Voorbereiding eener Reorganisatie van den Burgerlijken Geneeskundigen Dienst*, ed. J. Bijker (Batavia: Landsdrukkerij, 1908), 169–98.

provided care for prisoners, prostitutes, and members of chain gangs) and recommended the separation of the civil and military medical services.[15] Noting that a civilian medical service would require a significant increase in the number of Indies physicians, the committee made that its recommendation.

The committee hailed Indies physicians as the 'foundation of the building of the civil medical service'.[16] Their ethnic affiliations, facility with native languages, and awareness of the sensitivities of indigenous populations regarding health, disease, and the body were indispensable.[17] The indigenous population, the committee pointed out, was much more likely to follow the directives of Indies physicians because of the widespread distrust towards Europeans. Ideally, the Indies physician should be a 'cheerful, skilled practitioner able to treat the most common forms of disease and injury'.[18] A practical physician rather than a theorist would be preferable, the committee continued: 'Half-baked scientific knowledge would be fatal for our native physicians, [who should] not be encumbered by half understood or misunderstood scientific theories.'[19] A practical education was far better suited, the committee concluded, to the limited intellectual abilities of native students. They tended 'to forget a lot and to acquire little new knowledge' and should not be overburdened.[20] To generate a much larger number of Indies physicians the committee recommended abridging and simplifying the medical curriculum. Indies physicians only needed to be able to treat the most common tropical diseases under the supervision of their European colleagues.

To add insult to injury, the report further suggested that the health of the indigenous population was currently sacrificed to support the social ambitions of arrogant and over-educated Indies physicians who were distancing themselves from their native patients. The artificially high standards of the Batavia Medical College had unfortunately inspired students to adopt a modern, Western identity, so that the 'native physician no longer thinks he is a native and is treated by natives as a dissident and renegade'.[21] This, the committee contended, would interfere with the role they envisaged for them. 'To contribute to the elevation of the indigenous population', the Indies physician 'has to remain a native, not only in his worldview, but also in his everyday habits, his manners, his appearance, and in the way he dresses'.[22] The political activity

[15] J. Bijker, *Rapport der Commissie tot Voorbereiding eener Reorganisatie van den Burgerlijken Geneeskundigen Dienst* (Batavia: Landsdrukkerij, 1908).
[16] Bijker, *Rapport Reorganisatie BGD*, 21.
[17] Bijker, *Rapport Reorganisatie BGD*, 21.
[18] Bijker, *Rapport Reorganisatie BGD*, 72.
[19] Bijker, *Rapport Reorganisatie BGD*, 72, 70.
[20] Bijker, *Rapport Reorganisatie BGD*, 21.
[21] Bijker, *Rapport Reorganisatie BGD*, 75.
[22] Bijker, *Rapport Reorganisatie BGD*, 75.

of medical students, the recent appointment of Abdul Rivai as military medical officer, the ease with which Indies physicians could enrol in Dutch medical schools, and the countless speeches by Ethical politicians had created misguided ambitions in Indies physicians. They now thought, quite mistakenly, that the differences between Indies and European physicians could be overcome, and with relative ease.[23]

The report received extensive attention in the Indies press. The limited mental capacities and moral sensibilities of Indies physicians, as well as their alienation from the indigenous population, were discussed frequently. Kohlbrugge endorsed the report.[24] Colonel J. Haga, former director of the colonial medical service and an instructor at the Batavia Medical College, agreed that the colonies 'need *Dokters Djawa* with a shorter education'.[25] Upgrading the medical curriculum would be counterproductive: 'The education for native physicians, which is patterned far too much on European examples, is the greatest obstacle for an adequate or, preferably, for comprehensive medical care to the indigenous population.'[26] The semblance of scientific training and its associated fantasies of independent thinking had only produced vanity; Indies physicians should 'preferably [be] practitioners rather than native physicians with fake knowledge and a mere varnish of science'.[27]

The report infuriated Roll, who wrote an elaborate rebuttal arguing that the Indies needed 'full physicians, not half physicians'.[28] Moreover, Indies physicians studying at Dutch universities had been excellent students, as several Dutch professors attested.[29] Unsurprisingly, the report also enraged Indies physicians. Willem Karel Tehupeiory, then studying medicine at the University of Amsterdam, interjected that poorly educated Indies physicians would never be able to work independently, as was often required, and would irrevocably damage the reputation of Western medicine among the indigenous population.[30] Indies physicians had encountered opposition only from aristocrats, he suggested, never from the general population. A brochure written by eight

---

[23] Bijker, *Rapport Reorganisatie BGD*, 77.

[24] J. H. F. Kohlbrugge, 'Het Rapport der Commissie, tot Voorbereiding eener Reorganisatie van den Burgelijken Geneeskundigen Dienst in N.I., Critisch Beschouwd', *Indische Gids* 31 (1909), 312–25.

[25] J. Haga, 'Geneeskundige Dienst in Ned.-Indië', *Indische Gids* 30 (1908), 28.

[26] J. Haga, 'Reorganisatie van den Geneeskundigen Dienst in Ned.-Indië', *Indische Gids* 31 (1909), 463.

[27] Haga, 'Geneeskundige Dienst', 29.

[28] Roll, quoted by Jacob Samallo, 'Herinneringen uit het Leven van de Élèves der STOVIA 25 Jaar Geleden', in *Ontwikkeling van het Geneeskundig Onderwijs te Weltevreden, 1851–1926*, ed. A. de Waart (Weltevreden: Kolff, 1926), 291.

[29] H. F. Roll, *Is Reorganisatie van de School tot Opleiding van Inlandsche Artsen te Weltevreden Nogmaals Nodig?* (Dordrecht: Morks & Geuze, 1909), 15–16.

[30] W. K. Tehupeiory, 'Reorganisatie van het Onderwijs aan de School tot Opleiding van Inlandsche Artsen te Weltevreden', *Indische Gids* 31 (1909), 922–28.

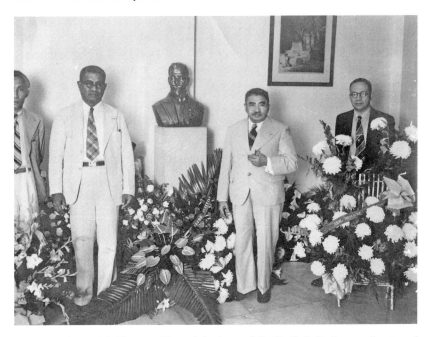

Figure 4.2 The unveiling of the bust of Dr H. F. Roll, former director of the Batavia Medical School (STOVIA), in the hall of the Batavia Medical School. The bust was made by the architect C. P. Wolff-Schoemaker for the Association of Indonesian Physicians. On the figure: unknown, J. Kayadoe, W. K. Tehupeiory, and Bahder Djohan. Figure: author's collection

Indies physicians enrolled at Dutch universities marshalled similar arguments and praised Roll for his efforts to increase the quality of medical education in the Indies (Figure 4.2).[31] This brochure marked the first time Indies physicians collectively expressed their opinions to protect their professional interests.

The Association of Native Physicians

Indies physicians were motivated by a powerful desire for social advancement and emancipation, which they saw as achievable only by eliminating all differences between themselves and their European colleagues. In 1908, Tehupeiory was the first Indies physician (and the first native) to address the august Indies Society [Indisch Genootschap], a group of politicians,

---

[31] H. J. D. Apituley, R. Tumbelaka, H. F. Lumentut, Radjiman, M. Brenthel, Moh. Salih, P. Laoh, and Abdul Rivai, *Eenige Opmerkingen naar Aanleiding van de Voorstellen tot Reorganisatie van den Civiel Geneeskundigen Dienst in Nederl. Oost-Indië* (Amsterdam: Eisendrath, 1910).

academics, and businessmen committed to the ideals of the Ethical Policy, based in The Hague. He discussed the position of Indies physicians within the colonial medical service and life at the Batavia Medical College. Tehupeiory argued against two speakers who had, on previous occasions, presented both in a damaging light: Kohlbrugge, invoking his psychological colonial policy, and a former STOVIA instructor who had denounced the overly intellectual focus of the medical curriculum and its neglect of students' moral development.[32]

Far from fostering alienation, mental derangement, or moral depravity, argued Tehupeiory, medical education provided native students with a superior moral compass. Older students provided support and moral direction to younger students, and medicine itself appealed to higher moral sensibilities:

Is there any science more morally instructive than medicine? So many virtues are imparted through medical education as every medical encounter is a search for truth. A desire for truth, charity, civility, and exemplary social behaviour is developed.[33]

Indies physicians suffered profound injustices, Tehupeiory suggested. After graduation, they were obliged to work for the colonial medical service for ten years at salaries far lower than those of less educated indigenous officials. They could not maintain a European lifestyle nor live in European neighbourhoods. They suffered the indignity of living near the *kampong*. There, 'decent social interaction is out of the question', he protested; 'we are not able to afford subscriptions to newspapers and magazines, let alone the membership of European social clubs'.[34] Tehupeiory discussed a number of other insidious forms of discrimination. Although he and his colleagues enjoyed the trust of their European and Indo-European patients, were often invited to their parties, and became close friends with their families, they still suffered galling exclusion at key junctures. Echoing Rivai's complaints, Tehupeiory claimed that Indies physicians were too often treated 'as plain natives'.[35] It was hardly a surprise that students abandoned their studies and careers for more lucrative paths, and that Indies physicians left the employ of the civil medical service as soon as they could to work in plantations, businesses, and private practice. Rather than revealing a lack of commitment to their indigenous brethren or a superficial desire for material success, these decisions reflected economic necessities.

---

[32] J. H. F. Kohlbrugge, 'Hygienische Toestanden in de Desa', *Indisch Genootschap*, 12 February 1907, 189–205; A. J. H. Scherp, 'De Inrichting der Gouvernements-Internaten voor Inlandsche Jonglieden in Nederlands-Indië in Verband met de Zedelijke Vorming der Leerlingen', *Indisch Genootschap*, 26 Maart 1907, 219–41.

[33] W. K. Tehupeiory, 'Iets over de Inlandsche Geneeskundigen', *Indisch Genootschap*, 28 January 1908, 107. For a translation, see W. K. Tehupeiory, 'The Native Physicians', in *Regents, Reformers, and Revolutionaries: Indonesian Voices of Colonial Days: Selected Historical Readings, 1899–1949*, ed. Greta O. Wilson (Honolulu: University of Hawaii Press, 1978), 48–59.

[34] Tehupeiory, 'Iets over de Inlandsche Geneeskundigen', 114.

[35] Tehupeiory, 'Iets over de Inlandsche Geneeskundigen', 100.

In the face of strong opposition, Indies physicians saw the need to create an organisation to represent their interests. Tehupeiory held extensive discussions with his colleagues on how to accomplish this.[36] The elite Association for the Advancement of Medical Research in the Dutch Indies rarely involved itself in mundane matters such as salaries, working conditions, and intra-professional rivalries. The Union of (European) Physicians had revealed itself as the main opponent of ambitious Indies physicians and was best avoided. Tehupeiory, a Christian Ambonese physician, suggested following the strategies embraced by educated Ambonese during the first part of the twentieth century: achieving 'equality with Europeans, through working within the system'.[37] Together with the inhabitants of the Minahasa, the Christian inhabitants of the Moluccan islands viewed themselves as a group standing between the Dutch and the rest of the population. Tehupeiory's initiatives were, in effect, an attempt to transfer the elite status of his privileged ethnic group to the Indies medical profession.

On 17 September 1909, a year and a half after the founding of Boedi Oetomo, in the same hall of the Batavia Medical College and with many of the same individuals present, Tehupeiory established the Association of Native Physicians [Vereeniging van Inlandsche Geneeskundigen] (VIG).[38] The Association aimed to further the interests of Indies physicians and to promote the health of the indigenous population.[39] Because Tehupeiory was about to be transferred to remote Bangka (Figure 4.3), Ambonese *Dokter Djawa* D. J. Siahaija was elected president. The reason for the Association, announced Tehupeiory, was the 'desire for equality with Europeans'.[40] Too often he had 'witnessed the attitude of Europeans towards the natives, how the latter were considered inferior irrespective of the education they had enjoyed'.[41] Invoking van Deventer's sleeping beauty parable, Tehupeiory declared that the founding

---

[36] In 1907, Tehupeiory and Raden Boenjamin, a *Dokter Djawa* who was in the Netherlands for further study, met with the minister of colonies to discuss the plight of Indies physicians. After that meeting, they wrote a long letter to their colleagues trying to convince them of the importance of founding an association. See Letter, W. K. Tehupeiory and R. Boenjamin to Indies physicians, 10 December 1907. Archive Willem Karel Tehupeiory, inventory number 6, International Institute of Social History, Amsterdam.

[37] Richard Chauvel, *Nationalists, Soldiers and Separatists: The Ambonese Islands from Colonialism to Revolt, 1880–1950* (Leiden: KITLV Press, 2008), 72.

[38] This Association was founded as the Association of Native Physicians [Vereeniging van Inlandsche Geneeskundigen] (VIG) in 1911; in 1918 it was renamed the Association of Indies Physicians [Vereeniging van Indische Geneeskundigen] (VIG) (I use this name throughout). In 1938, the name was changed to the Association of Indonesian Physicians [Vereeniging van Indonesische Geneeskundigen] (VIG).

[39] 'Vereeniging van Inlandsche Geneeskundigen', *Het Nieuws van den Dag in Nederlandsch Indië*, 16 July 1909, 2.

[40] W. K. Tehupeiory, 'Onze Vereening: De Voorgeschiedenis van Hare Oprichting en Hare Kleuterjaren', in *Jubileumnummer 1911–1936* (Batavia: Kolff, 1937), 4.

[41] Tehupeiory, 'Onze Vereening', 2.

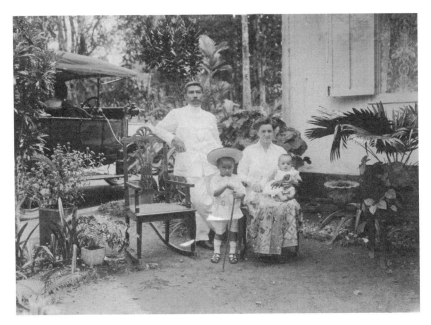

Figure 4.3 W. K. Tehupeiory, his wife, and his two children photographed while he was stationed on the island of Bangka, off the east coast of Sumatra. Figure courtesy of Herman Keppy

of the Association represented the awakening of Indonesian physicians, and that their emancipation would benefit the indigenous population as a whole.[42]

The first issue of the Association's journal, the *Organ of the Association of Native Physicians*, contained Tehupeiory's address to the Indies Association and a discussion of the report on the reorganisation of the colonial medical service.[43] During the following years, members submitted articles on the various locations they worked to provide useful insights to colleagues who might be transferred there in the future.[44] Numerous reports on everyday injustices also featured. One physician noted that he did not have access to the medicine cabinet at his clinic because the key was held by the local European physician. Another related how he was called to see a patient displaying the symptoms of acute malaria more than twenty kilometres away without being

---

[42] Tehupeiory, 'Onze Vereening', 4.
[43] This Bulletin appeared in July 1909. See 'Vereeniging Inlandsche Geneeskundigen', 2.
[44] The editor hoped that these reports could be compiled in a Guide for Native Physicians. See 'Gids for Inlandsche Geneeskundigen', *Orgaan der Vereeniging van Inlandsche Geneeskundigen* 2, no. 1 (1911), 1–2.

allowed to take a dose of quinine with him because a diagnosis had not yet been made. 'Again', this author concluded, 'the necessity of an Association has been demonstrated'.[45] The board of the Association frequently wrote to the Governor-General to highlight the plight of Indies physicians and to plead for adequate remuneration. The entry salary for native lawyers after completing a three-year course, they explained, was double the salary Indies physicians made after ten years' service.[46] The reimbursements for rent, travel, and time spent away from home did not even come close to covering actual expenses.[47] Irritations with high aristocrats featured.[48] Members also discussed the need to establish a fund to support the widows and orphans of deceased Indies physicians, since the colonial administration made no provision for them.[49]

Ambonese Indies physician P. L. Augustin expressed the concerns of the Association's members in a pamphlet written while he was stationed in Merauke, West Guinea.[50] He reiterated the complaints that had filled the pages of the *Organ*: the workload was too heavy, amenities too few, responsibilities too great, salaries too low, and expressions of respect rare or entirely absent. Moreover, Indies physicians were frequently transferred and the costs of relocation far exceeded any disbursement provided – the loss incurred, Augustin argued, was akin to the damage caused by a house fire.[51] Low remuneration meant that physicians had to live in less desirable neighbourhoods, which allowed for little socialisation with educated Europeans. When travelling by train, they were provided with second-class fares and were therefore forced to travel among 'dirty, stinking Arabs or slurping Chinese'.[52] Because

---

[45] 'Uit de Verslagen van de Vergaderingen van de Afdeeling West-Java', *Orgaan der Vereeniging van Inlandsche Geneeskundigen* 2, no. 1 (1910), 9–10.

[46] Roem, 'Nogmaals: Collega's Vereenigt U!', *Orgaan der Vereeniging van Inlandsche Geneeskundigen* 2, no. 3 (1911), 21–25.

[47] Soetomo, 'Een Gemotiveerde Grief', *Orgaan der Vereeniging van Inlandsche Geneeskundigen* 3, no. 3 (1912), 43.

[48] J. Westplat, 'Urgente Rangverbetering voor de Inlandsche Geneeskundigen', *Orgaan der Vereeniging van Inlandsche Geneeskundigen* 3, no. 2 (1912), 5–7. See also F. H. Wuller, 'Verslag van de Lotgevallen der Vereeniging van Inlandsche Geneeskundigen over het Jaar 1911', *Orgaan der Vereeniging van Inlandsche Geneeskundigen* 3, no. 3 (1912), 35–38.

[49] Hoofdbestuur, 'Geachte Collega's!', *Orgaan der Vereeniging van Inlandsche Geneeskundigen* 3, no. 3 (1912), 39–41; J. Westplat, 'Een Compensatie in het Moeilijke Bestaan in den Ouden Dag', *Orgaan der Vereeniging van Inlandsche Geneeskundigen* 4, no. 6 (1913), 77–79.

[50] Ambonese physician Paulus Lineus Augustin graduated from the STOVIA in 1911 and studied in the Netherlands from 1922 to 1926. His pamphlet was first given as a lecture to the Association of Indies Physicians during its monthly meetings in Batavia. Augustin was one of the more active members. P. L. Augustin, *Iets over Rechten en Plichten van den Inlandschen Arts* (Batavia: Kolff, 1914).

[51] On another occasion an Indies physician claimed he was 'saved by disease' because it obviated his transfer: Raden Soekardie, 'Uit het Leven van een Indisch Geneeskundige Nu 25 Jaar Geleden: Door Ziekte Gered', in *Ontwikkeling van het Geneeskundig Onderwijs te Weltevreden, 1851–1926*, ed. A. de Waart (Weltevreden: Kolff, 1926), 296–97.

[52] Augustin, *Rechten en Plichten*, 25.

they could not enjoy the lifestyle they were entitled to, Augustin concluded, it was not surprising that they loathed their jobs and left the colonial medical service as soon as they were able for the private sector or private practice.

During its first decade, the Association of Native Physicians functioned as a trade union, presenting its relatively modest demands in a reasoned, moderate manner. Board meetings took place in the outpatient department of the Batavia Medical College until a board member suggested requesting the teachers' meeting room for this purpose. This inspired extensive discussion: some members argued that it was not up to them to breach the line separating Indies and European physicians; others thought it unwise to make requests that could result in humiliation. The request was denied.[53] During these years, the Association maintained a moderate level of activity. It had about 200 members, and some twenty who were actively involved. The *Organ* was filled with reports of meetings, requests to the colonial administration, and grievances about the manifold issues that vexed members. The conditions under which Indies physicians worked slightly improved over this period, even though most of the petitions to the Governor-General went unanswered. The accomplishments of the Association's main rival, the Union of (European) Physicians, were jealously followed. All in all, the Association's activities were decidedly modest. Rather than mounting a critique of the colonial order, its members merely wanted to increase their social standing within it. Even if its demands were sometimes seen as radical by its opponents, the Association scrupulously avoided involvement in political affairs. Because Indies physicians were transferred regularly, it was difficult to sustain activity. Although the board frequently encouraged members to participate, little life was left in the Association by 1913.[54]

The Protest of the Union of (European) Physicians

In early 1913, the Batavia and Surabaya Medical Colleges (the latter about to be established) announced that they would accept students from all ethnic

---

[53] Djoehari and Asharie, 'Gewone Vergadering Gehouden op de 18e Juli 1915 in the Polikliniek Zaal der STOVIA', *Orgaan der Vereeniging van Inlandsche Geneeskundigen* 5–6, no. 6–1 (1916), 9–10. The issue was further discussed during the next meeting: Djoehari and Asharie, 'Gewone Vergadering Gehouden op de 1ste Augutus 1915 in the Polikliniek Zaal der STOVIA', *Orgaan der Vereeniging van Inlandsche Geneeskundigen* 5–6, no. 6–1 (1916), 11.

[54] Asharie, 'Stimulantia', *Orgaan der Vereeniging van Inlandsche Geneeskundigen* 4, no. 1–2 (1914), 1–5; 'Jaarverslag Betreffende den Bond van Inlandsche Geneeskundigen over 1913', *Orgaan der Vereeniging van Inlandsche Geneeskundigen* 4, no. 1–2 (1913), 19; W. J. Th. Tangkau, 'Woord van Opwekking', *Orgaan der Vereeniging van Inlandsche Geneeskundigen* 5, no. 1-2-3-4 (1915), 21–25; Abdul Hakim, 'Meditaties over Solidariteit en Broederzin Onder de Inlandsche Geneesheeren', *Orgaan der Vereeniging van Inlandsche Geneeskundigen* 5, no. 1-2-3-4 (1915), 33–35.

groups in the Indies. It provoked a vitriolic response from the Union of (European) Physicians. In a widely circulated pamphlet, the Union's board argued that Indo-Europeans and natives were unsuitable to become doctors because of their moral deficiencies. Removing obstacles for Indies physicians to enrol at Dutch universities had already disgraced those universities and been a 'slap in the face' to European physicians.[55] Permitting Indo-European and Chinese men to enrol in medical studies constituted an even greater offence, since it would mean that paupers could now become physicians. Colonial stereotypes were rehearsed: neither Indo-Europeans nor Chinese had any sense of duty, or service to humankind, or morality. They would only 'earn their bread with abortions and fill their spare time with adultery'.[56] Worse, the pamphlet suggested that these moral concerns were secondary to the main issue: the Javanese lacked the mental capacity for medical training. Opening these second-rate medical colleges to indigent students of inferior character and dismal mental ability spelled disaster: 'It is a mockery and revilement of the excellent education offered by our Dutch universities; the consequences of this measure for the public and the medical profession in the Dutch Indies are incalculable.'[57]

The pamphlet of the Union of (European) Physicians was unanimously condemned even in the more conservative European papers: 'Vile!' 'Scandalous!' 'False Diagnosis.'[58] Although most of its derogatory comments pertained to poor Indo-Europeans and the Chinese, the Union's opposition to a second medical school deeply offended Indies physicians. The Association's *Organ* simply reprinted one of the more outspoken passages from the pamphlet without commentary. In later years, Indies physicians often quoted from the pamphlet to invoke the reactionary attitudes of their European colleagues.[59] There were, however, few repercussions for the Union, and J. J. van Lonkhuijzen, the Union secretary, was appointed director of the civil medical service in 1921. Indeed, the bellicose pamphlet expressed publicly what many

---

[55] Hoofdbestuur, 'Het Indisch Ontwerp 1913', *Bond van Geneesheeren in N.-I.*, no. 52–53 (1912), 26.

[56] Hoofdbestuur, 'Indisch Ontwerp 1914', 28.

[57] Hoofdbestuur, 'Indisch Ontwerp 1914', 29.

[58] 'Infaam!', *Bataviaasch Nieuwsblad*, 7 September 1912, 1; 'Misplaatste Zelfverheffing!', *Javabode*, 9 September 1912, 1; 'Valse Diagnose', *De Locomotief*, 11 September 1912, 1; G. L. Topee, 'Rede', *Het Tijdschrift* 2, no. 4 (15 October 1912), 114–21.

[59] 'Infaam!', *Orgaan der Vereeniging van Inlandsche Geneeskundigen* 3, no. 4–5 (1912), 63–68. Abdul Rivai quoted the pamphlet in full during one of his speeches in the *Volksraad*: Abdul Rivai, 'Voorstel Betreffende de Voorbereiding der Stichting van een Universiteit in Indië, 9 Dec 1918', in *Handelingen van den Volksraad, Tweede Gewone Zitting* (Batavia: Volksraad van Nederlandsch-Indië, 1918), 571–72. The pamphlet was also cited during the first Congress of Indonesian Physicians in 1938: J. B. Sitanala, 'Beschouwt de Oosterling "Arbeid" als een "Vloek" Des Heeren?', in *Het Eerste Congress van de Vereeniging van Indonesische Geneeskundigen* (Batavia: Kenanga, 1938), 143–84.

Europeans had thought privately for years. At the first Congress on Education in the Colonies, held in The Hague in 1916, J. Boeke, professor of medicine at the University of Leiden and the founding president of the Batavia Medical School when it opened in 1927, openly expressed assimilationist sentiments:

If one aims to have indigenous individuals partake in Western civilisation, one has to guard oneself against cultivating imitation Europeans, who are hybrids without inner security and are useless both in the Netherlands and the East Indies, except in subordinate positions which would not provide them with a sufficient level of satisfaction and will not induce others to make efforts to obtain the same level of civilisation.[60]

Boeke called for an end to the cosmopolitan aspirations of Indies physicians. Natives, he argued, however educated they might be, should stay within their own cultural sphere.

Indies Physicians and Political Activism

The years between 1918 and 1921 were the most progressive the Dutch East Indies would ever experience. During the war years, communication between the Netherlands and its colonies was disrupted and the colonial administration had to act more or less independently.[61] Governor-General J. P. Count van Limburg Stirum, determined to realise the ideals of the Ethical Policy, was sympathetic to the demands of the nationalist movement.[62] In May 1918 the Volksraad commenced proceedings and a semblance of democracy appeared in the colonies. Van Limburg Stirum had appointed Tjipto Mangoenkoesoemo and other fierce critics of the colonial administration to the Volksraad; Abdul Rivai and Radjiman were elected. The presence of three Indies physicians in the Volksraad provided an unprecedented opportunity for native doctors to present their grievances. During the Volksraad's opening weeks, when members presented their ideas and perspectives, Rivai and Tjipto gave eloquent speeches full of optimism about the future and scathing about the past record of the colonial administration. Rivai harshly criticised the lack of educational opportunities for the great majority of the indigenous population.[63] Tjipto hailed the Governor-General's promises to eradicate racial differentiation in colonial

[60] J. Boeke, 'Prae-Advies', in *Prae-Adviezen van het Eerste Koloniaal Onderwijscongres* (The Hague: Korthals, 1916), 79.
[61] Kees van Dijk, *The Netherlands Indies and the Great War, 1914–1918* (Leiden: KITLV Press, 2007).
[62] For a biography of Governor-General van Limburg Stirum, see Bob de Graaff and Elsbeth Locher-Scholten, *J. P. Graaf van Limburg Stirum, 1873–1948: Tegendraads Landvoogd en Diplomaat* (Zwolle: Waanders, 2007).
[63] Abdul Rivai, 'Algemeene Beschouwingen, 19 Juni 1918', in *Handelingen van den Volksraad, Eerste Gewone Zitting* (Batavia: Volksraad van Nederlandsch-Indië, 1918), 136–40.

life.[64] Even the moderate and at times conservative Radjiman spoke of the abject poverty of the indigenous population, and the difficulty of access to education and medical care.[65]

In November 1918, a few days after the cessation of hostilities in Europe, revolutionary fervour swept the continent, alarming many colonial Dutchmen. The three physicians in the Volksraad became even more outspoken. Tjipto argued that the colonial administration had never been serious about the Ethical Policy.[66] Radjiman protested that colonial bureaucrats frequently abused their powers.[67] To prevent revolutionary agitation, van Limburg Stirum promised far-reaching reforms in colonial governance.[68] His statements, later named the November promises, encouraged nationalist leaders to express their demands still more forcefully. In the meantime, international shipping had resumed and demand for Indies exports rose dramatically, creating high revenues. This made reforms seem viable. The numerous small strikes protesting stagnant wages in the face of high post-war inflation were mostly settled amicably through mediation.[69]

The Association of Native Physicians also became more outspoken. It was sufficiently emboldened to address political issues not immediately related to the interests of its members. It became more visible in public life and was represented on various official committees dealing with health and medical care.[70] In 1919, Christian Ambonese physician Jeremias Kaijadoe became the Association's president, which renamed itself the Association of Indies Physicians [Vereeniging van Indische Artsen; the acronym remained VIG]. Kaijadoe had graduated from the Batavia Medical College in 1909 and had worked in remote Kalimantan combatting cholera. He had left the employ of the colonial administration as soon as he was allowed to and accepted a position with an oil company in another remote area, which was also not to his

[64] Tjipto Mangoenkoesoemo, 'Algemeene Beschouwingen, 19 Juni 1918', in *Handelingen van den Volksraad, Eerste Gewone Zitting* (Batavia: Volksraad van Nederlandsch-Indië, 1918), 124–30.

[65] Radjiman, 'Algemeene Beschouwingen, 19 Juni 1918', in *Handelingen van den Volksraad, Eerste Gewone Zitting* (Batavia: Volksraad van Nederlandsch-Indië, 1918), 153–58.

[66] Tjipto Mangoenkoesoemo, 'Algemeene Beschouwingen, 14 November 1918', in *Handelingen van den Volksraad, Tweede Gewone Zitting* (Batavia: Volksraad van Nederlandsch-Indië, 1918), 159–70.

[67] Radjiman, 'Algemeene Beschouwingen, 14 November 1918', in *Handelingen van den Volksraad, Tweede Gewone Zitting* (Batavia: Volksraad van Nederlandsch-Indië, 1918), 170–75.

[68] The declaration of the Governor-General was transmitted to the members of the People's Council by the government representative. See D. Talma, 'Regeeringsverklaring, 18 November 1918', in *Handelingen van den Volksraad, Tweede Gewone Zitting* (Batavia: Volksraad van Nederlandsch-Indië, 1918), 251–52.

[69] John Ingleson, *In Search of Justice: Workers and Unions in Colonial Java, 1908–1926* (Singapore: Oxford University Press, 1986), 94–149.

[70] J. Kaijadoe, 'Uit Roerige Jaren', in *Jubileumnummer 1911–1936* (Batavia: G. Kolff, 1937), 6–13.

liking either.[71] In 1918 he established a successful private practice in Batavia and soon became involved in various political associations.

Kaijadoe's nationalism proved much more outspoken than that of Tehupeiory. He was not convinced that the special status of the Moluccan islands (and the Minahasa) had resulted in real advancement. The Ambonese, suggested Kaijadoe, had been like

Mopie or Fidel, an excellent and watchful house pet, that plays, goes out, romps with the boss, the wife and the children, that now and then gets a titbit, a ribbon, a beautiful little chain around the neck, but however loyal and watchful he remains a house pet, is never taken up into the family.[72]

In 1920, Kaijadoe helped found the Ambonese Association [Sarekat Ambon], which advocated a closer association with other ethnic groups in the Indies, more education, and a greater voice in colonial affairs, but not independence. Its members were disappointed with the minor gains the Ambonese had made through their close association with their colonial overlords, and opted to relinquish their special status in the colonies. Although the Sarekat Ambon was hardly radical, its activities were closely followed by the secret police, which recorded Kaijadoe's more outspoken statements.[73] Kaijadoe had broad political interests. In 1925, he was elected to Batavia's city council and advocated sanitation and public health programs.

After 1918, the *Organ*'s tentative and cautious tone disappeared. Soetomo, for example, pointed out that Indies physicians were often transferred when wealthy European and Chinese families settled in their area to make room for a European colleague eager to supplement his income.[74] He also argued that Indies physicians had a central role in increasing the 'physical power of the population needed to attain greater welfare'.[75] Referring to the involvement of medical students in the national awakening of the Indies, Augustin hoped

---

[71] J. Kaijadoe, 'Enkele Medische Problemen Hier te Lande', in *Het Eerste Congres van de Vereeniging van Indonesische Geneeskundigen* (Batavia: Kenanga, 1938), 21–22; J. Kaijadoe, 'Waarschuwing', *Orgaan der Vereeniging van Inlandsche Geneeskundigen* 5–6, no. 6–1 (1916), 27–28.

[72] J. Kaijadoe in the Ambonese journal *Mena Moeria* in 1922. Quoted and translated by Chauvel, *Nationalists, Soldiers and Separatists*, 77.

[73] J. Kaijadoe's brother Erasmus Augustinus Kaijadoe was a member of the Volksraad. Their political views diverged on several important points. For the reports of the Indies secret police on the activities of the Sarekat Ambon, see Ch.F. van Fraassen and P. Jobse, eds., *Bronnen Betreffende de Midden-Molukken 1900–1942*, 4 vols. (The Hague: Instituut voor Nederlandse Geschiedenis, 1997). For an overview of Ambonese initiatives and the activities of several physicians within them (among them Tehupeiory, Kaijadoe, Westplat, and Apituley), see Chauvel, *Nationalists, Soldiers and Separatists*.

[74] Soetomo, 'Mijn Standpunt, I', *Orgaan der Vereeniging van Indische Geneeskundigen* 8, no. 1–2 (1918), 2–3.

[75] Soetomo, 'Mijn Standpunt, II', *Orgaan der Vereeniging van Indische Geneeskundigen* 8, no. 1–2 (1918), 6–8.

that the Volksraad's medical members would represent the interests of Indies physicians forcefully.[76] In 1918, the Association participated in a meeting protesting the stringent franchise requirements for Volksraad elections, which included the ability to speak Dutch and an annual salary which most natives could only dream of.[77] The Association branched out from health and medicine to wider concerns, and in 1923 the *Organ* reported that 'important issues, both politically and socially, whether or not they touched the direct interests of the Association, have had the full interest of the board.'[78]

The colonial administration's forbearance did not last. In 1919 several strikes were forcefully suppressed, and the administration stopped responding to the demands of the indigenous members of the Volksraad. In September, the military shot a farmer near Garut after he refused to sell his grain below market rates to the administration. Conservative politicians claimed that he had been inspired by a clandestine Communist branch of the Islamic Union [Sarekat Islam], at that time the largest political party in the Indies. Most Dutchmen concluded that the colonial state was under threat and that the administration had to take a more severe stance towards the nationalist movement. The relationship between the Association of Indies Physicians and the colonial administration became increasingly fraught. Rivai successfully presented a motion to the Volksraad to increase the salaries of Indies physicians but it was twice put aside by the minister of colonies.[79] Despite its lauded status as the harbinger of democracy in the colonies, the Volksraad's recommendations were often ignored.

Years of campaigning to improve the professional status of Indies physicians had produced negligible results. In October 1919 members of the Association of Indies Physicians demanded 'forceful action'.[80] A physicians' strike was proposed, but rejected, because it would affect patients adversely.[81] A second bold proposal was accepted: all Indies physicians in the employ of the civil medical service would tender their resignation. A resistance fund was

---

[76] P. L. Augustin, 'De Oud-Leerlingen van de STOVIA en de Volksraad', *Orgaan der Vereeniging van Indische Geneeskundigen* 8, no. 1–2 (1918), 9–12.

[77] 'Vergadering van de Vereeniging van Ind. Geneeskundigen Gehouden den 27en Januari 1918', *Orgaan der Vereeniging van Indische Geneeskundigen* 8, no. 1–2 (1918), 15; 'Protestmeeting Decapark', *Bataviaasch Nieuwsblad*, 18 February 1918, 2–3.

[78] 'Mededeelingen van de Redactie', *Orgaan der Vereeniging van Indische Geneeskundigen* 12, no. 1 (1923), 1.

[79] 'Teleurgestelde Indische Artsen', *Het Nieuws van den Dag voor Nederlandsch-Indië*, 29 May 1919, Section II, 1.

[80] 'Ontevreden Indische Artsen', *Het Nieuws van den Dag voor Nederlandsch-Indië*, 28 October 1919, Section IV, 1.

[81] Physicians have not often gone on strike. A famous example is the Saskatchewan physicians' strike; see Robin F. Badgley and Samuel M. Wolfe, *Doctors Strike: Medical Care and Conflict in Saskatchewan* (New York: Atherton, 1967).

established and quickly raised a considerable sum. In November, the board instructed the Surabaya branch to organise a protest at a large convention of the Sarekat Islam, several small political parties, and a number of trade unions.[82] The Sarekat Islam had at that time close to a million members and its president, H. O. S. Tjokroaminoto, was a member of the Volksraad.[83] Abdul Moeis, a former STOVIA student and also a Volksraad member, was a board member and editor of its newspaper, *The Young Generation* [*Kaum Moeda*]. Communists were seeking to radicalise the organisation.

On the final evening of the convention, the Surabaya branch of the Association invited representatives of the participating political parties to a lavish dinner. Afterwards, in a series of speeches, all delegates declared their support for a physicians' protest action.[84] Representatives of the Association assured guests that their action would not affect patients in any way – its members would continue to care for the ill. On Sunday morning, the convention hall was crowded. Several political leaders were seated on the podium: Tjokroaminoto, members of the board of the Sarekat Islam, former STOVIA student Soewardi Soerjaningrat with other members of the board of the Sarekat Hindia (a moderate version of the former Indies Party), and three members of the Surabaya branch of the Association of Indies Physicians. In the front rows of the audience, a group of Indies physicians was seated next to Dr L. S. A. M. von Römer, inspector for East Java of the civil medical service. J. A. Latumeten, Tehupeiory's brother-in-law and a young Christian Ambonese Indies physician working at the mental asylum at Lawang near Surabaya, rose and spoke of the contempt in which the colonial administration held Indies physicians and the indigenous population as a whole – the same contempt seen in the 1912 Union of (European) Physicians pamphlet. The strike would go ahead, and if the Indies physicians were prevented from private practice after their collective resignation, 'they would establish themselves as traditional healers [*dukun*]!

---

[82] 'Ontevreden Indische Artsen, II', *Het Nieuws van den Dag voor Nederlandsch-Indië*, 28 October 1919 Section II, 2.

[83] On the Sarekat Islam, see A. P. E. Korver, *Sarekat Islam, 1912–1916: Opkomst, Bloei en Structuur van Indonesië's Eerste Massabeweging* (Amsterdam: Historisch Seminarium, Universiteit van Amsterdam, 1982). For the relationship between Islam and politics in the Indies more generally, see Michael F. Laffan, *Islamic Nationhood and Colonial Indonesia: The Umma below the Winds* (London: Routledge, 2007).

[84] Present were representatives of the Islamic Union [Sarekat Islam], the Sarekat Hindia (a reincarnation of Douwes Dekker's Indies Party, also led by him), Boedi Oetomo, the Minahasa Association [Perserikatan Minahassa], the Ambonese Study Fund [Ambonsch Studiefonds], Djowo Dipo (a group advocating the simplification of Javanese, in particular the elimination of the various registers indicating social class), a federation of labour unions in the process of organising (Vakcentrale), and the Union of Native Civil Servants [Inlandsche Ambtenarenbond]. See 'Een Feestmaaltijd', *Bataviaasch Nieuwsblad*, 3 November 1919, 1; 'De Indische Artsen', *Het Nieuws van de Dag in Nederlandsch-Indie*, 3 November 1919, Section II, 4.

They do not need permits!'[85] Latumeten's speech was followed by thunderous applause.

Soewardi also rose to speak, welcoming the Association's protest as an example of the vigorous activity of indigenous unions. The poor treatment of Indies physicians stemmed from the racial discrimination fundamental to colonial life – it was deeply offensive, for instance, that European nurses earned more than Indies physicians. In the colonial dialectic between rulers and ruled, Indies physicians were lumped with indigenous clerks, tram conductors, and plantation workers.[86] Von Römer, an energetic high official of the civil medical service nicknamed 'the Napoleon of medicine', grew increasingly vexed.[87] When he tried to address the audience, he was heckled with demands to speak Malay. Von Römer continued, in Dutch, by arguing that the salaries of Indies physicians were already slated to increase, and that the Association had already been informed. Physicians could never be mere labourers because they followed a higher calling to serve humankind, and, finally, it was unfathomable that the Association had sought the cooperation of a radical group like the Islamic Union.[88] Von Römer failed to sway the audience. The final word was given to Tjokroaminoto, the charismatic leader of the Sarekat Islam, who declared that while his heart did not ache for the Indies physicians, he vehemently opposed the racial policies of the colonial administration.[89] A motion in support of the physicians' action passed unanimously.

The motion divided the Volksraad. A conservative administrative official noted curtly that it was simply further evidence of the radicalisation of the Sarekat Islam.[90] Tjipto defended the proposed actions with impressive verve, expounding on the significance of Indies physicians for the nationalist movement and invoking the founding of Boedi Oetomo and the leading roles Indies physicians had played in colonial politics (including himself and Soewardi Soerjaningrat). Enlisting the assistance of political associations, he argued, was a natural and important step: 'history itself prescribed to Indies physicians the road they have now chosen to

---

[85] J. A. Latumeten, quoted in Adviseur voor Inlandsche Zaken [G. A. J. Hazeu], *Sarekat Islam Congres (4e Nationale Congres), 26 Oct–2 Nov. 1919, Soerabaja* (Batavia: Landsdrukkerij, 1919), 43. The events during the congress of the Islamic Union were reported extensively in the press. Hazeu's report is the most comprehensive one. See also 'Het S. I. Congres', *Nieuws van den dag voor Nederlandsch Indië,* 3 November 1919, Section II, 1–2.

[86] Soewardi Soerjaningrat, quoted in Adviseur voor Inlandsche Zaken [G. A. J. Hazeu], *Sarekat Islam 4e Congres,* 44.

[87] Adviseur voor Inlandsche Zaken [G. A. J. Hazeu], *Sarekat Islam 4e Congres,* 44.

[88] L. S. A. M. von Römer, quoted in Adviseur voor Inlandsche Zaken [G. A. J. Hazeu], *Sarekat Islam 4ᵉ Congres,* 44–45.

[89] Tjokroaminoto, quoted in Adviseur voor Inlandsche Zaken [G. A. J. Hazeu], *Sarekat Islam 4e Congres,* 45.

[90] M. B. van der Jagt, 'Algemeene Beschouwingen, 22 November 1919', in *Handelingen van den Volksraad, Tweede Gewone Zitting* (Batavia: Volksraad van Nederlandsch-Indië, 1919), 94–95.

take.'[91] There were two reasons, continued Tjipto, why Indies physicians occupied an exceptional position in the indigenous world. Their education, first, meant that they experienced the injustices of colonial society acutely: 'because of his intellectual development, he vividly feels the burdens of the life of a dominated people.'[92] Second, the indigenous population followed their plight with great interest: 'the capacities of the indigenous population as a whole were measured by appraising Indies physicians' who had been permitted to 'drink from the cup containing the holy bread [*manna*] called Western science'.[93] Tjipto was sceptical about the speed with which the new salary scales were being implemented, and proposed several amendments.[94]

In the weeks following the Sarekat Islam convention, members of the Association of Indies Physicians continued to be active. The resistance fund continued to grow.[95] Several branches supported the proposed strike action and promised to assist physicians who lost their jobs.[96] A well-attended meeting in Batavia expressed full support.[97] Then, in the second week of November, the colonial administration unexpectedly inundated the members of the Volksraad with numerous new proposals regarding the 1920 budget, the proposed regency councils, and the principles of a new remuneration system.[98] Among the many proposals were significant salary increases for Indies physicians. The administration planned to implement these increases retroactively, from 1904, providing senior Indies physicians with a significant and unexpected financial windfall. It was a transparent attempt to appease them, and it succeeded. The Association lost its appetite for political action, and the board reverted to polite requests to the colonial administration for details of proposals and suggesting amendments on matters from the size of annual increments and their spacing, rent indemnity, reimbursement for travel expenses, and so on.[99]

---

[91] Tjipto Mangoenkoesoemo, 'Rede, Algemeene Aanvullingsbegrooting voor het Dienstjaar 1919', in *Handelingen van den Volksraad, Tweede Gewone Zitting* (Batavia: Volksraad van Nederlandsch-Indië, 1919), 319.

[92] Mangoenkoesoemo, 'Voordracht', 99.

[93] Mangoenkoesoemo, 'Voordracht', 99.

[94] Mangoenkoesoemo, 'Rede', 489–90.

[95] 'De Indische Artsen, II', *Het Nieuws van den Dag voor Nederlandsch-Indië*, 11 November 1919, Section II, 2.

[96] 'De Actie der Indische Artsen', *Het Nieuws van den Dag voor Nederlandsch Indië*, 17 November 1919, 3.

[97] 'Actie Ind. Artsen', *Het Nieuws van den Dag voor Nederlandsch Indië*, 19 November 1919, 2.

[98] 'Bij Overrompeling', *Bataviaasch Nieuwsblad*, 22 November 1919, 1.

[99] Several papers emphasised that the action had been entirely unnecessary since these improvements had been conveyed to the board of the Association of Indies Physicians in June. It is likely that the board of the Association did not trust the promises of the colonial administration and therefore organised the protest. See 'De Actie der Indische Artsen', *Het Nieuws van den Dag voor Nederlandsch Indië*, 14 November 1919, Section II, 1; 'De Positie-Regeling der Indische Artsen', *Bataviaasch Nieuwsblad*, 21 November 1919, 1. See also 'Actie der Indische Artsen', *Het Nieuws van den Dag voor Nederlandsch Indië*, 29 December 1919, 2.

Even though the Association of Indies Physicians had been successful in raising its members' salaries, its public image was in tatters. Its actions were widely criticised in the European press, and declared frivolous. The proposed physicians' strike had, nevertheless, stimulated members' interest in political action. In 1923, Kaijadoe suggested that the Association should become a member of the Radical Concentration [Radicale Concentratie], a group of political parties critical of the colonial administration. He was convinced that union activity, including that of the Association, was 'not conceivable without political action at its roots'.[100] Soetomo declared that Indies physicians could not be expected to remain loyal to the colonial administration unconditionally.[101] Protests against low remuneration and poor working conditions continued. The *Organ* reprinted a highly critical address by Rivai to the Volksraad complaining of that body's ineffectiveness. The Association passed a motion supporting Rivai's disapproval, and appointed him as its official representative in the Volksraad.[102] When the colonial administration finally tabled the administrative reforms promised in November 1918, they had been dramatically revised and acted to severely curtail the already limited powers of the Volksraad.

Conclusion

The central position of Indies physicians in debates about the Ethical Policy and the nature of the Dutch colonial project in the Indies made their profession a symbolic index of the successes and failures of the Policy. For indigenous populations, conservative Europeans, and progressive Europeans, the shifting social status of Indies physicians represented the quality and progress of the colonial administration's long-promised reforms. Indies physicians themselves interpreted their success by the concrete outcomes for their profession. Bahder Djohan, the tireless organiser of student life at the Batavia Medical College, reflected on their struggles late in his life:

As a homogeneous group of intellectuals, Indonesian physicians dealt head-on with colonial society. Several of them had to face ridicule and contempt, not only in official matters, but also in everyday life, as Indonesians were considered second-class people.

---

[100] Marzoeki, 'Notulen van de Ledenvergadering, Gehouden in de Conferentiekamer van het Nieuwe Stoviagebouw, Salemba, op 19 Nov 1922', *Orgaan der Vereeniging van Indische Geneeskundigen* 12, no. 1 (1923), 8.

[101] R. Soetomo, 'Ter Overweging', *Orgaan der Vereeniging van Indische Geneeskundigen* 12, no. 1 (1923), 11–12.

[102] Abdul Rivai, 'Rede over het "Kostbaar Geschenk"', *Orgaan der Vereeniging van Indische Geneeskundigen* 12, no. 2 (1923), 19–26; the original speech appeared as Abdul Rivai, 'Rede over het "Kostbaar Geschenk", 10 November 1922', in *Handelingen van den Volksraad, Tweede Gewone Zitting* (Batavia: Volksraad van Nederlandsch Indië, 1922), 8–15.

It stands to reason that Indonesian physicians as major intellectual exponents [among their people] were subject to and had to fend off attacks.[103]

According to leading Indonesian historian Taufik Abdullah, the Indonesian nationalist movement did not originate with the founding of Boedi Oetomo, nor with the moment the *Bintang Hindia* commenced publication. It 'was set in motion when the small number of educated "natives", the colonized people, began to reflect on their places in the plural society of the colonial towns'.[104] Because of their ambiguous, contested, and sometimes paradoxical social position, Indies physicians reflected obsessively on their place in colonial society. Their reflections hardened into grievances, which fuelled their professional and political initiatives.

In the history of medicine, it is not difficult to find instances in which medical theories have been employed to mark difference, inscribing it in race, constitution, physiology, brain configuration, or genetic inheritance, mediated, or not, by climate, nutrition, disease, or culture. Biologists and physical anthropologists did likewise, with their own disciplinary vocabulary. A number of cultural anthropologists and sociologists, however, have analysed the pervasive influence of culture, social organisation, and ritual to account for the differences between Western and primitive society. Kohlbrugge offered an unusual blend of psychiatric diagnosis, psychological theory, mental analysis, and cultural anthropology to explain the backwardness of the archipelago's population, and on this basis advocated association rather than integration and assimilation. Indies physicians used their status as members of the cosmopolitan medical profession to erase the assumed differences between themselves and their European colleagues and, by implication, between the Europeans and indigenous populations. To this end they deployed the universalism inherent in science and medicine, and the egalitarianism of the medical profession, which tends to discount ethnic distinctions amongst practitioners and favour skill, training, and accomplishment as differentiators. By conducting medical research and publishing the fruits of their investigations, Indies physicians demonstrated their commitment to rationality and objectivity, and by implication, their capacity to restrain emotion and subjectivity. By doing so they worked against the assumptions of primitivism and emotionalism which permeated colonial discourse. Their links with the global medical profession enabled them to criticise such racial distinctions as contingent, historical, and, indeed, irrational.

---

[103] Bahder Djohan, 'Segi-Segi Sosial Politik dalam Perkembangan Dunia Kedoktoran Indonesia', in *125 Tahun Pendidikan Dokter di Indonesia 1851–1976*, ed. M. A. Hanafiah, Bahder Djohan, and Surono (Jakarta: FKUI, 1976), 80.

[104] Taufik Abdullah, *Indonesia: Towards Democracy* (Singapore: Institute of Southeast Asian Studies, 2009), 4.

5   The Insults of Colonial Psychiatry and the Psychological Damage of Colonialism

After the heady months following the November promises of Governor-General van Limburg Stirum, which constituted the high point of the Ethical Policy, the conservative forces in the Dutch East Indies organised and gained in strength. Many colonial Dutchmen viewed the increasingly vocal and restive nationalist movement with mounting apprehension. After a short economic boom following the end of World War I, an international recession commenced and the colonial budget recorded growing deficits. With the appointment of conservative politician Dirk Fock as Governor-General in 1921, it was clear that the tide had turned. His rule, which lasted until 1926, prioritised law and order, strict budgetary measures, and curbing the nationalist movement. Strikes were brutally repressed, thousands of workers were fired, and several nationalist leaders were exiled.[1] In reaction, indigenous political leaders launched a policy of non-cooperation, refusing to participate in the quasi-democratic institutions of the colonial state and establishing banks, clinics, and shops for the indigenous population instead of waiting for the colonial state to do so. Rather than engaging in strikes and protest actions, they focused on educating and preparing nationalist cadres, and building the infrastructure of the future independent state. Nationalists now preferred preparation to political agitation. Fock's repressive policies fuelled the political career of a young nationalist named Sukarno, who would become the first president of independent Indonesia.

Advocates of the Ethical Policy had characterised the indigenous population as children: smart, eager to learn, even precocious, and intent on developing their society along a trajectory which followed the Dutch example. Although children could be hard to comprehend and difficult to deal with, they were family, and would eventually mature.[2] Very different images of the indigenous

---

[1] John Ingleson, *In Search of Justice: Workers and Unions in Colonial Java, 1908–1926* (Singapore: Oxford University Press, 1986), 210–65. An interesting portrait of Fock is given in D. M. G. Koch, *Batig Slot: Figuren uit het Oude Indië* (Amsterdam: De Brug/Djambatan, 1960), 27–34.

[2] For an incisive analysis of family metaphors used in describing the relationship between colonisers and colonised in the Dutch East Indies, see Frances Gouda, 'Good Mothers, Medeas, or Jezebels: Feminine Imagery in Colonial and Anticolonial Rhetoric in the Dutch East Indies,

population came to dominate Dutch colonial discussions during the 1920s. The natives were now seen as difficult and disruptive adolescents who bore the semblance of Europeans – of adults – but who were, at the core, impulsive and egotistical children with rudimentary intellectual capacities and negligible moral sensitivities. When two Dutch colonial psychiatrists presented medical theories that reinforced these opinions, their views were welcomed by colonial Dutchmen. Indies physicians were understandably outraged. In reaction to the changed political climate, the Association of Indies Physicians transformed itself from a physicians' union into an organisation promoting medical research. This change also reflected the influence of the growing elite among Indies physicians comprising Indonesian doctors with European medical degrees.

Colonial Psychiatry and Theories on the Nature of the Native Mind

The members of the Volksraad were either elected or formally appointed for three-year terms. Between 1918 and 1921, members included outspoken advocates of the Ethical Policy and several radical indigenous politicians. Conservative voices had ignored the Volksraad elections of 1918 because they doubted that it would exert any influence, but when it proved to offer a platform for radical, even revolutionary opinions, they established several political parties in anticipation of the 1921 elections. The Political-Economic Association [Politiek-Economischen Bond] (PEB) and the Indo-European Association [Indo-Europeesch Verbond] (IEV) were the most prominent. The reactionary and rhetorically gifted Surabaya-based Indo-European lawyer Arnold van Gennep, representative of the PEB, became one of the most influential representatives of the new conservatism in colonial politics. Van Gennep was closely associated with the sugar syndicate, the organisation representing the interests of the owners of sugar factories. He was fond of using Ethical ideals to cloak his deeply conservative proposals, which infuriated the indigenous members of the Volksraad and enraged their progressive European colleagues.[3] The inauguration of Fock as Governor-General in March 1921 and the opening of the new Volksraad two months later signalled the death of the Ethical Policy, and an era of colonial conservatism commenced.

1900–1942', in *Domesticating the Empire: Race, Gender, and Family Life in French and Dutch Colonialism*, ed. Julia Clancy-Smith and Frances Gouda (Charlottesville: University Press of Virginia, 1998), 236–54.

[3] Van Gennep regularly quoted from his 'Verplichte Rechtsbijstand in Civiele Zaken bij de Landraden en Residentiegerechten op Java en Madoera in Verband met Deunificatie van Recht', *Indisch Genootschap*, 27 December 1910, 59–112.

During the first two sitting months, the members of the new Volksraad presented their views in their opening speeches. Several indigenous members attacked a PEB proposal to establish a committee 'to conduct scientific research on the nature of the native'.[4] Its insights would further guide the further development of the indigenous population by strengthening its morality, intellect, and other capacities required for participating in the colonial economy and in civil society. Rivai was deeply suspicious of this proposal, since the PEB bluntly favoured business interests, advocating free competition, low taxation, and the strengthening of law and order; it opposed unions, rejected increasing the political rights of indigenous individuals, and favoured reduced spending on initiatives that would benefit them. In his opening speech, Rivai argued that this scientific committee would merely provide 'a theoretical justification through PEB psychology and sociology for the exploitation of the Indonesian population'.[5] Regent Achmad Djajadiningrat, an erudite Javanese member of the Volksraad, said that investigating the indigenous population would mean studying its language, religion, literature, art, morals, and culture, and that a committee was unnecessary because 'we can provide everything that is required.'[6] Despite his kind offer, it was clear that the PEB delegates and other conservative Dutchmen would value the results of the scientific research of the proposed scientific committee more highly than the informed opinions of educated Indonesians.

Two days later, Arnold van Gennep gave his maiden speech and revealed that the maligned proposal was his. The scientific committee he envisioned would, he argued, provide the insights necessary for the successful implementation of the Ethical Policy.[7] He continued by characterising Java's *adat* as primitive and poorly suited to the modern world, Javanese art as primitive and underdeveloped, and Javanese religion as superficial and amoral. Van Gennep referred to the writings of colonial psychiatrist P. H. M. Travaglino, superintendent of the Lawang mental hospital near Surabaya, for impartial, scientific insights into the nature of the Javanese. Travaglino thought natives were poorly evolved, 'very emotional, highly imaginative, and strikingly childish and infantile, unduly pleasure-loving, and morbidly egoistic'.[8] Importantly, van Gennep did not cite Travaglino's publications in scientific or medical

---

[4] 'Wetenschappelijke Grondslag eener Ontwikkelingspolitiek', in *Handelingen van den Volksraad* (Batavia: Landsdrukkerij, 1921), Onderdeel 1, Afdeeling 1, stuk 6, 12.
[5] Abdul Rivai, 'Rede, 13 June 1921', in *Handelingen van de Volksraad, Eerste Gewone Zitting* (Batavia: Landsdrukkerij, 1921), 32.
[6] R. Achmad A. A. Djajadiningrat, 'Rede, 13 June 1921', in *Handelingen van de Volksraad, Eerste Gewone Zitting* (Batavia: Landsdrukkerij, 1921), 61.
[7] Arnold van Gennep, 'Voordracht, 15 June 1921', in *Handelingen van den Volksraad, Eerste Gewone Zitting* (Batavia: Landsdrukkerij, 1921), 133–42.
[8] Van Gennep, 'Voordracht', 138–39.

journals, but an article he had published in the *PEB Magazine*.[9] Travaglino was obviously aware of the political purchase of his ideas, and van Gennep saw it too. When Kohlbrugge had advocated the benefits of a psychological colonial politics in 1907 he had been ignored.[10] Society had changed by the 1920s. Psychological and psychiatric perspectives on colonial governance were becoming increasingly common and colonial psychiatrists found a receptive audience for their professional views.

Van Gennep's speech was a clear indication that the political tide in the Indies had turned – 'the reaction' was becoming increasingly influential – but in 1921, Van Gennep's views were still too extreme for most. Even the founder and chairman of the PEB, who had hoped to reconcile the different ethnic groups in the Indies, quickly announced that the PEB neither shared nor supported his ideas.[11] Newspaper editors, social commentators, and many members of the Volksraad were outraged by van Gennep's 'racial speech'.[12] In a highly unusual move, the Governor-General expressed his disapproval: his representative relayed, in typical understated fashion, that speeches like these increased distrust between Europeans and natives by assuming the former's racial superiority.[13] Van Gennep's cantankerous nature precluded his nomination for the Volksraad elections in 1924, even though his views on the childlike and overly emotional nature of the indigenous population were by then widely accepted. In December 1923 and February 1924, two colonial psychiatrists, Travaglino and F. H. van Loon, expressed views similar to van Gennep's in public speeches; a psychological colonial policy no longer seemed outlandish. Unlike the silence following the publication of Kohlbrugge's articles in 1907, these lectures provoked outspoken reactions from progressive forces. Indies physicians were acutely aware of the political implications of these views and disputed them vigorously by deconstructing their theories.

---

[9] P. H. M. Travaglino, 'Het Karakter van den Inlander', *PEB* 5, no. 27, 28 (1920), 343–47, 357–60.

[10] J. H. F. Kohlbrugge, *Blikken in het Zieleleven van den Javaan en Zijner Overheerschers* (Leiden: Brill, 1907); 'Psychologische Koloniale Politiek', *Vereeniging Moederland en Koloniën* 8, no. 2 (1907), 1–44; 'Zielkunde als Grondslag van Koloniaal Beleid', *Militaire Gids* 27 (1908), 229–51.

[11] A. J. N. Engelenberg, 'Voordracht, 15 June 1921', in *Handelingen van den Volksraad, Eerste Gewone Zitting* (Batavia: Landsdrukkerij, 1921), 133.

[12] C. G. Cramer, for example, stated that van Gennep's address 'has unleashed a storm of outrage'. The phrase 'racial speech' [*rassenrede*] was first used by A. Salim (*Handelingen van den Volksraad, Eerste Gewone Zitting* [Batavia: Landsdrukkerij, 1921], 397, 402) and repeatedly used by others after that.

[13] W. Muurling, 'Voordracht door de Regeeringsgemachtigde voor Algemeene Zaken, 22 June 1921', in *Handelingen van den Volksraad, Eerste Gewone Zitting* (Batavia: Landsdrukkerij, 1921), 320. With the phrase 'racial conceit [*rassenwaan*]', Muurling was referring to Thomas Karsten, 'Rassenwaan en Rassenbewustzijn', *De Taak* 1, no. 18 (1 December 1917), 205–06.

Travaglino's Psychological Colonial Politics

In December 1923, van Gennep, in his position as chairman of the Surabaya branch of the PEB, introduced a lecture by Travaglino on politics and psychology at a branch meeting.[14] Travaglino, a gifted and entertaining speaker, began by stating that it was necessary for governments to have a thorough understanding of the mind of the people they governed.[15] The effort to outlaw prostitution in several Dutch cities and Prohibition in the United States had been decisive failures, he continued, because neither had taken the population's psychological characteristics into account. Governing effectively and justly required scientific insight into the mentality of the governed. The increased political turbulence in the Indies indicated that a psychological colonial policy was urgently needed. Travaglino said that the psychoses of his native patients were strongly emotional in nature, and that the incidence of this type of psychosis was seven to ten times higher in the Indies than in Europe.[16] These psychoses were generally preceded by emotionally jarring events and were accompanied by highly charged emotional expressions. Assuming that emotional individuals suffered from emotional psychoses, Travaglino concluded that natives were highly emotional.

Travaglino went on to discuss the active imagination of natives, evident in the games village children played, the improvised dancing during *gamelan* playing, and the elaborate confabulations of servants caught out telling white lies or engaging in petty theft. European fairy tales featured dragons with two or three heads; dragons in Eastern sagas had a hundred heads, even a thousand. A powerful imagination and a strong emotionality were, argued Travaglino, indicative of the infantile nature of the native mind; instinct and emotion prevailed over reasoning and planning, and moral functions were undeveloped, if not entirely absent. Natives were driven by strong vital functions and sensual pleasure, and were consequently highly egocentric, which was why they could pay close and enduring attention to matters that were of interest to them while ignoring everything else. Natives were fully absorbed, for instance, by *gamelan* music, shadow puppet shows, and ox races. Once, said Travaglino, when he was driving his car and wanted to pass a group watching a parade, he found it impossible to gain their attention. On another occasion a group watching a *wayang kulit* performance failed to notice him and a noisy hunting party. In

---

[14] P. H. M. Travaglino, 'Politiek en Psychologie', *PEB*, 21 February 1924, 86–93.

[15] Travaglino, 'Politiek en Psychologie', 87.

[16] Travaglino had reported these ideas in medical publications: P. H. M. Travaglino, 'De Psychose van den Inlander in Verband met zijn Karakter', *Geneeskundig Tijdschrift voor Nederlands Indië* 60 (1920), 99–111; 'De Sociale Beteekenis der Schizophrenie voor de Inlandsche Samenleving', *Mededeelingen van den Dienst der Volksgezondheid in Nederlandsch-Indië* (1925), 125–31; 'De Schizophrenie en de Javaanse Psyche', *Psychiatrische en Neurologische Bladen* 31 (1927), 416–25.

both cases it was in the interest of the locals to pay attention and to make way. Proponents of the Ethical Policy had assumed mental isomorphism: native and Western minds were essentially alike; differences between them could be explained by referring to various external factors, the effect of which could be overcome by progressive colonial governance. Travaglino instead advocated a mental polymorphism: native and Western minds were essentially different. In order to be effective, colonial governance had to take these differences into account.

The obvious conclusion for Travaglino was that the indigenous population of the Indies remained in a primitive evolutionary phase, and this had significant implications for colonial governance. Political opportunists could easily mislead audiences because native minds were imaginative and suggestible, which meant that protective measures including censorship and jailing political agitators were justified. Trade schools and agricultural programs were preferable to Western-style education, which, he argued, was incompatible with the Javanese mind. The colonial administration could best stimulate the development of the indigenous population by maintaining law and order, and by guiding it with a strong paternal hand. Nearing the end of his lecture, Travaglino added a caveat: Eastern culture was neither inferior nor superior to Western culture, only different, as men and women were different. There was no reason to assume that the archipelago's development would follow a Western trajectory. Indeed, it was imperative that colonial administrators understood and appreciated the specific characteristics and mental traits of the indigenous population, and patiently guided it to its ultimate, as-of-yet-unknown destination.

The following day, a critical reaction to Travaglino's speech appeared in the *Indies Courant*.[17] Its editor, left-leaning journalist D. M. G. Koch, argued that Travaglino merely repeated outdated and clichéd assertions, and that his conclusions were 'as superficial as they were wrong'.[18] The political motivation behind the speech was all too clear and it was hardly surprising that the PEB appreciated his superficial theories. 'If the native is, with respect to his psychic predisposition, completely different in comparison to us', wrote Koch, 'then all attempts for his advancement can be given up as hopeless' and more sharply: 'Dr. Travaglino is the psychologist of colonial conservatives.'[19] And the reasoning was flawed. Travaglino assumed that the mental characteristics of a specific population at a particular stage of its development were racial

---

[17] The *Indische Courant* was the newspaper of the sugar syndicate; Koch's editorship did not last long because of the political differences between him and the representatives of the Indies sugar factories. For Koch's autobiography, see D. M. G. Koch, *Verantwoording: Een Halve Eeuw in Indonesië* (The Hague/Bandung: Van Hoeve, 1956).

[18] [D. M. G. Koch], 'Psychologie en Politiek, I', *De Indische Courant*, 15 December 1923, 1.

[19] [Koch], 'Psychologie en Politiek, I', 1.

in nature and therefore static, but these characteristics were, Koch argued, largely produced by social and cultural factors and therefore amenable to change. Unlike their rural counterparts, Indonesians in urban environments had successfully learned to stay out of the way of moving cars. Similarly, it was specious to equate the mental characteristics of insane individuals with those of ethnic groups as Travaglino had.[20]

Four weeks later, a satirical account of the lecture was published in progressive magazine *The Task* [*De Taak*], under the suggestive title 'Psychiatric Fascism'.[21] Its anonymous author criticised Travaglino for his unwarranted generalisations, and suggested that the Dutch in the Indies could be diagnosed in a similar way: they were highly egocentric, focused on pleasure, and had established their colonial empire with the exclusive aim to make money. In subsequent issues of the *PEB Magazine*, a few indigenous PEB members praised Travaglino for his interest in the native mind but suggested that it was impossible to draw conclusions about normal minds from observations of the insane.[22] The Madurese, they argued, might be extremely cheerful when their team won the ox races, but similar behaviour was common among Europeans as well – one only needed to attend a soccer match. And Europeans were also frequently absent-minded. Travaglino's critics did not argue against studying native minds scientifically, but thought that a grasp of local language, culture, religion, and history would be indispensable, so that only Indies intellectuals were qualified to conduct this research.

Van Loon on the Mental Characteristics of the Malay

Travaglino was not the only psychiatrist in the Dutch East Indies convinced that his discipline's insights could contribute to colonial governance. In February 1924, F. H. van Loon, instructor in psychiatry and neurology at the STOVIA and director of Batavia's psychiatric clinic, addressed a meeting of the Indies Society in The Hague.[23] He had previously argued that the colonies were unusually fascinating to psychiatrists, since 'nowhere else in this world can we observe so many serious neurological disturbances as in the Dutch East

---

[20] See also [D. M. G. Koch], 'Psychologie en Politiek, II', *De Indische Courant*, 19 December 1923, 1.

[21] 'Psychiatrisch Fascisme', *De Taak* 7, no. 311 (15 January 1924), 1809–11. The architect Thomas Karsten was a member of the editorial board. About Karsten and *De Taak*, see Joost Coté, 'Thomas Karsten's Indonesia: Modernity and the End of Europe, 1914–1945', *Bijdragen tot de Taal-, Land- en Volkenkunde* 170 (2014), 66–98; Joost Coté and Hugh O'Neill, *The Life and Work of Thomas Karsten* (Amsterdam: Architectura & Natura, 2017).

[22] 'Politiek en Psychologie, *Vervolg*', *PEB*, 28 February 1924, 99–100.

[23] After returning to the Netherlands, Feico Herman van Loon extended his last name and became known as F. H. Glastra van Loon.

Indies.'[24] Van Loon contradicted earlier medical notions that the 'primitive' races rarely suffered from mental illness. In fact, there was much more insanity in the colonies than in the West, but its nature and symptomatic expression differed markedly from those in Europe. Life in the Indies bordered on the pathological, argued van Loon, and the 'normal' native mind had distinctly abnormal characteristics. This was especially true in the tropics, where the pathological always threatened to engulf the normal.[25]

It was perhaps telling that van Loon regretted how little was known about the physiology and psychology of the Malay, a term he used interchangeably with 'native' and 'Javanese'. Observing that tensions between racial and ethnic groups were steadily increasing, van Loon staked his claim: 'only pure scientific research can rescue us out from the swamp in which the whole colonial question is about to sink.'[26] Harmonious relationships could be realised only through mutual understanding, trust, love, and the desire to cooperate. Understanding the specific characteristics of the Malay was a prerequisite. Naturally, van Loon contended that the Malay were not inferior, only different. Like Kohlbrugge and Travaglino, he advocated a psychological colonial policy before elaborating on the slowness, indolence, lack of initiative, underdeveloped reasoning capacity, and inability to plan ahead commonly observed among the Malay. They were overly emotional and impulsive, lacked concern for others, and were often cruel. They were highly suggestible and therefore vulnerable to political agitators. They were sensual, superstitious, and gullible, but also very practical. Melancholia was rare, while strongly emotional psychoses and acute confusional states were common.[27] The Malay mind was infantile, concluded van Loon, and their remarkable success in adopting Western language, technology, and knowledge indicated not strong intellectual capacity but superb imitative skills.

Van Loon did not impress everyone at the meeting. Influential missionary physician H. Bervoets said that 'nobody currently present recognises the

[24] F. H. van Loon, 'Het Onderwijs in de Zenuw- en Zielziekten', in *Ontwikkeling van het Geneeskundig Onderwijs te Weltevreden, 1851–1926*, ed. A. de Waart (Weltevreden: Kolff, 1926), 209.

[25] For similar observations in an entirely different colonial context, see Jonathan Sadowsky, 'Psychiatry and Colonial Ideology in Nigeria', *Bulletin of the History of Medicine* 71, no. 1 (1997), 94–111.

[26] F. H. van Loon, 'De Psychische Eigenschappen der Maleische Rassen', *Indisch Genootschap*, 22 February 1924, 23.

[27] Van Loon elaborated on these findings in his many other articles, among them F. H. van Loon, 'Acute Verwardheidstoestanden in Nederlands-Indië', *Geneeskundig Tijdschrift voor Nederlandsch-Indië* 62 (1922), 658–90; F. H. van Loon, 'Amok and Lattah', *Journal of Abnormal & Social Psychology* 4 (1927), 434–44; F. H. van Loon, 'Rassenpsychologische Onderzoekingen', *Psychiatrische en Neurologische Bladen* 32 (1928), 190–26; 'Protopathic-Instinctive Phenomena in Normal and Pathological Malay Life', *British Journal of Medical Psychology* 8, no. 4 (1928), 264–76.

native as portrayed by the speaker', and chided him for dwelling exclusively on the negative characteristics of the Malay mind.[28] Several audience members cited the loyalty, friendliness, spirituality, and endurance they had observed in the Indies. Batak law student Alinoeddin Enda Boemi argued that van Loon's views were flawed generalisations: more than seventy ethnic groups populated the Indies and each had its own nature, habits, and cultural heritage. Studying these groups required familiarity with local language and *adat*, and living in situ for long periods. Another audience member noted that distasteful displays of sexual behaviour were often seen in the Netherlands and that, by comparison, the people of the archipelago tended to be modest and demure. It 'would be most interesting to have an Indonesian lecture on the psychological characteristics of the Dutch races', suggested another: a promising form of reverse anthropology.[29]

The views of both colonial psychiatrists were remarkably derivative. Physicians, sociologists, and anthropologists had long expressed similar views while describing various non-Western populations. Lucien Lévy-Bruhl's characterisation of the primitive mind as pre-logical and mystical was widely known at the time.[30] Herbert Spencer's social Darwinism had already suffused sociological theories on the development of modern society with evolutionary ideas.[31] Advocates of the Ethical Policy had used these theories to argue that Javanese society was at a lower evolutionary stage than the West but that it would catch up in due time. After 1920, conservative colonial commentators employed anthropological, sociological, and psychological theories to portray Eastern and Western minds as essentially different. They argued that only arrogant Westerners assumed that the evolutionary processes of different racial and ethnic groups would eventually lead to the same, Western endpoint. The archipelago's various ethnic groups would instead evolve according to their own principles, which would lead them in different directions. These conservative and relativist views entailed a policy of association, organising colonial society in separate spheres to allow each group to chart its unique path unobstructed.

After his return to the Netherlands in 1913, Kohlbrugge was appointed professor of ethnology at the University of Utrecht. In the 1920s, his views on colonial governance gained more prominence. In 1927, his university established a

---

[28] Van Loon, 'Psychische Eigenschappen', 43.
[29] Van Loon, 'Psychische Eigenschappen', 45. This speaker was an engineer, P. J. Ott de Vries, an expert on irrigation in the Dutch East Indies.
[30] See, for example, Lucien Lévy-Bruhl, *How Natives Think* (London: George Allen & Unwin, 1926 [1910]); *Primitive Mentality* (London: George Allen & Unwin, 1923); and *The Soul of the Primitive* (London: George Allen & Unwin, 1928 [1927]).
[31] See, for example, Robert Richards, *Darwin and the Emergence of Evolutionary Theories of Mind and Behavior* (Chicago: University of Chicago Press, 1987).

department of Indologie (the study of Indonesian history, language, literature, and culture as a preparatory course for future civil servants) with generous funding from Dutch business interests in direct competition with its progressive counterpart at the University of Leiden, the bastion of the Ethical Policy.[32] During the opening ceremonies, Kohlbrugge presented his views on the current unrest in the Indies unapologetically, reprising his statements from twenty years earlier. He welcomed the fact that politicians were, finally, considering a psychological colonial policy.[33] Megan Vaughan argues that the significance of colonial psychiatry in Africa lay primarily in reinforcing colonial ideologies, since the number of colonial subjects admitted to mental hospitals was only ever exceedingly small. 'The power of colonial medicine' lay, then, in 'its ability to provide a "naturalized" and pathologized account of [African] subjects'.[34] This conclusion applies with equal force to the Dutch East Indies.

Indies Physicians Protest

Many Indies physicians receiving advanced medical training in the Netherlands joined the Indies Association [Indische Vereeniging], which organised lectures and social events for expatriate students.[35] In 1921, Soetomo became chairman and moved it in a more political direction. Two years later, after Mohammad Hatta joined the board, the association became even more radical. The Association's insight into the nature of colonialism increased as connections were made with students from other Asian regions. Indies physicians began articulating Asian identities, emphasising positive characteristics such as spirituality and communitarianism.[36] Their cosmopolitan identities, now comprising modern, Western components as well as newly affirmed traditional, Eastern ones, enabled these students to articulate identities which transcended the status of colonial subject and imagined a future beyond subjugation. The association explicitly and

---

[32] Cees Fasseur, *De Indologen: Ambtenaren voor de Oost, 1825–1950* (Amsterdam: Bert Bakker, 1993).

[33] J. H. F. Kohlbrugge, *De Inlandsche Beweging en de Onrust in Indië* (Utrecht: Oosthoek, 1927), 30.

[34] Megan Vaughan, *Curing Their Ills: Colonial Power and African Illness* (Stanford, CA: Stanford University Press, 1991), 10, 25.

[35] On the history of the Indische Vereeniging, see Harry A. Poeze, *In het Land van de Overheerser I: Indonesiërs in Nederland, 1600–1950* (Dordrecht: FORIS, 1986); John Ingleson, *Perhimpunan Indonesia and the Indonesian Nationalist Movement, 1923–1928* (Melbourne: Centre of Southeast Asian Studies, Monash University, 1975); Sunario, *Perhimpunan Indonesia dan Peranannja dalam Perdjuangan Kemerdekaan Kita* (Djakarta: Departemen Pendidikan dan Kebudajaan, 1970); and Abdul Rivai, *Student Indonesia di Eropa* (Jakarta: Gramedia, 2000 [1928]).

[36] For the contacts between Indonesian students and those from other Asian colonies, see Klaas Stutje, 'Indonesian Identities Abroad: International Engagement of Colonial Students in the Netherlands, 1908–1931', *BMGN: Low Countries Historical Review* 128, no. 1 (2013), 151–72.

defiantly advocated Indonesian independence and formulated a policy of non-cooperation which would inspire Indonesian nationalists.[37] It renamed itself the Indonesian Association [Dutch: Indonesische Vereeniging] in 1922; two years later it took the Malay name of Perhimpunan Indonesia. Its periodical took the name *Free Indonesia* [Malay: *Indonesia Merdeka*].

In 1924, the Dutch branch of the Association of Indies Physicians, founded by Soetomo in 1922 and now chaired by Latumeten, published a pamphlet attacking van Loon's views and deconstructing his arguments.[38] Latumeten had been Travaglino's assistant at the Lawang mental hospital and had moved to the Netherlands for advanced medical training. Like a small number of his fellow medical students, he had joined the Perhimpunan Indonesia (Figure 5.1). The same year, four long articles appeared in *Indonesia Merdeka* criticising van Loon's speech.[39] The company of radicals had sharpened the political sensitivities of the medical student members, and after van Loon held his speech, students in other disciplines could not fail to notice the ideological role of colonial psychiatry. In June 1924, the radical student association invited van Loon to discuss his views, and he accepted, with reservations. The atmosphere during the ensuing meeting was tense. After briefly repeating his main arguments, van Loon abruptly left to catch a non-existent train.[40] Those present beamed with delight at this minor victory.

The articles in *Indonesia Merdeka* and the pamphlet published by the Netherlands branch of the Association of Indies Physicians argued that van Loon's political convictions had clouded his scientific judgement. At a time when the colonial administration was enacting increasingly repressive measures against the nationalist movement and brutally repressing strikes by Indonesian workers, it was expedient to portray Indonesians as unreliable children in need of firm guidance. The critics also noted that neither van Loon nor Travaglino spoke more than passing Malay and had little insight into local customs, cultural conventions, or the history of the ethnic groups upon which

---

[37] The radicalisation of this organisation is clearly reflected in the book memorialising the fifteenth anniversary of the association. See Indonesiche Vereeniging, *Gedenkboek 1908–1923* (The Hague: Indonesiche Vereeniging, 1924).

[38] Afdeeling Nederland Bond van Indonesische Artsen, *Verweerschrift Tegen de Rede van Dr. F. H. van Loon over 'De Psychische Eigenschappen der Maleische Rassen'* (Amsterdam: Hesse, 1924). The pamphlet was issued anonymously but it is clear that Latumeten was the author. Latumeten's role is mentioned in Ali Sastroamijoyo, *Milestones on My Journey: The Memoirs of Ali Sastroamijoyo, Indonesian Patriot and Political Leader* (Brisbane: University of Queensland Press, 1979), 25.

[39] 'Dilettantisme of Wetenschap?', *Indonesia Merdeka* 2 (1924), 48; 'Enkele Opmerkingen naar Aanleiding van de Rede van Dr. F. H. van Loon', *Indonesia Merdeka* 2 (1924): 51–66; 'Modern Evangelie: Penneprikjes naar Aanleiding van Loon's Rede', *Indonesia Merdeka* 2 (1924): 66–68; 'Verdere Opmerkingen naar Aanleiding van de Rede van Dr. F. H. van Loon', *Indonesia Merdeka* 2 (1924): 79–91.

[40] Reported in 'Enkele Opmerkingen', and 'Verdere Opmerkingen'.

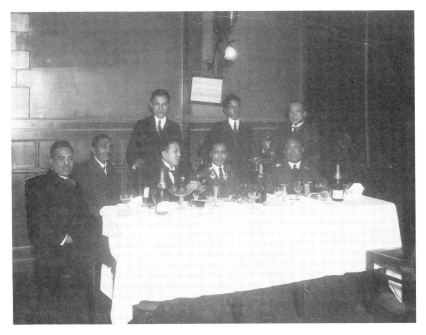

Figure 5.1 Several Indonesians studying in the Netherlands sit down for dinner. From left to right: J. B. Sitanala, J. A. Latumeten, Darnawan Mangoenkoesoemo, Iwa Koesoema Soemantri, H. D. J. Apituley. Standing: Mohamad Amir (?), Soekiman, Alinoeddin Boemi. Figure courtesy of Herman Keppy

they were passing judgement. Van Loon was 'obsessed', they argued, 'with the flaws of a small group and exploited these to characterise the mind of a nation consisting of millions'.[41] When van Loon commented on the high level of physical activity and spontaneous dancing of the Menadonese, his critics pointed out that similar behaviour could be observed at Dutch trade fairs, farmers' markets, and sporting events. The critics also addressed the condition of running amok, a mental state during which indigenous men suddenly embarked upon a murderous rage after suffering severe public embarrassment. Van Loon had cited this condition as evidence for Indonesians' highly charged emotional nature. His critics supplied a dozen Dutch newspaper clippings reporting fights involving weapons, knives, and blunt objects taking place at sporting matches, near bars, or at home. It was not that sudden explosions of aggression were uncommon in the Netherlands, but that they were interpreted

---

[41] Bond van Indonesische Artsen, *Verweerschrift*, 13.

differently: 'With us it is called "amok", here [in the Netherlands] it is called an affable expression of "*über Kultur*", isn't it?'[42]

The Great War itself could be characterised as European nations running amok. Further clippings were used to counter the allegedly deceptive nature of Indonesians, detailing examples of Dutch fraud and embezzlement. One critic even quoted a historical study describing nineteenth-century colonial Dutchmen as 'lazy, unreliable, treacherous, larcenous, incompetent, [and] vain'.[43] The negative qualities colonial psychiatrists identified as evidence of primitivism among Indonesians were also pervasive in European populations, and pointedly, in the Dutch. And more might be thrown at the metropolitans – the critics presented a fictional Indonesian study on the Dutch mind, enumerating its unique unfavourable characteristics: crude materialism, insensitivity, allegiance to Bacchus, and unhygienic behaviour. The Dutch intellect certainly appeared highly developed but was sadly applied exclusively to material pursuits.[44] It was relatively easy, the critics suggested, to present subjective censure as psychological theory.

Van Loon's critics attacked the fundamental assumptions underlying his arguments. It was impossible to draw a distinction between 'East' and 'West', they argued. With respect to 'the East', 'the Malay', or 'the native', they cited the latest census of the Indies which listed more than fifty-six ethnic groups speaking more than 500 languages. It would be virtually impossible to identify features they held in common. Nor was it any easier to identify which social, ethnic, or racial group represented the Western mind, generally known as an 'ideal psychic quantity, absolutely free of failings and unpleasant characteristics'.[45] Was the West best represented by the 'inhabitants of the Balkans, the Russians, the Scandinavians, the French, the Italians, etc. etc.?'[46] Even if the Dutch were chosen as a representative group, it was still not clear which subgroup qualified: 'the Freezian, the Hollander, or the Limburger, or maybe the tropical-Dutch?'[47] Should researchers focus on the 'psyche of the Amsterdam street youth, the Rotterdam dock worker, or the typical inhabitant of the Jordaan [a workers' neighbourhood in Amsterdam, known as a hotbed of political radicalism]?'[48] Neither the Eastern nor the Western mind was homogeneous, which made the identification of defining characteristics impossible. Comparisons were out of the question.

The critics conceded that van Loon had correctly identified a number of symptoms characterising the Malay but that his diagnosis was mistaken.[49] The

---

[42] Bond van Indonesische Artsen, *Verweerschrift*, 9.
[43] Quoted in Bond van Indonesische Artsen, *Verweerschrift*, 11.
[44] 'Enkele Opmerkingen', 64.
[45] 'Verdere Opmerkingen', 81.
[46] Bond van Indonesische Artsen, *Verweerschrift*, 3.
[47] Bond van Indonesische Artsen, *Verweerschrift*, 3.
[48] Bond van Indonesische Artsen, *Verweerschrift*, 3.
[49] 'Enkele Opmerkingen', 60.

lack of intellectual development observed in some Indonesians, they argued, was readily explained by the absence of educational opportunities, a state of affairs which had persisted through more than three centuries of Dutch colonial rule. The slowness and lack of initiative van Loon had observed could be the effect of malaria and other tropical diseases, which were still common in the Indies despite the presence of the colonial medical service – or it might be explained by the strictures of colonial society, which allowed them only subordinate roles and failed to reward achievement. Van Loon had unwittingly invoked the pervasive effects of colonialism: a 'colonial society like ours is simply pathological'.[50] The theories of colonial psychiatrists about the people of the Indies replicated the 'tragedy of an unfree people'. One could 'with impunity and haphazardly say just about anything' about them.[51] Further, both mad doctors were profoundly insane: they were 'scientific maniacs' and van Loon, in particular, had 'a smugness and prudency bordering on morbidity'.[52] The board of the Association of Indies Physicians followed the debate; the Association's journal devoted several pages to it.[53] The board wrote an official letter to the director of the colonial Public Health Service and the Governor-General expressing its doubts about van Loon's suitability as instructor at the Batavia Medical College.[54]

Non-Cooperation

Mohammad Hatta extended the critique of colonial psychiatry formulated by Latumeten and his colleagues by attributing the apparent lethargy of the indigenous population to colonialism itself. The armoury of the colonial state included not only the colonial army, police, bureaucracy, and control of the means of production, but psychology:

One of the means [to ensure Dutch supremacy in the Indies] is mass-suggestion: the injection of the idea of the superiority of the white race in Indonesian consciousness and the suggestion of national impotence. Each emerging idea or initiative is systematically and artificially paralysed by the forced hypnosis of ignorance with the psychological consequence of doubt in one's own abilities.[55]

Hatta argued that the perceived lack of initiative perceived amongst Indonesians was the result of an inferiority complex implanted by the colonial state. In 1928,

---

[50] Bond van Indonesische Artsen, *Verweerschrift*, i, 1.
[51] Bond van Indonesische Artsen, *Verweerschrift*, 1, i.
[52] Bond van Indonesische Artsen, *Verweerschrift*, i, 1.
[53] 'De Psychische Eigenschappen der Maleische Rassen', *Orgaan der Vereeniging van Indische Geneeskundigen* 13, no. 1 (December 1924), 36–40.
[54] 'Nogmaals Dr. van Loon!', *Orgaan der Vereeniging van Indische Geneeskundigen* 13, no. 1 (December 1924): 41–46.
[55] [Mohammad Hatta], 'Het Psychologische Conflict', *Hindia Poetra* 1 (1923), 67. *Hindia Poetra* was the journal by the *Indonesische Vereeniging* in 1923. In 1924, the name was changed to

Hatta and three other members of the Perhimpunan Indonesia were arrested for disturbing the public order and inciting political unrest. His defence was delivered in a now-famous speech, 'Free Indonesia'. He spoke of the psychological effects of being a colonial subject: 'The spiritual structure of the nation has been changed [and its] personality is temporarily broken.'[56] The masses were kept in ignorance by limiting educational opportunities, repressing political activity, and censoring the vernacular press. Medical theories of white superiority drawing upon the authority of science helped bolster Dutch hegemony. 'Day in day out, it has been emphasized that the Indonesians do not possess the capacities for leadership and that they are not capable of initiative', said Hatta, 'so that really they are predestined from the day of their birth to work under European leadership'.[57] For Hatta such failings were instead proof of the destructive work of colonialism.

Members of the Perhimpunan Indonesia joined Hatta to propose a policy of non-cooperation to rectify the damaging psychological effects of colonialism. Non-cooperation would result in 'a systematic destruction of the psychological foundations on which the authority and respect of the ruler are, in part, based'.[58] According to Hatta and his fellow nationalists, Indonesians should no longer wait for favours from the colonial administration and must rely on their own capacities instead.[59] They exhorted Indonesians to withdraw from the political bodies created by the colonial administration, and to take responsibility for their own development. Non-cooperation would, said Hatta, promote self-confidence, self-help and auto-activity, and result in improvements in the everyday life of Indonesians. Talk of the psychological flaws of the indigenous population was a smokescreen, deflecting attention away from the Netherlands' continuing exploitation. 'Under the guise of "immaturity" and "gradual development" hide the real policies', warned Hatta, 'which are readily influenced by the demand of *selfishness* and *covetousness*, the *Leitmotiv* of Dutch colonial statesmanship'.[60] Hatta's critique of the damaging psychological effects of colonisation was clearly influenced by the analysis of colonial psychiatry by the physician members of the Perhimpunan Indonesia. This critique formed one of the earliest sustained analyses of the role of psychological and psychiatric theories in colonial society as well as the psychological consequences

---

Indonesia Merdeka. This article appeared anonymously but is attributed to Hatta in Mohammad Hatta, *Verspreide Geschriften*, 2 vols. (Jakarta: Balai Buku Indonesia, 1952).

[56] Mohammad Hatta, 'Indonesia Free', in *Portrait of a Patriot: Selected Writings* (The Hague: Mouton, 1972 [1927]), 245.

[57] Hatta, 'Indonesia Free', 266.

[58] Hatta, 'Indonesia Free', 272.

[59] Hatta, 'Indonesia Free', 246.

[60] Hatta, 'Indonesia Free', 251 (italics in original).

of colonisation. Thirty years later, these issues would become familiar to a broader public through the writings of Franz Fanon.[61]

Non-Cooperation in the Indies

When it became clear that Arnold van Gennep would not be nominated for a seat in the Volksraad for the 1924 elections, the Surabaya city council appointed him as a member and assigned him the portfolio of public works, an area in which he had no experience or expertise. In 1923, Soetomo (Figure 5.2) had returned to the Indies as a lecturer in dermatology at Surabaya's Medical College. He had also been elected to the city council but found that the European council members consistently opposed his proposals for *kampong* improvements and public health initiatives. Soetomo interpreted van Gennep's appointment as an unequivocal indication that Surabaya was not interested in improving the living conditions of its indigenous population. Together with two other Indonesian members, he relinquished his seat in protest.[62] Soetomo subsequently founded the Surabaya study club which focused on instructing and preparing Indonesian leadership cadres.[63] In Bandung, a second study club was established by Tjipto Mangoenkoesoemo and E. F. E. Douwes Dekker. Here, one young member stood out for his radical political views: Sukarno.

Over the next several years, Soetomo built various institutions including a bank, an insurance company, cooperatives of many kinds, and labour unions.[64] He also established medical clinics and supported various public health projects in Surabaya and its surrounds. Soetomo subscribed to the policy of non-cooperation and refused to participate in the political institutions established by the Dutch. Instead, he encouraged Indonesians to take their fate into their own hands. He aimed to prepare them for independence by building a viable infrastructure and by training Indonesians to run it. At this time, most Indonesian political leaders turned away from strikes and demonstrations, and towards the archipelago's future. Some poured their energies into Indonesian

---

[61] Frantz Fanon, *Black Skin, White Masks*, trans. Charles Lam Markmann (New York: Grove Press, 1967); Frantz Fanon, *The Wretched of the Earth*, trans. Constance Farrington (New York: Grove Press, 1965).

[62] 'Uit den Gemeenteraad van Soerabaja', *De Indische Courant*, 14 March 1925, 3. Soetomo provided an explanation later: 'Het Standpunt van Soetomo c.s.', *Bataviaasch Nieuwsblad*, 23 March 1925, 1. See also D. M. G. Koch, 'Dr. Tjipto Mangoenkoesoemo', in *Batig Slot: Figuren uit het Oude Indië* (Amsterdam: De Brug/Djambatan, 1960), 141; and Soetomo to J. E. Stokvis, 7 November 1924. Collection J. E. Stokvis, inventory number 19, International Institute of Social History, Amsterdam.

[63] 'De Inlandsche Studieclub', *De Indische Courant*, 23 February 1925, section III, 2.

[64] See Savitri Scherer, 'Soetomo and Trade Unionism', *Indonesia*, no. 24 (1977), 27–38; John Ingleson, 'Sutomo, the Indonesian Study Club and Organised Labour in Late Colonial Surabaya', *Journal of Southeast Asian Studies* 39, no. 1 (2008), 31–57.

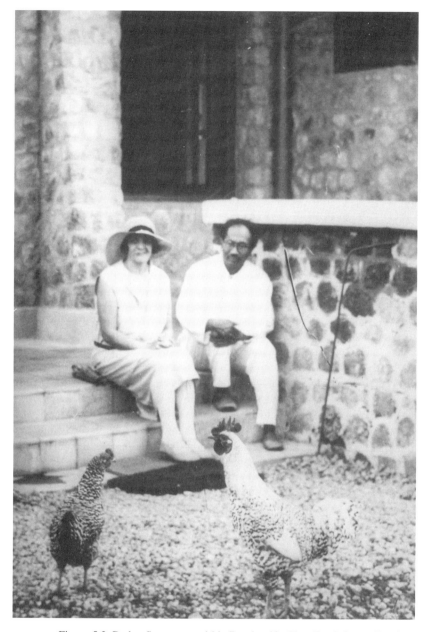

Figure 5.2 Raden Soetomo and his Dutch wife, Everdina Johanna Bruring, near their house near Lawang, south of Surabaya. They married in 1917. Figure courtesy of the NIAS Museum, Faculty of Medicine, Airlangga University

scouting associations, which provided training in a variety of skills, taught discipline and physical endurance, and built strong personal bonds. In 1930, Soetomo founded the Indonesian National Union [Persatoean Bangsa Indonesia]. In 1935, he was co-founder of the Great Indonesia Party [Partai Indonesia Raja] (Parindra), which proposed moderate social and political reforms, by uniting his own party and Boedi Oetomo.[65] He served as president until his early death in 1938. The funeral procession, which numbered some 50,000 people, was testimony to Soetomo's profound significance within the nationalist movement.

Goenawan Mangoenkoesoemo, Tjipto's younger brother and one of the founders of Boedi Oetomo, consistently modelled his political views on those of his closest friend, Soetomo. During Goenawan's first sojourn to the Netherlands, from 1918 to 1920, he touted radical political opinions.[66] In 1927, he received a fellowship from the colonial administration for advanced medical training in the Netherlands and spent two years there with his wife, Raden Ajeng Srijati, Soetomo's sister. Goenawan's research focused on tuberculosis, which was then endemic in the Indies. He continued to associate with members of the Perhimpunan Indonesia but disliked their increasing radicalisation – the association had become, by this point, a communist front.[67] Goenawan decided to refrain from political activism to focus on his research in the conviction that he and his medical colleagues could best contribute to the welfare of their compatriots through medicine. He could best help usher in an independent Indonesia by educating enough Indonesian medical specialists to staff a national medical infrastructure. After his return to the Indies, Goenawan was appointed to the Semarang Civil Hospital and initiated research projects ascertaining the prevalence of tuberculosis. Sadly, he died within a year of receiving this appointment.

The Association of Indies Physicians and Science

In 1914, the editors of the *Organ for Indies Physicians* had stated that the periodical would primarily discuss issues of professional interest and refrain from publishing scientific articles, which were best submitted to the *Journal for Indies Physicians* edited by instructors at the Batavia Medical College. The 'general desire is to consider the *Organ* as the only "social advocate"

---

[65] See Susan Abeyasekere, 'Partai Indonesia Raja, 1936–42: A Study in Cooperative Nationalism', *Journal of Southeast Asian Studies* 3, no. 2 (1972), 262–76.

[66] See, for example, Goenawan Mangoenkoesoemo, 'De Geboorte van Boedi-Oetomo', in *Soembangsih: Gedenkboek Boedi-Oetomo 1908 – 20 Mei – 1918* (Amsterdam: Nederlandsch-Indië Oud en Nieuw, 1918), 9–14.

[67] Soetomo, *Towards a Glorious Indonesia* (Athens: Ohio University Center for International Studies, 1987), 80.

of the interests of native physicians', wrote the editors.[68] In 1925, the *Organ* was renamed the *Bulletin* and started to appear monthly.[69] That same year, Mohamad Amir, ardent Theosophist, former president of Young Sumatra, student at the University of Amsterdam, and member of the Perhimpunan Indonesia, submitted a proposal to transform the *Bulletin* into a scientific journal. The *Journal for Indies Physicians* had ceased publication because of financial cutbacks, and it was as a scientific journal that the *Bulletin* would further the professional development of all Indonesian physicians, and play a leading role in 'intensifying medical life in Indonesia [as] this country is gradually becoming a centre for medical research'.[70] Although increasing numbers of Indonesian physicians were conducting medical research, argued Amir, their work had not attracted significant attention. A professional journal edited and published by Indonesian physicians showcasing their research would increase its visibility and lead to greater appreciation of their abilities and skills. 'Our own professional journal', he wrote, 'will place the activities and aspirations, and the medical knowledge and abilities of Indonesians, in the forefront of public attention, which could lead to a higher moral and material appreciation on the part of general public and the government'.[71] In an editorial entitled 'The Association and Science', the *Bulletin*'s editors observed that labour unions had become ineffective and that union activities were perhaps inappropriate for physicians. The Association should instead 'increase its scientific level to achieve the same ends'.[72]

Amir hoped to stimulate Indies physicians to engage in medical research. They could continue to read medical periodicals written and produced by their European and North American colleagues, but this would not inspire 'productive scientific work, initiative, and self-confidence'.[73] He exhorted his colleagues to stop deferring to foreign authority: 'The time has passed that Indonesian physicians are completely silent or merely beg for a modest place for [their] intellectual products in a periodical created by others for [them], the immature pupil[s]'.[74] With the *Journal for Indies Physicians* discontinued, it was an opportune time to gear the *Bulletin* towards medical research. The *Bulletin*'s editors supported Amir's position, arguing that it 'could not be ruled out that, if

---

[68] Asharie and D. J. Siahaija, 'Gewone Vergadering op Zondag den 7en Juni 1914 in het Polikliniek Lokaal van de STOVIA', *Orgaan der Vereeniging van Inlandsche Geneeskundigen* 4, no. 4–5 (1914), 4–5.
[69] 'Het Nieuwe Kleed', *Bulletin van den Bond van Indische Geneeskundigen* 14, no. 2 (1925), 1.
[70] Mohamad Amir, 'Prae-Advies Dr. Amir: Een Eigen Vaktijdschrift voor den Indonesischen Arts', *Bulletin van den Bond van Indische Geneeskundigen* 14, no. 3 (1925), 9.
[71] Amir, 'Prae-Advies', 9.
[72] 'De Bond en de Wetenschap', *Bulletin van den Bond van Indische Geneeskundigen* 14, no. 3 (1925), 12.
[73] Amir, 'Prae-Advies', 9.
[74] Amir, 'Prae-Advies', 10.

the scientific accomplishments of the Indies physician is driven to new heights, his social position will also improve accordingly'.[75] Everybody in the Indies was engaged in battles for increased rank and status, and these battles were 'often fought in the political domain, which appears to us not the correct way for all parties, least of all for a party of physicians'.[76] Kaijadoe endorsed Amir's proposal and rejoiced that the *Bulletin* would soon become the first medical journal published 'by ourselves and for ourselves'.[77] 'The time has passed in which we are guided in everything by foreigners', he declared; 'in the medical domain we have to exercise independence and autonomy.'[78] Publishing a scientific journal was a deeply political act: it demonstrated that Indies physicians were taking 'our medical fate in our own hands'.[79] It constituted medical non-cooperation, and implied a new professional self-confidence.

For the next six years, the *Bulletin* exclusively published articles detailing the medical research conducted by Indonesian physicians. As an affirmation of sorts, advertisements for pharmaceutical products and medical equipment started to appear in its pages. Most articles were written by those Indonesian doctors who had obtained Dutch medical degrees and earned medical doctorates. Upon their return to the Indies, they were appointed as medical researchers, department heads or vice directors in leading hospitals, instructors at the two medical colleges, or directors of smaller hospitals. By focusing on research, they demonstrated that they were able to function independently and no longer needed the guidance of their Dutch colleagues. Apart from being an interesting statement on medical non-cooperation, Amir's initiative indicated that a new medical elite had emerged among Indies physicians, consisting of Indonesian doctors with advanced medical training and Dutch medical degrees. Holding Western medical qualifications, they earned the same salary as their Dutch colleagues, since the colonial administration discriminated on the basis of degrees obtained rather than ethnicity. In the 1920s, this elite was still relatively small and never comprised more than thirty individuals. Nonetheless, they presented a powerful scientific image for the Indonesian medical profession, and together began shaping the future development of Indonesian medicine. Under their guidance, the Association of Indies Physicians had become a scientific organisation and it would soon rival the (European) Association for the Advancement of Medical Sciences in the Dutch Indies.

---

[75] 'De Bond en de Wetenschap', 12.
[76] 'De Bond en de Wetenschap', 12.
[77] K. [Kaijadoe], 'Ons Tijdschrift', *Bulletin van den Bond van Indische Geneeskundigen* 14, no. 3 (1925), 21.
[78] K., 'Ons Tijdschrift', 21–22.
[79] 'Berichten uit Nederland', *Bulletin van den Bond van Indische Geneeskundigen* 14, no. 3 (1925), 13.

Conclusion

The advocates of the Ethical Policy held that the ultimate aim of social development was a modernity in which race, ethnicity, and religious belief would disappear. This promised equality, however, was deferred time and again and at times was even repudiated outright. The Dutch colonial administration, to repeat the medical metaphor possibly used unintentionally by Dipesh Chakrabharty, consigned natives to the 'waiting room' of history.[80] According to the conservative ideas that became dominant in the 1920s, Indonesians and Europeans were essentially different. Both were evolving, albeit in a different way, and following different trajectories. This made it impossible to predict the future of the Indies. These relativist and culturalist views inspired the formulation of a policy of association, which relegated Europeans and Indonesians to separate spheres. Providing a Western-style education or trying to move the indigenous sphere towards the European sphere would be counterproductive, as it led to cultural dislocation, to social disintegration, or worse, to violent insurrection. At the same time, Indonesian intellectuals and political leaders, including Indies physicians, were seen as estranged from their ethnic communities.

The debate on the nature of the native mind indicated a decisive turn in the political orientation of Indonesian nationalist physicians. In their critiques, they argued against psychiatric views on *our* mental characteristics and claimed that *we* were offended by them. During the 1920s, Indonesian intellectuals no longer aspired to become Europeans, and instead identified with the indigenous population. This had two profound correlative effects. First, Indonesian nationalists and Indies physicians ceased lauding the West and the promises of modernity, and began to elaborate on Eastern spirituality, communitarianism, and the strength of indigenous cultural traditions. Second, Indies physicians, in particular the highly educated elite of Indonesian doctors with Dutch medical degrees among them, started to focus on research and to publish their findings. This demonstrated their rationality and protested against the notion that science was the exclusive property of white men. In their critique of colonial psychiatry, Indonesian physicians argued that they themselves were best placed to conduct this research. In this way, the insults of colonial psychiatry instigated the decolonisation of Indonesian medicine.

---

[80] Dipesh Chakrabarthy, *Provincializing Europe* (Princeton, NJ: Princeton University Press, 2000), 8. Colonial deferral (of bestowing equal rights and privileges, attaining relative autonomy, or reaching a sufficient level of maturity to become equal partners in administrative matters) has also been discussed by Warwick Anderson in *Colonial Pathologies: American Tropical Medicine, Race, and Hygiene in the Philippines* (Durham, NC: Duke University Press, 2006), 3, 71, 178, 205; and Ann Laura Stoler, for example, in 'On Degrees of Imperial Sovereignty', *Public Culture* 18, no. 1 (2006), 139–42.

Before the 1920s, the Dutch East Indies had a two-tier medical profession, with both European and Indies physicians. Both tiers were frequently at odds but coexisted, despite a strong mutual distrust and, at times, outright hostility. In the 1920s, Indies physicians were divided into two groups: an elite tier of Indonesian doctors with Dutch medical degrees and a much larger group consisting of the remaining Indies physicians. The former did not participate in the activities of the Association, but used its *Bulletin* to publish their articles. They appeared to be apolitical, unlike the large group of Indies physicians. Despite their small number, they dominated the image of the Association.

6   The Great Depression: Rockefeller Initiatives and Medical Nationalism

The Great Depression decimated the export-based economy of the Dutch East Indies, causing hardship for Europeans and Indonesians alike. By 1935, the total value of exports had dropped to one third of 1929 levels. Many sugar factories, plantations, and mines closed, while the few businesses that kept operating greatly reduced staff numbers. Unemployment rose dramatically. The revenue of the colonial administration decreased significantly, leading to painful salary reductions for civil servants.[1] Since the majority of Indies physicians were employed by the Public Health Service, they suffered economic hardship. The political climate deteriorated further during the Depression years and became ruthlessly oppressive and authoritarian.[2] The reactionary Fatherland Club [Vaderlansche Club], Arnold van Gennep's new political home, dominated the Volksraad.[3] B. C. de Jonge, Governor-General from 1931 to 1936, once quipped that the Dutch had ruled the Indies for more than 300 years with whip and club in hand, and would continue to do so for at least another 300 years. De Jonge relied on the police, the military, and the ever-expanding intelligence services to control and repress the nationalist movement. Sukarno toured the colonies and kept audiences spellbound with his powerful rhetorical skills until his arrest, together with all the leaders of his Indonesian National Party [Partai Nasional Indonesia] (PNI), in December 1929. The colonial administration had exiled several nationalist leaders to Upper-Digul, a notorious internment camp in a swamp-ridden, malarial area in New Guinea. With virtually all nationalists exiled, jailed, or silenced, most colonial Dutchmen were convinced that peace and quiet reigned in the colonies.

---

[1] *Vaststelling van de Herziene Bezoldigingsregeling voor Burgerlijke Landsdienaren ('HBBL 1934')* (Batavia: Landsdrukkerij, 1934). For the salary measures taken during the Depression, see H. W. van den Doel, 'Indianisatie en Ambtenarensalarissen', *Tijdschrift voor Geschiedenis* 100, no. 4 (1987), 556–79.

[2] John Ingleson, *Road to Exile: The Indonesian Nationalist Movement 1927–1934* (Singapore: Heinemann, 1979).

[3] Pieter Joost Drooglever, *De Vaderlandse Club, 1929–1942: Totoks en de Indische Politiek* (Franeker: Wever, 1980).

The Association of Indies Physicians lay dormant during these years, until the late 1930s when it was revived by Indies physician and Volksraad delegate Abdul Rasjid, a Batak aristocrat from Sumatra's Tapanuli highlands with a strong interest in *adat*. In 1935, Rasjid visited a health demonstration project of the Rockefeller Foundation in the Banyumas regency and enthusiastically adopted its principles as the foundation of his own medical nationalism. The aim of the Rockefeller initiative was to demonstrate how the health of poor and rural populations could be improved through health education and the provision of basic medical care in modest clinics. Legal scholars argued that *adat* principles had to be implemented at a local level in accordance with local customs, preferences, circumstances, and family configurations. Rasjid similarly argued that public health measures were best implemented locally by individuals with a thorough knowledge of local *adat* regulations, particularly those relating to health, disease, hygiene, and the body. On the basis of these insights, Rasjid formulated a program for the organisation of health care benefiting the indigenous population. He successfully revived the Association of Indies Physicians with his medical nationalism, which was guided by the idea that health accelerated economic productivity and improved national strength.

The Opening of the Batavia Medical School

In 1927, the Batavia Medical School [Geneeskundige Hoogeschool] (GH), which conferred medical degrees equivalent to those in the Netherlands, opened in the new STOVIA buildings (Figure 6.1). Indies physicians had long advocated transforming both medical colleges into full-fledged medical schools; earning full medical degrees assisted their emancipation. Whereas the STOVIA's medical curriculum had been organised in a highly structured fashion with compulsory lecture attendance, supervised study, and regular examinations, the program of the Batavia Medical School adhered to the German academic model, which emphasised student agency. Lecture attendance was voluntary, students studied at their own pace, and scheduled their exams when they felt prepared. General examinations were held annually. Students were required to pay tuition, although a small number received bursaries that obligated them to work for the Public Health Service for ten years. As a consequence, the composition of the student body changed significantly, with Dutch, Indo-European, and Indo-Chinese students dominating and Indonesians in the minority. For medical research, the opening of the Batavia Medical School was a positive development; for Indonesians wishing to study medicine, it was not.

The Batavia Medical School's opening caused a crisis at the Surabaya Medical College (NIAS). Teachers and students alike were convinced that it would collapse if it was not transformed into a full medical school. Director A. E. Sitsen did not want his institution to become a second-class teaching

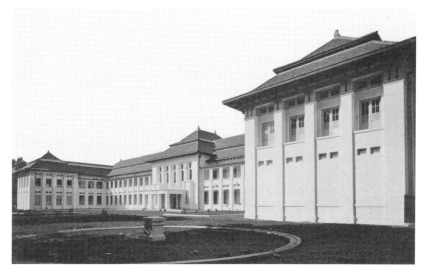

Figure 6.1 The building of the Batavia Medical School [Geneeskundige Hoogeschool]. This building housed the Batavia Medical College or STOVIA (1919–26), the Batavia Medical School (1926–42), and the Faculty of Medicine at the University of Indonesia from 1950. Figure courtesy of the Dutch National Museum of Ethnology, Leiden (TM-60036529)

institution and resigned in protest.[4] After the onset of the Great Depression, it appeared increasingly likely that the Surabaya Medical College would close, inspiring vehement protests by students. Against all expectations, the colonial administration eventually decided against closure, but cuts were made. From 1933, matriculating students no longer received stipends and graduates were released from the obligation to work for the Public Health Service. Student numbers nevertheless continued to increase, slightly. The 1934 yearbook, which marked the twentieth anniversary of the Surabaya Medical College, explicitly declared its continuing social and political significance. At the elitist Batavia Medical School, enrolling a greater proportion of students from wealthy, non-Indonesian backgrounds, student political culture declined. The NIAS, in contrast, remained a centre of political activity – it had become the medical school for Indonesians and the spirit of Indonesian nationalism continued to thrive.[5]

---

[4] Bestuur, 'De NIAS Vereeniging', in *NIAS Jaarboek 1932* (Surabaya: Kolff, 1932), 99.

[5] S., 'The Positie van de Medische Scholen in Indonesië', in *NIAS Lustrum Almanak 1933–1934* (Batavia: Kolff, 1934), 20–26. See also, for example, a selection of former NIAS student Hario Kecik's autobiography: Suhario 'Kecik' Padmodiwiryo, *Student Soldiers: A Memoir of the Battle That Sparked Indonesia's National Revolution* (Jakarta: Yayasan Pustaka Obor Indonesia, 2015) and the ample writings of NIAS students in the 1930s.

In 1940, a new hospital opened across the road, placing the medical laboratory, hospital, and medical school in close proximity.

During the Depression years, the Public Health Service continued to be the main employer of Indies physicians, but it hired fewer and fewer medical graduates, and released the remainder from their ten-year obligation to it.[6] What had been a burdensome, exploitative arrangement was now a highly coveted, secure position, out of reach for most. In 1932, rumours abounded that newly hired Indonesian doctors with European medical degrees would receive the much lower starting salary of Indies physicians. For many, the 'attractiveness [of obtaining a European medical degree], for which we previously spared neither expense nor effort, has disappeared'.[7] The Association of Indies Physicians established a fund to assist those who had lost their jobs to establish private practices. In an overly optimistic vein, it asserted that 'nationalist perspectives [were] opened up with a forceful class of free [i.e., self-employed] Indies physicians, from which the national medical services will be born later.'[8] Under the prevailing economic conditions, this initiative was bound to fail. In the past, only a few Indies physicians had been able to make a living by running a private practice. The Association's board joined with a trade union to fight the salary reductions imposed by the colonial administration.[9]

The Rockefeller Foundation Comes to the Dutch East Indies

In 1909, the immensely wealthy and notorious entrepreneur John D. Rockefeller, then president of the Standard Oil company, established a number of philanthropic organisations to 'promote the well-being and to advance the civilization' of humankind, stimulating activities 'in the acquisition and dissemination of knowledge, in the prevention and relief of suffering, and in the promotion of any and all the elements of human progress'.[10] From the beginning, the Foundation focused on education and health, as its officers viewed disease

---

[6] 'De Verbreking van het Dienstverband', *Orgaan der Vereeniging van Indische Geneeskundigen* 21, no. 1–2 (1933), 5–7.

[7] 'De Kwestie van het Doctoraal-Examen', *Orgaan der Vereeniging van Indische Geneeskundigen* 21, no. 3–4 (1932), 28.

[8] 'Het Steunfonds', *Orgaan der Vereeniging van Indische Geneeskundigen* 21, no. 1–2 (1933), 3–4; Hoofdbestuur, 'Verslag over 1932', *Orgaan der Vereeniging van Indische Geneeskundigen* 21, no. 3–4 (1932), 13; 'Het Steunfonds', *Orgaan der Vereeniging van Indische Geneeskundigen* 21, no. 5–6 (1933), 33–34.

[9] 'Verslag over 1934', *Orgaan der Vereeniging van Indische Geneeskundigen* 24, no. 1–2 (1936), 2–4; 'Verslag over 1935', *Orgaan der Vereeniging van Indische Geneeskundigen* 24, no. 1–2 (1936), 13–14; Hoofdbestuur, 'De Salaris-Vermindering', *Orgaan der Vereeniging van Indische Geneeskundigen* 19, no. 3–4 (1931), 47.

[10] Deed of trust establishing the Rockefeller Foundation, quoted in John Farley, *To Cast Out Disease: A History of the International Health Division of the Rockefeller Foundation (1913–1951)* (New York: Oxford University Press, 2004), 3.

as 'the supreme ill of human life and … the main source of almost all other human ills' including poverty, crime, vice, and inefficiency.[11] They saw disease as one of the main causes of poverty and economic stagnation, and improving health as one of the most important conditions for further economic development. The Foundation's first successful health project demonstrated how hookworm disease, prevalent in the American South, could be treated and how reinfection could be prevented.[12] Hookworm disease, the outcome of an intestinal infestation, induced severe anaemia and listlessness, thereby reducing labour productivity. Vermifuge treatment effectively dislodged worms wedged in an individual's intestines. Because reinfection generally occurred when individuals stepped in human faeces containing hookworm larvae, it could be prevented if people wore shoes and used latrines; preventing reinfection required effective public health education. The Foundation's officers held that public health education was essential to the success of its health projects, because it made individuals active participants in the prevention of disease and the maintenance of health.

The International Health Board, established by the Rockefeller Foundation in 1913, funded a number of public health demonstration projects in the Dutch East Indies in the 1920s.[13] While successful, these did not initially receive much attention. Surveys established that in some areas more than 90 per cent of the population suffered from hookworm infestation (Figure 6.2). In regions where malaria was also endemic, the population suffered from severe anaemia. In 1924, Rockefeller physician John L. Hydrick arrived in the Indies to establish the Medical-Hygiene Propaganda Division within the Indies Public Health Service.[14] European physicians remained suspicious of these American

---

[11] Frederick Gates, one of the most important advisors to John D. Rockefeller Sr., quoted in Farley, *To Cast Out Disease*, 3.

[12] John Ettling, *The Germ of Laziness: Rockefeller Philanthropy and Public Health in the New South* (Cambridge, MA: Harvard University Press, 1981).

[13] Farley, *To Cast Out Disease*; William H. Schneider, *Rockefeller Philanthropy and Modern Biomedicine: International Initiatives from World War I to the Cold War* (Bloomington: Indiana University Press, 2002); Marcos Cueto, 'The Cycles of Eradication: The Rockefeller Foundation and Latin American Public Health, 1918–1940', in *International Health Organizations and Movements, 1918–1939*, ed. Paul Weindling (Cambridge: Cambridge University Press, 1995), 222–43; and Anne-Emanuelle Birn and Armando Solorzano, 'The Hook of Hookworm: Public Health and the Politics of Eradication in Mexico', in *Western Medicine as Contested Knowledge*, ed. Andrew Cunningham and Bridie Andrews (Manchester: Manchester University Press, 1997), 147–71. For the activities of the Rockefeller Foundation in Southeast Asia, see Liew Kai Khiun, 'Wats and Worms: The Activities of the Rockefeller Foundation's International Health Board in Southeast Asia (1913–1940)', in *Global Movements, Local Concerns: Medicine and Health in Southeast Asia*, ed. Laurence Monnais and Harold J. Cook (Singapore: Singapore University Press, 2012), 43–61.

[14] On Hydrick's experiences in Java, see Terence H. Hull, 'Conflict and Collaboration in Public Health: The Rockefeller Foundation and the Dutch Colonial Government in Indonesia', in *Public Health in Asia and the Pacific: Historical and Comparative Perspectives*, ed. Milton Lewis and Kerrie L. MacPherson (New York: Routledge, 2007) and Han Mesters, 'J. L. Hydrick

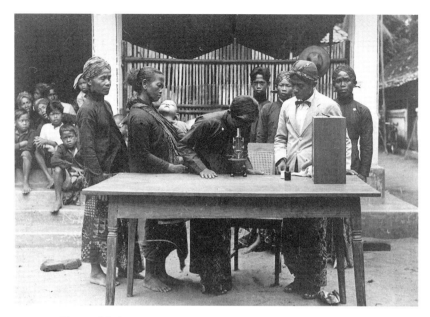

Figure 6.2 A Javanese man from the Banyumas region views the worms found in his stool through a microscope. Figure courtesy of the National Museum of Ethnology, Leiden (TM10014113)

initiatives, and Hydrick repeatedly encountered resistance, obstruction, and even sabotage.[15] The European physicians assigned to assist him were either unsuitable or disinterested in public health work. Despite this, the Medical-Hygiene Propaganda Division produced large numbers of health films. These contained enlarged images of hookworms and the mosquitos which transmitted malaria and greatly impressed indigenous audiences.[16] Indonesian physicians were appreciative of Hydrick's initiatives because they addressed the endemic ill health of the Indonesian population, and several participated in the Rockefeller projects.

in the Netherlands Indies: An American View of Dutch Public Health Policy', in *Health Care in Java: Past and Present*, ed. Peter Boomgaard, Rosalia Sciortino, and Ines Smyth (Leiden: KITLV Press, 1996), 51–62.

[15] See Hull, 'Conflict and Collaboration', and Letter by John Lee Hydrick to Wilbur A. Sawyer, 17 December 1935. Rockefeller Archive Centre, Rockefeller Foundation, Record Group 1.1, Project 655 Java.

[16] John Lee Hydrick, 'Health Education by the Public Health Service of the Netherlands East Indies', *Mededeelingen van den Burgelijken Geneeskundigen Dienst* 16 (1927), 476–89; Eric Andrew Stein, 'Colonial Theatres of Proof: Representation and Laughter in 1930s Rockefeller Foundation Hygiene Cinema in Java', *Health and History* 8, no. 2 (2006), 14–44.

In the early 1930s, Hydrick established comprehensive health demonstration projects in several villages around Purwokerto, in Banyumas regency – a poor, rural area in Central Java.[17] He first surveyed health conditions, the state of households, and the availability of fresh drinking water. Local civil servants assisted by drawing elaborate maps and numbering households. Indies physicians established a population census which included births, deaths, and marriages. From these data, a region's health could be gauged and health interventions assessed. Hydrick aimed to motivate the indigenous population to actively participate in public health. He addressed local ideas and habits, and sought to impart modern, hygienic habits which would improve health and labour productivity. Programs emphasised simple everyday measures to promote health, such as boiling water before drinking it, sweeping yards, washing hands, and defecating in latrines. Indies physicians trained hygiene assistants [*mantris*] to visit households and instruct families in making toothbrushes and other tools from cheap materials, and latrine construction (Figure 6.3). These assistants were familiar with local conditions, attitudes, religious beliefs, and status differences as well as indigenous sensitivities towards health, disease, and the body (Figure 6.4). Indies physicians instructed schoolteachers, who incorporated the principles of hygiene in their teaching. They also trained traditional birth attendants [*dukun bayi*] to practise their craft in a hygienic manner.[18] Assisted by nurses, birth attendants provided maternal and child care in modest clinics constructed from bamboo. In 1936, a Hygiene Mantri School was founded in Purwokerto.

In 1937, the Rockefeller Foundation initiated a hygiene demonstration project in the densely populated Tanah Tinggi neighbourhood near the Batavia Medical School. This neighbourhood had 26,000 residents of whom 22,000 were Indonesian. The project afforded medical students experience in public health projects, thereby supporting instruction at the Wilhelmina Institute of Hygiene and Bacteriology, which had been established in 1933.[19] Hygiene

---

[17] On the Purwokerto program, see Eric Andrew Stein, 'Hygiene and Decolonization: The Rockefeller Foundation and Indonesian Nationalism, 1933–1958', in *Science, Public Health, and the State in Modern Asia*, ed. Liping Bu, Darwin H. Stapleton, and Ka-Che Yip (New York: Routledge), 2012), 51–70, and Eric Andrew Stein, 'Vital Times: Power, Public Health, and Memory in Rural Java' (PhD, University of Michigan, 2005). My discussion of Hydrick's activities and the Banyumas health demonstration projects have been informed by Stein's excellent scholarship. For Hydrick's own account, see J. L. Hydrick, *Intensive Rural Hygiene Work and Public Health Education of the Public Health Service of Netherlands India* (Batavia: Author, 1937).

[18] A school for midwives in Batavia existed at various times; its graduates had difficulty finding a place in small villages and preferred to stay in urban settings. See Liesbeth Hesselink, *Healers on the Colonial Market: Native Doctors and Midwives in the Dutch East Indies* (Leiden: KITLV Press, 2011).

[19] Johan W. Tesch, *The Hygiene Study Ward Centre at Batavia: Planning and Preliminary Results, 1937–1941* (Leiden: Universitaire Pers, 1947); see also Terence H. Hull, *Looking Back to the*

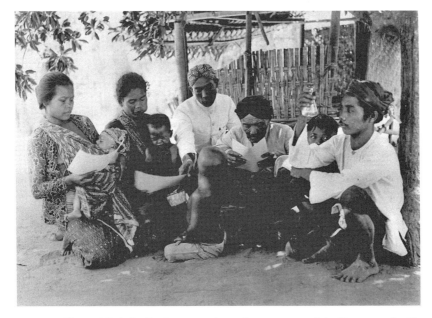

Figure 6.3 A family demonstration at home as part of the Banyumas health demonstration project. Figure courtesy of the National Museum of Ethnology, Leiden (TM60012961)

assistants and local civil servants completed a census and made comprehensive surveys of dwelling types, the availability and quality of the drinking water, the location and nature of privies, the composition of households, and the state of health of every resident. They also provided public health education in hygiene centres and made house visits. Indies physicians coordinated the activities of the clinics that were already operating in the neighbourhood and organised an infant welfare centre. Students and staff of the Batavia Medical School undertook research projects on tuberculosis and diphtheria.[20] Both the Banyumas and Tanah Tinggi health projects aimed to demonstrate how public health measures could be organised and implemented in the Dutch East Indies.

Throughout his stay in the Indies, Hydrick found it difficult to interest European physicians in public health. The professors at the Batavia Medical

---

Hygiene Study Ward: A Brief Guide to the Literature (Canberra: Australian National University, Research School of Social Sciences, 1995).

[20] The results of the diphtheria project were reported in J. E. Dinger, R. Soekonto, and J. W. Tesch, 'Investigation into the Epidemiology of Diphtheria in the Hygiene Study War at Batavia', *Documenta Neerlandica et Indonesica de Morbis Tropicis* 1, no. 1 (1949), 3–33.

School were only mildly interested.[21] Because they shared general stereotypes about the backwardness of the indigenous population, most were convinced that teaching them the principles of health and hygiene was futile. Indies physicians, in contrast, were keenly interested. Hydrick employed several, and some worked their way up to key positions. Arifin, for example, directed the Medical-Hygiene Propaganda Division from 1935 to 1938 and the Purwokerto demonstration unit from 1938 to 1942. He had been a member of the Volksraad and had praised the Banyumas demonstration project in that capacity.[22] Raden Mochtar, from Purwokerto, took over the Medical-Hygiene Propaganda Division following Hydrick's departure in 1938. He received a Master of Public Health from Harvard University in 1951 and was appointed professor of public health at the University of Indonesia, where he continued to oversee both health demonstration projects.[23]

By emphasising public health initiatives, the officers of the Rockefeller Foundation provided a viable alternative to the principles informing the organisation of medical care in the Indies, which was curative in orientation, and relied on well-equipped hospitals and the direct ministration of physicians. Historian Eric A. Stein argues that 'the coming of the Rockefeller Foundation rural hygiene projects on Java in the 1920s enabled indigenous physicians to break with the orthodoxy of Dutch clinical practice and engage directly with vast rural publics.'[24] For a number of Indies physicians, public health projects like Hydrick's realised their nationalist ideals – they served the Indonesian population far more effectively than the hospitals and the clinics of the Public Health Service. Hydrick's projects were recognised as successful both within and without the Dutch East Indies, and were seen as models for future initiatives. They catapulted a number of Indies physicians into prominence on an international stage, and several started to participate in international health organisations and shaped debates on the optimal organisation of health care. J. Offringa, head of the Indies Public Health Service from 1931 to 1938, considered the Banyumas project the 'centre of rural hygiene' in the colony and hoped that similar projects were implemented in all regencies.[25]

[21] W. S. Carter, Report of March 1928 on the University Faculty of Medicine. Archives of the Rockefeller Foundation, Record Group 1.1, Projects: 655 Java, Box 1, Folder 3, File 655A 'Medical Education in Java', JAV-1.

[22] Arifin, 'Begroting, Dienst der Volksgezondheid, 19 July 1934', in *Handelingen van den Volksraad, Zittingsjaar 1934–1935* (Batavia: Landsdrukkerij, 1934), 306.

[23] Hull, *Looking Back to the Hygiene Study Ward*.

[24] Stein, 'Hygiene and Decolonization', 55.

[25] Letter, J. Offringa (head of the Dutch East Indies Public Health Service) to the Minister of Colonies, dated 3 January 1936, quoted in Stein, 'Vital Times', 48. See also Letter, John Lee Hydrick to Victor G. Heiser, dated 29 June 1932; Letter, John Lee Hydrick to Victor G. Heiser, dated 8 July 1932; Letter, John Lee Hydrick to Victor G. Heiser, dated 1 September 1932. Rockefeller Foundation Archives, Record Group 1.1. Projects 655 Java, Box 1, Folder 4, File 655J Public Health Demonstrations, 1932–1934.

Hydrick's demonstration projects received much attention at the 1937 Intergovernmental Conference of Far Eastern Countries on Rural Hygiene, which was held in Bandung, a new and modern city close to Batavia known as the 'Paris of the East'.[26] The conference was organised by the League of Nations Health Organisation (LNHO) and hosted many physicians and colonial administrators from Southeast Asia. Partly sponsored by the Rockefeller Foundation, the LNHO was established in 1920 to promote international collaboration in health. Hydrick had chaired the preparatory committee on Health and Medical Services and his influence is apparent from its report.[27] Conference attendees went on an excursion to Purwokerto to observe the Rockefeller project themselves. Hydrick set out its principles in a booklet, including photographs, which was widely disseminated by the Foundation.[28] The report of the Bandung conference lauded prevention and public health education as the most economic methods of improving the health of rural populations, something which involved 'enrolling the local people themselves to cooperate in the task of their own improvement'.[29] According to historian Sunil Amrith, the Bandung conference was a pivotal moment in the formation of transnational alliances in public health work, and Hydrick's project was a prime example of the transformation of 'local expertise into a global discourse on health'.[30] Rural hygiene initiatives in Southeast Asia 'provided space', argues Amrith, 'for unlikely intellectual alliances between colonial officials, scientists, and Asian nationalists'.[31]

The participants of the Bandung conference advocated a comprehensive and holistic perspective on health which took local social, economic, political, and cultural factors into account.[32] Interestingly, Hydrick had not addressed the adverse economic conditions in the region, where most sugar mills had closed and inhabitants had, of necessity, returned to subsistence farming.[33] Villagers

[26] On the importance of the Bandung conference, see Theodore M. Brown and Elizabeth Fee, 'The Bandoeng Conference of 1937: A Milestone in Health and Development', *American Journal of Public Health* 98, no. 1 (2008), 40–43. See also Annick Guénel, 'The 1937 Bandung Conference on Rural Hygiene: Toward a New Vision of Healthcare?', in *Global Movements, Local Concerns: Medicine and Health in Southeast Asia*, ed. Laurence Monnais and Harold J. Cook (Singapore: Singapore University Press, 2012), 62–80; Sunil S. Amrith, *Decolonizing International Health: India and Southeast Asia, 1930–1965* (Basingstoke: Palgrave Macmillan, 2006), 36–42.

[27] League of Nations Health Organisation, *Intergovernmental Conference of Far-Eastern Countries on Rural Hygiene: Report of the Preparatory Committee* (Geneva: League of Nations Health Organisation, 1937).

[28] Hydrick, *Intensive Rural Hygiene Work.*

[29] League of Nations Health Organisation, *Report Preparatory Committee*, 442.

[30] Amrith, *Decolonizing International Health*, 36–42, 29.

[31] Amrith, *Decolonizing International Health*, 29.

[32] Guénel, 'The 1937 Bandung Conference', 70–72.

[33] Stein, 'Colonial Theatres of Proof', 32.

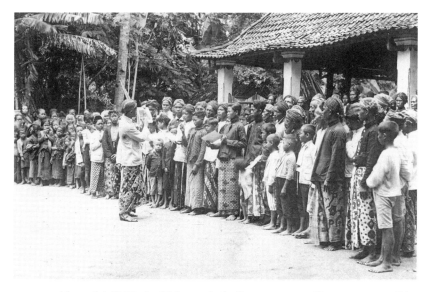

Figure 6.4 Public health lesson in the Banyumas area. Figure courtesy of the
National Museum of Ethnology, Leiden (TM10014114)

often went hungry and physicians frequently observed children with hunger
oedema. Hydrick's project was based on the naïve idea that good health would
eventually stimulate economic productivity. This same naiveté was present in
the arguments of both the colonial administration and Indies physicians: the
idea that health could be had on the cheap if only the population could be
motivated to desire it was appealing during the Great Depression. The concep-
tion that unfavourable economic conditions adversely effected health was not
present in their deliberations.

Abdul Rasjid: *Adat* Enthusiast and Advocate of
Medical Nationalism

Abdul Rasjid (whose full name was Abdul Rasjid *gelar* Maharadja Mahkota
Soangkoepon) was a scion of a Batak aristocratic family. His uncle was chief of
the largest district [*kuria*] near Sipirok, in the South Tapanuli area of the Batak
highlands in northern Sumatra. Rasjid graduated from the STOVIA in 1914
and worked for the colonial medical service in Sumatra for eleven years, except
in 1919, when he was placed at the Batavia Medical College as an assistant
instructor in surgery. During his employment by the colonial medical service, Rasjid was involved in malaria eradication campaigns, which eliminated
breeding sites for the mosquito larvae that transferred the disease. In 1926,

he established a private practice in Padang Sidempuan and, subsequently, in Sipirok – both in South Tapanuli. He was the first chairman of the Batak Association [Batakkersbond] and set up the Batak Study Fund. In 1931, he was elected to the Volksraad; his brother had already been a member for three years. Both remained members until the Japanese annexation of the Indies in 1942. The Soangkoepon brothers were moderate and pragmatic nationalists who were able to work within the confines of the repressive colonial administration. They aligned themselves, most of the time, with Husni Thamrin's national faction.[34] Rasjid was known as a soft-spoken parliamentarian who filled his lengthy and convoluted speeches with philosophical wisdom, similes and metaphors, and Islamic teachings – subtly but sharply critical of the colonial administration. One commentator characterised him as 'a *whispering baritone*, or, at least a *whispering tenor*, using flowery language and graciously smiling while, at the same time, hiding the disagreeable prickliness of the bouquet of roses he appeared to offer'.[35] Rasjid once characterised the Batak, his ethnic group, as profoundly intractable; many thought him a perfect example.

During the Depression years, the colonial administration embarked on an ambitious decentralisation program to acquaint Indonesians with democratic institutions at the local level. Aceh-veteran and arch-conservative future prime minister Hendrikus Colijn and other leading conservative politicians were convinced that the archipelago's various ethnic groups were governed most effectively at the local level because each group had its own *adat* and was at a different level of development.[36] Pivotal to decentralisation was the implementation of codified versions of *adat*, containing traditional and often implicit prescriptions with respect to land tenure, marriage, the entitlement and responsibilities of local rulers, and conflict resolution.[37] Ethical politicians had previously tried to develop a unified legal code for the whole archipelago, but leading legal scholar Cornelis van Vollenhoven argued that Indies law should prioritise local custom, and that introducing a uniform and necessarily alien

---

[34] A number of their speeches were published on the occasion of Soangkoepon's tenth anniversary as a member of the Volksraad: Soangkoepon and Abdul Rasjid, *Redevoeringen van de Leden van den Volksraad de Heeren: Abdul Firman gelar Maharadja Soangkoepon en Abdul Rasjid gelar Maharadja Mahkota Soangkoepon over het Zittingsjaar 1936–1937* (Buitenzorg: Buitenzorgsche Drukkerij, 1937). As Susan Abeyasekere has argued, cooperating and moderate Indonesian nationalists have mostly escaped historical attention. See Susan Abeyasekere, *One Hand Clapping: Indonesian Nationalists and the Dutch, 1939–1942* (Melbourne: Centre of Southeast Asian Studies, Monash University, 1976).

[35] 'Van de Tribune', *Nieuws van den dag voor Nederlandsch Indië*, 14 July 1937, 1. Italics in the original; italicised words in English in the original. See also ' "Oosterse Poezie": Bloemrijk Betoog van Dr. Rasjid', *Sumatra Post*, 24 July 1939, Section IV, 1.

[36] Hendrikus Colijn, *Koloniale Vraagstukken van Heden en Morgen* (Amsterdam: Standaard, 1928).

[37] See the historical chapters in Jamie S. Davidson and David Henley, *The Revival of Tradition in Indonesian Politics: The Deployment of Adat from Colonialism to Indigenism* (London, New York: Routledge, 2007).

legal code would be counterproductive.[38] Van Vollenhoven was inspired by German Romanticism and the legal philosophy of Friedrich Karl von Savigny, the main advocate of the German Legal-Historical School, which held that each ethnic group [*Volk*] was a living organism with its own legal system [*Recht*], and that legal codes should reflect these intuitive legal understandings.[39]

In the 1920s, European scholars, colonial administrators, and Indonesian nationalists began to emphasise the profound differences between East and West. They praised the authenticity, spirituality, and vibrancy of the archipelago's indigenous traditions, and idealised its organic, peaceful village communities, which they contrasted with the bureaucratic, atomised, anonymous, materialistic, and individualistic culture dominant in urbanised and industrialised Western societies.[40] Many used the popular sociological distinction between community [*Gemeinschaft*] and society [*Gesellschaft*], coined by the German sociologist Ferdinand Tönnies, to express their disenchantment with modern life.[41] In a similar vein, economist J. H. Boeke emphasised the fundamental differences between modern Western economies and the cooperative and self-sufficient life of Eastern traditional communities.[42] Theosophists were fascinated by Eastern mysticism and by Javanese spirituality, which had been obliterated elsewhere by rampant materialism. Advocates of these various forms of modernist orientalism warned of the social disintegration and cultural dislocation which inevitably followed the exposure of traditional communities to Western influences. Turning away from earlier impulses towards development and modernity, many now emphasised the importance of protecting and reviving precious indigenous traditions.

Colonial administrators engaged in *adat* restoration by resurrecting long-forgotten and discredited aristocratic lineages, often appointing unknown individuals as traditional chiefs in places where none had existed before. To paraphrase Ernest Gellner's analysis of the interest in traditional cultures

---

[38] For an overview of these developments, see Cees Fasseur, 'Colonial Dilemma: Van Vollenhoven and the Struggle between Adat Law and Western Law in Indonesia', in *The Revival of Tradition in Indonesian Politics: The Deployment of Adat from Colonialism to Indigenism*, ed. Jamie S. Davidson and David Henley (London, New York: Routledge, 2007), 50–67, and Peter Burns, *The Leiden Legacy: Concepts of Law in Indonesia* (Leiden: KITLV Press, 2004). See also David Bourchier, *Illiberal Democracy in Indonesia: The Ideology of the Family State* (New York: Routledge, 2014). For Van Vollenhoven's most influential writings, see Cornelis van Vollenhoven, *De Indonesiër en zijn Grond* (Leiden: Brill, 1919); *De Ontdekking van het Adatrecht* (Leiden: Brill, 1928).

[39] Peter Burns, 'Custom, That Is before All Law', in *The Revival of Tradition in Indonesian Politics: The Deployment of Adat from Colonialism to Indigenism*, ed. Jamie S. Davidson and David Henley (London, New York: Routledge, 2007), 72.

[40] Hans Pols, 'Anomie in the Metropolis: The City in American Sociology and Psychiatry', *OSIRIS*, no. 18 (2003), 194–211.

[41] Ferdinand Tönnies, *Gemeinschaft und Gesellschaft: Grundbegriffe der Reinen Soziologie*, 2nd edn (Berlin: Karl Curtius, 1912).

[42] J. H. Boeke, *Dualistische Economie* (Leiden: Van Doesburgh, 1930).

commonly found in modernising agrarian societies, this interest in *adat* resembled creating botanical gardens in which all plants native to specific areas were represented in carefully tended flowerbeds organised according to a European classificatory scheme. Trained personnel optimised their inherent features by using fertiliser, regulating environmental conditions, administering the optimal amount of water, and regularly pruning the precious plants in their care.[43] The *adat* revival in the Indies was led by the educated and westernised Indonesian elite and the colonial administration, and did not represent the awakening of a long-dormant indigenous soul. Critics argued that it acted against the nationalist program, which hoped to unite all ethnic groups on the basis of their shared identity as colonial subjects. They resented the fact that Dutch politicians and *adat* scholars were turning the Indies into a vast *adat* museum, forestalling further development. For others, however, including a number of leading Indonesian nationalists, *adat* was something precious. It represented the unique communal spirit of cooperation, consensus-seeking, and mutual assistance inherent in Indonesia's traditional communities. It was precisely this spirit that needed to be protected against self-serving incursions by colonising powers. In addition to providing arguments against colonialism, traditional culture was central to building social solidarity, indigenous pride, and political resistance against the Dutch colonial administration.

In his speeches to the Volksraad, Rasjid endorsed the decentralisation policies of the colonial administration. Only traditional local leaders had an intuitive and holistic understanding of the cultural traditions of their ethnic group, he argued, and only they were aware of local conditions and concerns as well as local religious and cultural sensitivities. Like van Vollenhoven, Rasjid used biological metaphors to describe traditional communities as organisms, and recommended 'a medical way of thinking on a social and political level', which meant that 'the further development of organic communities should be based on the principles that already govern them.'[44]

We have to conclude that each ethnic group in which all members are bound by a psychological bond and all are animated by a common spirit as well as common interests and desires, constitutes a living organism, and is therefore subject to the laws of life, such as those relating to growth, revival, and decay. It then also follows that each ethnic group has to follow its own line of experience on the basis of its own institutions, which are rooted in the life of that community itself.[45]

---

[43] Ernest Gellner, *Nations and Nationalism*, 2nd edn (Malden, MA: Blackwell, 2006), 48–51.

[44] Abdul Rasjid, 'Algemeene Beschouwingen, 9 November 1940', in *Handelingen van den Volksraad, Zittingsjaar 1940–41* (Batavia: Landsdrukkerij, 1940), 801. See also Abdul Rasjid, 'Algemeene Beschouwingen, 9 July 1931', in *Handelingen van den Volksraad, Zittingsjaar 1931–1932* (Batavia: Landsdrukkerij, 1931), 93–95.

[45] Rasjid, 'Binnenlandsch Bestuur, 7 August 1931', 819. See also Abdul Rasjid, 'Algemeene Beschouwingen, 15 July 1932', in *Handelingen van den Volksraad, Zittingsjaar 1932–1933* (Batavia: Landsdrukkerij, 1932), 360–65.

Only the traditional leaders of each ethnic group were able to 'listen to the beating heart of the people'.[46] Because traditional communities were best viewed as organisms, Rasjid argued, a medical approach was most suited to understanding their internal dynamics, and physicians were their natural leaders. Rasjid criticised medical researchers for their exclusive interest in theoretical knowledge of disease rather than diseased individuals, and urged his fellow Indies physicians to work in their own communities. He was critical of those physicians who disparaged their cultural heritage in their eagerness to imitate Europeans, living Western lives in urban centres where lucrative private practices could be sustained. Instead, Rasjid urged them to become leaders in their communities and opt for a simpler and more authentic lifestyle.[47]

At first, Rasjid's idealistic and evocative visions were not accompanied by practical suggestions for their translation into Indonesian medical care. This changed in 1935, when he visited the Rockefeller demonstration project around Purwokerto and saw 'all the public hygiene ideas I had cherished for a long time applied in their full glory'.[48] From that moment, Rasjid became one of the most enthusiastic and persistent advocates of the Rockefeller health programs. In the Volksraad, he praised the 'powerful impulses that continuously emanate from the Rockefeller Foundation, which have demonstrated that it has a keen eye for the interests of the silent masses'.[49] He continuously promoted the Foundation's health demonstration projects and called for their multiplication across the archipelago. To accomplish this, he favoured splitting the Public Health Service into two: a minor branch devoted to curative care and a more substantial one to 'the realisation of ideas presented in the booklet of Dr. Hydrick'.[50] Prevention was better than cure, Rasjid announced, and all who recognised 'this fundamental truth will have to accede that the fundamental work of Dr. Hydrick at Purwokerto has to be regarded as the correct one, considered from the perspective of the interest of the people'.[51] Rasjid incorporated the principles behind the Rockefeller projects into his medical nationalism: public health programs were the most efficient way to improve the health and physical strength of the Indonesian population. It was a striking appropriation. A number of historians of medicine have interpreted Rockefeller initiatives in the non-Western world as efforts to make indigenous populations more productive – efforts which served exploitative colonial economic

---

[46] Rasjid, 'Algemeene Beschouwingen, 9 July 1931', 513.
[47] Abdul Rasjid, 'Dienst der Volksgezondheid, 21 July 1936', in *Handelingen van den Volksraad, Zittingsjaar 1936–1937* (Batavia: Landsdrukkerij, 1936), 285–55.
[48] Abdul Rasjid, 'Dienst der Volksgezondheid, 17 February 1936', in *Handelingen van den Volksraad, Zittingsjaar 1935–1936* (Batavia: Landsdrukkerij, 1936), 1774.
[49] Rasjid, 'DVG 17 February 1936', 1773.
[50] Rasjid, 'DVG 21 July 1936', 387.
[51] Rasjid, 'Dienst der Volksgezondheid, 20 August 1936', 1139.

interests.[52] Here, however, Rockefeller initiatives met with apathy in the colonial Public Health Service but inspired Indies physicians who saw their medicine as a means of nation-building.

Abdul Rasjid and the Association of Indonesian Physicians

The Association of Indies Physicians languished during the Great Depression. Members wishing to publish their research were encouraged to submit their articles to the *Medical Journal of the Dutch Indies* after the Association's *Bulletin* folded.[53] In 1936, members of the Semarang branch founded a new journal, *Medical Reports* [*Medische Berichten*]. It was edited by Mas Sardjito, who had studied at the University of Amsterdam and, with support from the Rockefeller Foundation, at the Johns Hopkins University. He held a position at the Semarang Central Civil Hospital and was a rising star in the Association – after independence, he became the founding president of the University of Gadjah Mada. The following year, the Association celebrated its twenty-fifth anniversary with a reception for 200 at a fashionable restaurant in Batavia.[54] Kaijadoe commemorated the Association's efforts towards greater appreciation of Indies physicians and presented a memorial volume to the director of the Public Health Service.[55] Members responded with several laudatory speeches praising Kaijadoe and Tehupeiory. Three months later, Kaijadoe received a knighthood in the Order of Orange-Nassau.[56]

---

[52] E. Richard Brown, 'Public Health in Imperialism: Early Rockefeller Programs at Home and Abroad', *American Journal of Public Health* 66, no. 9 (1976), 897–903. For a more elaborate analysis, see E. Richard Brown, *Rockefeller Medicine Men: Medicine and Capitalism in America* (Berkeley: University of California Press, 1979). Similar views can be found in more recent works. See, for example, Howard Waitzkin, *Medicine and Public Health at the End of Empire* (New York: Routledge, 2015). More recent scholarship on the health initiatives of the Rockefeller Foundation has painted a more nuanced picture while remaining critical of some aspects; see, for example: Marcus Cueto, *Missionaries of Science: The Rockefeller Foundation and Latin America* (Bloomington: Indiana University Press, 1994); Anne-Emmauelle Birn, *Marriage of Convenience: Rockefeller International Health and Revolutionary Mexico* (Rochester, NY: University of Rochester Press, 2006); Schneider, *Rockefeller Philanthropy*. John Farley explicitly argues against the interpretation of Rockefeller health initiatives as imperialist in nature: Farley, *To Cast Out Disease*.

[53] 'Hoofdbestuursmededeelingen', *Orgaan der Vereeniging van Indische Geneeskundigen* 21, no. 1–2 (1933), 2.

[54] 'De Bond van Indische Artsen: Onder Groote Belangstelling der Medische Wereld Heeft het Bestuur een Drukbezochte Receptie Gehouden', *Het Nieuws van den Dag voor Nederlandsch-Indië*, 30 August 1937, Section II, 3; 'Jaarverslag over 1937', *Orgaan der Vereeniging van Indische Geneeskundigen* 25 (1937), 1–4.

[55] Hoofdbestuur, 'Verslag over de Viering van het 25-Jaar Bestaan Onzer Vereeniging te Batavia-Centrum', *Orgaan der Vereeniging van Indische Geneeskundigen* 26, no. 1–2 (1938), 2; *Jubileumnummer 1911–1936: Orgaan Vereeniging van Indische Geneeskundigen* (Batavia: Kolff, 1937).

[56] 'J. Kayadoe', *Het Nieuws van den Dag voor Nederlandsch-Indië*, 16 October 1937, Section IX, 3.

In the late 1930s, Rasjid revived the moribund Association as a vehicle for the realisation of his medical nationalism. In 1937, he criticised the low remuneration of Indies physicians in a speech to the Volksraad, helping him gain their confidence.[57] The following year, 'the most restless one in the life of our Association', Rasjid rewrote the Association's constitution, and worked behind the scenes to oust the board and instal a new one under his leadership.[58] He was elected president during the Association's first congress, held in December 1938, at which it was renamed the Association of Indonesian Physicians. Rasjid's energetic leadership ushered in a period of unprecedented activity. Two large congresses were held in quick succession (Christmas 1938 and Easter 1940; a third congress, planned for 1942, was cancelled after the Japanese annexation). Chapters were established in several cities and a small congress with chapters' delegates was held over Easter in 1941 at Purwokerto. The Association's journal was renamed the *Medical Tribune* [*Medisch Tribune*] and appeared monthly. Membership rose from around 100 in 1938 to more than 500 in 1940 with less than a dozen Indies physicians in the archipelago opting out. At the end of 1940, the Association opened its own headquarters in Batavia.

In his presidential address to the Association's first conference, Rasjid claimed that Indies physicians were crucial mediators between East and West, and had an important role in the archipelago's future: 'Indies physicians will have to be one of the levers for the development of the Indonesian population.'[59] Although it was unfortunate that they did not receive the respect they deserved, he emphasised that the Association was primarily a professional group focused on the health of the Indonesian people rather than the remuneration of its members: Indies physicians should focus their attention on building the health and physical strength of the future nation and abstain from political activity. Tehupeiory, honorary chairman, agreed: Indies physicians should 'retreat to the pure and scientific medical terrain, especially as there is still so much to do to achieve the goal of a healthy and strong population'.[60] Kaijadoe, the outgoing chairman, added that public health was one of the main pillars of Indonesian society.[61] Rasjid's medical nationalism allowed physicians averse

[57] Abdul Rasjid, 'Dienst der Volksgezondheid, 15 Sep 1937', in *Handelingen van den Volksraad, Zittingsjaar 1937–1938* (Batavia: Landsdrukkerij, 1937), 1413–15.
[58] Bahder Djohan, 'Verslag over 1938', *Medisch Tribune* 27, no. 3 (1939), 17.
[59] Abdul Rasjid, 'Beschouwingen over de Positie van den Ind.-Arts', in *Het Eerste Congres van de Vereeniging van Indonesische Geneeskundigen* (Batavia: Kenanga, 1938), 10; Abdul Rasjid quoted in *Medisch Tribune* 27, no 3 (March 1939), 10. As Rasjid could not attend the congress, his speech was read by Bahder Djohan.
[60] W. K. Tehupeiory, 'Openingsrede', in *Het Eerste Congres van de Vereeniging van Indonesische Geneeskundigen* (Batavia: Kenanga, 1938), 14.
[61] J. Kaijadoe, 'Enkele Medische Problemen Hier te Lande', in *Het Eerste Congres van de Vereeniging van Indonesische Geneeskundigen* (Batavia: Kenanga, 1938), 16.

to political involvement to join hands with their nationalist colleagues. The Association's name change was fuelled by a desire to welcome the graduates of the Batavia Medical School and Indonesian physicians with European medical degrees.[62] Only Kaijadoe objected – he wanted the Association to remain an interest group for Indies physicians only. In a politically astute move, Rasjid insisted that no one should be excluded from membership on the basis of ethnicity or race, and that the 'Indonesian' in the Association's name referred to the territory and not to ethnicity or race.[63]

The Public Health Service's decentralisation program was discussed by a number of speakers.[64] Rasjid was in favour because he thought that effective health projects were best organised at a local level. Raden Mochtar argued that it was necessary in bringing the benefits of modern medicine to the great majority of Indonesians living in the countryside:

We only have to fly with our modern automobiles over the asphalt of the Lord's highways to realise that, within a mere twenty-five meters to the left and right of our roads, are located the miserable huts of *Kromo* [the common Indonesian villager], whose backwardness and sterile culture has caused many severe headaches to educated individuals.[65]

He unreservedly praised public health education as an essential part of a larger mission stimulating development and nation-building. Other speakers encouraged their colleagues to open and run their own hospitals and clinics.[66] Closing the first congress, Bahder Djohan exclaimed: 'Out of the old association a new one is born, imbued with new vigour and new ideas. Let us all gather under the new banner: the elevation of our Country and People.'[67]

---

[62] Djohan, 'Verslag over 1938', 18.

[63] Moewardi, 'Verslag van het Secretariaat, Uitgebracht aan het Congres te Solo', *Medisch Tribune* 28, no. 5 (1940) 136; Abdul Rasjid, 'Rede, Uitgesproken op de in Sept j.l. Gehouden Vergadering van de Afdeeling Batavia', *Medische Tribune* 28, no. 10 (1940), 269.

[64] S. B. Zahar, 'Over den Positie van den Regentschapsarts', in *Het Eerste Congres van de Vereeniging van Indonesische Geneeskundigen* (Batavia: Kenanga, 1938), 56–68; R. Poerwosoewardjo, 'De Organisatie van den Regentschapsgezondheidsdienst', in *Het Eerste Congres van de Vereeniging van Indonesische Geneeskundigen* (Batavia: Kenanga, 1938). 74–90; R. M. Wirasmo Partaningrat, 'Positie en Instructie van den Regentschapsgeneeskundige', in *Het Tweede Congres van de Vereeniging van Indonesische Geneeskundigen* (Batavia: Kenanga, 1940), 64–95; Soemedi, 'De Noodzakelijkheid van een Goede Opleiding bij het Intensief Hygiënewerk', in *Het Tweede Congres van de Vereeniging van Indonesische Geneeskundigen* (Batavia: Kenanga, 1940), 125–43.

[65] R. Mochtar, 'De Decentralisatie van den Dienst der Volksgezondheid', in *Het Eerste Congres van de Vereeniging van Indonesische Geneeskundigen* (Batavia: Kenanga, 1938), 45.

[66] R. Kodijat, 'Specialistische Kliniek', in *Het Tweede Congres van de Vereeniging van Indonesische Geneeskundigen* (Batavia: Kenanga, 1940), 5–18; R. Seno [Sastroamidjojo], 'Algemeen Ziekenhuis', in *Het Tweede Congres van de Vereeniging van Indonesische Geneeskundigen* (Batavia: Kenanga, 1940), 19–34.

[67] Bahder Djohan, 'Verslag over het 1e Congres van de Vereeniging van Indonesische Geneeskundigen op 24, 25 en 26 December 1938 te Semarang', *Medisch Tribune* 27, no. 3 (1939), 16.

Boentaran Martoatmodjo, later Indonesia's first minister of health, declared that the Association was 'only at the beginning – from December 1938 – of its *organised* thinking and working'.[68]

In July 1939 Rasjid gave his most eloquent, powerful, and controversial Volksraad address. He commenced by declaring that he would discuss the activities of the Public Health Service as an Indonesian nationalist, taking the perspective of the Indonesian population with special attention to its cultural heritage. It was clear, in other words, that he viewed health and medicine from the perspective of an *adat* scholar.[69] Rasjid argued that the Public Health Service should focus on public health initiatives and leave curative care to private initiative. Unfortunately, European physicians with their elaborate scientific training and Western orientation were poorly equipped for this work. Graduates of the Surabaya Medical College were much better suited than those of the Batavia Medical School because Indies physicians maintained much closer ties with their various ethnic groups. It followed, then, that the Public Health Service should be run by Indies physicians, and that the two-tier medical system should be abolished.[70] Rasjid was calling for the decolonisation of the Public Health Service.

Over the next three years, the *Medisch Tribune* published numerous articles about initiatives realising Rasjid's medical nationalism, and the Rockefeller health programs featured regularly. Raden Mochtar, for example, argued that such initiatives were capable of realising the 'full reconstruction … of the spiritual and social constellation of the village-based population'.[71] It was self-evident for Mochtar that 'the Hygienic Organisation essentially forms [one of] the pillars on which, in the distant future, the complete edifice of the state will rest.'[72] The profound influence of Hydrick's health demonstration projects on Rasjid's medical nationalism can be gauged from Rasjid's comments upon his departure from the Indies in 1938: 'Unconsciously, perhaps, you have made, through your science, an important contribution to the establishment of the foundation of Indonesian society.'[73] Rarely has an officer of the Rockefeller Foundation received such high praise.

[68] R. Boentaran Martoatmodjo, 'Openingsrede', *Medisch Tribune* 29, no. 5 (1941), 121.
[69] Abdul Rasjid, 'Dienst der Volksgezondheid, 25 July 1939', in *Handelingen van den Volksraad, Zittingsjaar 1939–40* (Batavia: Landsdrukkerij, 1939), 418–19. This speech was reprinted in full in the *Medisch Tribune* as: 'Uit den Volksraad', *Medisch Tribune* 27, no. 8 (1939), 11–24.
[70] Rasjid, 'DVG 25 July 1939', 420.
[71] R. Mochtar, 'Intensief Hygiënewerk en Medisch-Hygiënische Propaganda, I', *Medisch Tribune* 27, no. 10 (1939), 18.
[72] R. Mochtar, 'Intensief Hygiënewerk en Medisch-Hygiënische Propaganda, III', *Medisch Tribune* 27, no. 12 (1939), 8.
[73] Quoted in 'John Lee Hydrick, M.D.', *Medisch Tribune* 27, no. 8 (1939), 4.

Two speakers at the Association's 1940 Congress added a surprising and novel element to Rasjid's program of medical nationalism by calling for the integration of indigenous herbal medicine [*jamu*] in medical practice. Demonstrating the efficacy of herbal medicine, they believed, would enable Indonesian physicians to revive and modernise age-old healing traditions which the population had relied on from time immemorial. It had the potential to bolster nationalist sentiment since it encouraged Indonesian physicians to use Indonesia's own medicines in preference to expensive, imported pharmaceutical products. Goelarso Hadikoesoemo, formerly a member of the Medical-Hygiene Propaganda Division, opened his address by reviewing generally accepted views on the history of modern Western medicine as the progressive liberation from superstition, religious beliefs, astrology, and alchemy, leading to the triumph of modern science. He lamented that the great majority of the Indonesian population still lived in the Stone Age and was guided by irrational traditions and superstitions. The most pressing dilemma Indonesian physicians faced, argued Goelarso, was the great expense of modern pharmaceutical compounds, which made providing medical care to the whole population unaffordable. By investigating traditional herbal concoctions, researchers could 'eliminate what is superfluous … and retain and possibly modernise what is cheap and what turns out to be good'.[74] The exhibition of several ingredients used in traditional herbal medicine was viewed with great interest by congress attendees. The second speaker, Kanjeng Raden Toemenggoeng Saleh Mangoendiningrat, Radjiman's successor as Solo's court physician, suggested that, by embracing traditional herbal medicine, Indonesian physicians might enjoy the confidence in which the population held traditional healers while providing them with remedies they knew actually worked.[75]

Rasjid enthusiastically endorsed both speakers and urged the Public Health Service to investigate traditional herbal medicine, preferably by Indonesian physicians working in small hospitals.[76] He also presented an elaborate plan for a central research institute, echoing his earlier plans for the systematic investigation of *adat*.[77] In April 1941, the colonial administration established a special

---

[74] Goelarso Astrohadikoesoemo, 'Sedikit Pemandangan tentang Obat-Obat Kita oentoek Diselidiki', in *Het Tweede Congres van de Vereeniging van Indonesische Geneeskundigen* (Batavia: Kenanga, 1940), 219. See also Goelarso Astrohadikoesoemo, 'Onze Eigen Geneesmiddelen', *Medisch Tribune* 28, no. 2 (1940), 35–36.

[75] K. R. T. Saleh Mangoendiningrat, 'Ketabiban didalam Bangsa Indonesia ditanah Djawa', in *Het Tweede Congres van de Vereeniging van Indonesische Geneeskundigen* (Batavia: Kenanga, 1940), 222–47.

[76] Rasjid, 'Dienst der Volksgezondheid, 18 November 1940', 1000–01. Reprinted as 'Uit den Volksraad', *Medisch Tribune* 29, no. 3 (1941), 73–83.

[77] Abdul Rasjid, 'Dienst der Volksgezondheid, 28 July 1941', in *Handelingen van den Volksraad, Zittingsjaar 1941–42* (Batavia: Landsdrukkerij, 1941), 478–82. Reprinted as 'Uit den Volksraad', 245–56.

committee for the study of indigenous herbal medicine featuring Rasjid, Raden Mochtar, and Goelarso as members. After the war, Seno Sastroamidjojo, the Association's vice chairman, published a book which included several traditional prescriptions drawn from research conducted by Dutch physicians more than fifty years prior.[78] Indonesian physicians interested in traditional herbal medicine did not rely on traditional healers; they preferred the insights of Dutch physicians. From Rasjid's perspective, herbal medicine was a form of *adat* – a tradition that deserved careful study by Western-educated physicians who could preserve, transform, improve, systematise, and codify it for use in the modern world. As he argued in a speech to the Volksraad: 'When we assume that the Indonesian population has a cultural heritage, it is reasonable to assume that it is in possession of a science of healing as well.'[79] To return to Gellner's botanical metaphors, the interest of Indonesian physicians in the medicinal fruits of Indonesia's gardens resembled the exploration of a carefully planted botanical garden rather than an intrepid foray into untouched wilderness. Rather than going out into the field, then, Indonesian physicians explored the library of the Batavia Medical School.

In the Dutch East Indies, herbal medications were generally prepared by poor and illiterate women, and traditional healers. Even though Indonesians already used traditional herbal medications on a daily basis and indigenous healing traditions were therefore strong and vibrant, practitioners did not have the social position, financial resources, or political connections to present their craft as a viable alternative to Western medicine. Unlike *Ayurveda* practitioners in India and traditional Chinese physicians, they did not rely on extensive written sources detailing distinct medical philosophies, theories on health and disease, or appropriate treatment methods. *Jamu* peddlers were unable to present themselves as superior medical practitioners or their craft as rivalling Western medicine. Indonesian physicians became the final authorities on *jamu* concoctions since they could assess their efficacy, by the methodology they had learned from Western science.

Despite the Association of Indonesian Physicians adopting a program of medical nationalism, its members continued to speak Dutch at the Association's functions and to write their medical publications in that language (the two presentations on traditional herbal medicine were exceptions; a Dutch translation appeared in the conference proceedings). When a prominent member

---

[78] Seno Sastroamidjojo, *Obat Asli Indonesia* (Djakarta: Kebangsaan Pustaka Rakjat, 1948). For an overview of the Dutch research, see Hans Pols, 'European Botanists and Physicians, Indigenous Herbal Medicine in the Dutch East Indies, and Colonial Networks of Mediation', *East Asian Science, Technology, and Society: An International Journal* 3, no. 2–3 (2009), 245–59.

[79] Abdul Rasjid, 'Eerste Buitengewone Zitting, 18 November 1941', in *Handelingen van den Volksraad, Zittingsjaar 1940–41* (Batavia: Landsdrukkerij, 1941), 1000; reprinted in 'Uit den Volksraad', 73–84.

opted to speak in Dutch at a meeting of the Batavia chapter, he felt the need to justify this by arguing that only a few members could understand Malay.[80] Rasjid noted that a small number of members had a 'volcanic interest' in adopting Malay as the Association's official language.[81] Although he saw that this adhered to the Association's principles, he suggested that Malay should not be introduced hurriedly. Bahder Djohan emphasised the need for preparatory work: an Indonesian medical language still needed to be developed and he expected that this would take several years.[82] He lauded the two physicians for speaking in Malay at the Congress but thought it better for the time being to stick to Dutch.[83] Despite their strengthening nationalism, most Indonesian physicians continued to speak Dutch and remained westernised. This is not altogether surprising; their medical education had profoundly influenced their personalities, cultural preferences, and linguistic abilities. They retained the Dutch ideas and language they acquired in their formative years, then, but their outlook on the role of medicine in Indonesian society had fundamentally changed.[84]

Conclusion

Rasjid's leadership transformed the political orientation and professional outlook of Indonesian physicians. The increased interest in *adat* of European academics and Indonesian administrative officials, the attentiveness towards Indonesia's cultural heritage among Indonesian nationalists, and the Rockefeller Foundation's health demonstration projects inspired a reorientation of Indies physicians' professional philosophy and interests. Instead of concentrating on modernity, politics, medical research, and the many inequities between Indies and European physicians, they now looked to the humble backwaters of the rural villages where most Indonesians lived – to the places that modern life had passed by. Rasjid encouraged his colleagues to focus on the plight of the Indonesian population and to see medicine as a vital means of nation-building.

Dutch *adat* scholars idealised Indonesia's organic communities and exalted the spiritualism inherent in Eastern cosmologies. Dutch conservative politicians appropriated these ideas by advocating a policy of association under

---

[80] Abu Hanifah, 'Gedachten over den Indonesischen Arts en de Maatschappij', *Medisch Tribune* 28, no. 11 (1940), 278.

[81] Abdul Rasjid, 'Oproep', *Medisch Tribune* 28, no. 5 (1940), 124.

[82] Bahder Djohan, 'Indonesich-Medische Taal', *Medisch Tribune* 27, no. 12 (1939), 17.

[83] Bahder Djohan, 'Beknopt Verslag van het 2e Congres', *Medisch Tribune* 28, no. 4 (1940), 101.

[84] Dutch remained the preferred language among the Indonesian educated elite in the 1950s. In his interviews with elderly residents of Batavia who once were part of the educated elite conducted in the 1980s and 1990s, Rudolf Mrázek found that their Dutch roots were still apparent. See Rudolf Mrázek, *A Certain Age: Colonial Jakarta through the Memories of Its Intellectuals* (Durham, NC: Duke University Press, 2010).

which education and health budgets could be drastically reduced. Indonesian nationalists appropriated these ideas as well, using them to indict Dutch colonialism for destroying Indonesian organic communities for monetary gain and to mobilise Indonesians to resist further incursions into their unique cultural life. Addressing a meeting tasked with preparing Indonesia's independence in 1945, Sukarno made mutual assistance [*gotong royong*] one of the five pillars of his *Pancasila* ideology, which provided the philosophical foundation of the Indonesian nation.[85] The 1945 constitution of the Republic of Indonesia, formulated by Soepomo, an Indonesian lawyer who had studied with van Vollenhoven in Leiden, was suffused with similar ideas. Rasjid creatively combined his interest in *adat* with the public health approaches advocated by the Rockefeller Foundation to formulate his medical nationalism. He argued that the social calling of Indonesian physicians was a natural expression of the deep sense of mutual assistance and solidarity prevalent in Indonesian village life.[86]

The health demonstration projects implemented throughout the world by the Rockefeller Foundation have frequently been criticised as preparing rural and backward populations to participate in capitalism by focusing on increasing manpower and labour productivity. During the last few years of the Dutch reign over Indonesia, when the possibility of a Japanese invasion appeared increasingly likely, several Dutch members of the Volksraad argued that social development, economic resilience, physical strength, and the collective health of the indigenous population were inextricably related. Rasjid subscribed to these views, noticing that all these factors were necessary components in the defence of the Indies.[87] Health and national strength went hand in hand and were now of vital interest. Nationalists held strong reservations about the economic exploitation of the archipelago – both its people and its natural resources – and at times doubted the motives for the colonial state's health initiatives. With an eye to the future Indonesian nation, however, the imperatives of health, national strength, and economic productivity made perfect sense. Many colonial health projects could therefore be continued and even strengthened in independent Indonesia.

---

[85] Sukarno gave his famous speech on the birth of *Pancasila* on 1 June 1945 to the Investigating Committee for the Preparation of Independence [Badan Penyelidik Usaha Persiapan Kemerdekaan Indonesia] (BPUPKI), which was meeting in the building formerly used by the Volksraad. See Soekarno, *Lahirnja Pantjasila: Filsafah Indonesia Tertjakup dalam Pantjasila* (Bandung: Duar-r, 1961).

[86] Rasjid, 'Rede Batavia', 265. See also Sn. [Seno Sastroamidjojo], 'De Indonesische Geneeskundige en zijn Gemeenschap', *Medisch Tribune* 29, no. 7 (1941), 187–97; and Hanifah, 'Gedachten', 277–88.

[87] Rasjid, 'Eerste Buitengewone Zitting, 18 November 1941', 999–1003.

7   Indonesian Physicians in the Greater East-Asia Co-Prosperity Sphere

In March 1942, Japanese troops landed on Java. Within a week, the colonial army had surrendered, ending Dutch colonial rule over the archipelago. Large groups of jubilant Indonesians welcomed the triumphant Japanese, who had defeated the much-hated Dutch and promised prosperity and independence through extensive radio propaganda campaigns. But Indonesians were soon disenchanted with the Greater East Asia Co-Prosperity Sphere. They came to detest the arrogance and abuse of the Japanese soldiers, the cruelty of the notorious secret police, the Kenpeitai, the shortage of food and basic necessities, and the forced recruitment of young men to serve in militias and as labourers on defence projects. During the final two years of the war, poverty, starvation, and disease were commonplace. Far from bringing prosperity to the archipelago, the Japanese brought Indonesia to the brink of catastrophe.

The Japanese imperial forces were accompanied by a cadre of physicians who impressed their Indonesian colleagues with appealing views on the role of medicine in nation-building. They urged Indies physicians to abandon their imperialist, Western, and now outdated model of health and medicine, and adopt their superior Asian vision characterised by holism, communitarianism, and a commitment to public health and social medicine. The Japanese model of medical care promised to benefit all Indonesians rather than only a wealthy elite, as had medicine during the Dutch colonial era. The Japanese vision echoed Abdul Rasjid's medical nationalism. The Indonesian medical community reacted to the call of the Japanese doctors in strikingly different ways. The majority of Indies physicians embraced Japanese medical idealism, though their enthusiasm waned during the later years of the annexation. The reaction of Indonesia's small medical elite was mostly opportunistic, consolidating its position by replacing the European incumbents in the archipelago's leading medical institutions. In contrast, Indonesian medical students sided with other disillusioned youth groups to vehemently oppose the new colonial power. The medical student strike in October 1943 was one of the first acts of resistance against the Japanese administration.

The Japanese Conquest of the Dutch East Indies

The armed forces of the Japanese Empire invaded the Dutch East Indies to secure access to the archipelago's rich natural resources, including oil, tin, and rubber.[1] Landing on Java, the Japanese encountered little resistance, and calmly peddled their bicycles to Batavia – soon to be renamed Jakarta – after overwhelming the disorganised Dutch forces. Enthusiastic crowds of Indonesians welcomed the Japanese, expecting deliverance.[2] The Dutch surrendered after one week, and the official capitulation was signed eight days after the first landing.[3] The hopes of Indonesians were promptly quashed. The Japanese administration banned the Indonesian national anthem, the Indonesian flag, and all discussion of independence. Indonesia was partitioned into three administrative zones: Sumatra, Java, and the remaining islands (Kalimantan, Sulawesi, and the eastern Indonesian islands). Contact between these three zones was restricted, precluding Indonesia-wide nationalist activity.[4] The natural resources of Sumatra and Kalimantan required full military control, but since Java was viewed principally as a labour reservoir, its governance was less repressive.[5] The Japanese quickly removed all residue of the Dutch colonial era. The use of Dutch was prohibited and all Europeans were interned. Dutch administrative arrangements, however, were retained, and the Japanese relied on the traditional aristocracy to collect taxes and maintain order. Nationalists were recalled from exile or freed from detention, and invited to lead several propaganda organisations to garner support for Japan and to build the Greater East Asia Co-Prosperity Sphere.[6]

Indonesian nationalists had taken Japan's 1905 victory over Russia as a sign that the supposedly dormant, oppressed peoples of Asia were not inferior to

---

[1] Ken'ichi Gotō, 'Cooperation, Submission, and Resistance of Indigenous Elites of Southeast Asia in the Wartime Empire', in *The Japanese Wartime Empire, 1931–1945*, ed. Peter Duus, Ramon Hawley Myers, and Mark R. Peattie (Princeton, NJ: Princeton University Press, 1996), 274–76. For background information on the Japanese occupation of the Indies, see George Sanford Kanahele, 'The Japanese Occupation of Indonesia: Prelude to Independence' (PhD, Cornell University, 1967); Peter Post, William H. Frederick, Iris Heidebrink, and Shigeru Sato, eds., *The Encyclopedia of Indonesia in the Pacific War* (Leiden: Brill, 2010); the scholarship of Shigeru Sato, Ken'ichi Gotō, and several others.

[2] Kanahele, 'Japanese Occupation', 23–26; a number of students, intellectuals, and journalists had positive experiences with Japanese representatives; a few even visited Japan. See Kanahele, 'Japanese Occupation', 1–18; Ken'ichi Gotō, *Tensions of Empire: Japan and Southeast Asia in the Colonial and Postcolonial World* (Singapore: Singapore University Press, 2003), 107–48.

[3] For details, see P. C. Boer, *The Loss of Java: The Final Battles for the Possession of Java Fought by Allied Air, Naval and Land Forces in the Period of 18 February–7 March 1942* (Singapore: NUS Press, 2011); Kanahele, 'Japanese Occupation', 19–23.

[4] Kanahele, 'Japanese Occupation', 37–40.

[5] Kanahele, 'Japanese Occupation', 35–36.

[6] Aiko Kurasawa, 'Propaganda Media on Java under the Japanese, 1942–1945', *Indonesia*, no. 44 (1987), 59–116.

those of Europe and North America.[7] In the following decades, a number of Indonesian intellectuals came to view Japan as the embodiment of an alternate, Asian path to modernity. It had successfully incorporated European technological progress and fused it with its own cultural heritage without losing its unique, Asian identity. Japan appeared to have become a superior harmonious society in which the more destructive elements of Western civilisation, such as individualism, materialism, and exploitative colonialism, had been eliminated. Japan's pan-Asian ideology strongly resonated with notions of the communitarian nature of Indonesian village life advocated by Rasjid and other leading Indonesian intellectuals, many of whom viewed colonialism as a natural outgrowth of capitalism which necessarily oppressed non-Western populations. The alternative path led by Japan seemed immeasurably more appealing.

Before the Japanese annexation, only a few nationalists had expressed misgivings about the fascist regime to the north. The most prominent were Tjipto Mangoenkoesoemo and Sutan Sjahrir, a close associate of Mohammad Hatta who had spent more than ten years in the Netherlands studying law. They had anticipated a Japanese military incursion and called on Indonesians to cooperate with the Dutch colonial administration in resisting it.[8] Moderate nationalists suggested that indigenous militias might be established in exchange for greater participation in colonial governance. Their advances were rebuffed.[9] After the archipelago's annexation by the Japanese imperial armed forces, most leading nationalists, motivated by a mixture of conviction and opportunism, participated in the Japanese military administration. After Japan's capitulation they would be forced to answer uncomfortable questions about their collaboration with its brutal military regime, and many disappeared from public life. Sukarno, however, was able to reinforce his position as Indonesia's nationalist leader despite his open collaboration with the Japanese.

In the years before the Japanese annexation, both Sjahrir and the left-wing lawyer and political activist Amir Sjarifuddin were popular among the

---

[7] For the views of Indonesian intellectuals on the Asian nature of Indonesian society and their perspectives on both India and Japan, see Ethan Mark, '"Asia's" Transwar Lineage: Nationalism, Marxism, and "Greater Asia" in an Indonesian Inflection', *Journal of Asian Studies* 65, no. 3 (2006), 461–93; and 'The Perils of Co-Prosperity: Takeda Rintaro, Occupied Southeast Asia, and the Seductions of Postcolonial Empire', *American Historical Review* 119, no. 4 (2014), 1184–206. For a historical approach to pan-Asian ideas, see Prasenjit Duara, 'The Discourse of Civilization and Pan-Asianism', *Journal of World History* 12, no. 1 (2001), 99–130; and 'Asia Redux: Conceptualizing a Region for Our Times', *Journal of Asian Studies* 69, no. 4 (2010), 963–83.

[8] Another political activist who held strong reservations towards the Japanese regime because of its fascist nature was Amir Sjarifuddin. For Sjahrir (as well as Sjarifuddin), see Rudolf Mrázek, *Sjahrir: Politics and Exile in Indonesia* (Ithaca, NY: Southeast Asia Program, Cornell University, 1994).

[9] D. M. G. Koch, *Om de Vrijheid: De Nationalistische Beweging in Indonesië* (Jakarta: Jajasan Pembangunan Djakarta, 1946), 130–39.

few students who maintained political interests.[10] After the annexation, they attempted to establish an underground resistance in covert cooperation with Sukarno and Hatta. Amir was arrested in January 1943. Sjahrir continued to travel across Java building the resistance.[11] Sjahrir's popularity and influence among medical students grew steadily during the occupation.[12] The resistance movement was, however, relatively modest, and mostly confined to heated discussions and minor symbolic acts of defiance. Nonetheless, the networks established between young people in these years were of decisive importance during the Indonesian revolution, and afterwards in independent Indonesia. Their leaders became politicians, army generals, senior administrators, business leaders, and influential academics.

Re-establishing Medical Care during the Japanese Occupation

Within weeks after Japan annexed Java, all institutions of higher education closed, including the Surabaya Medical College (NIAS) and the Batavia Medical School (GH). Advanced medical students were permitted to continue their residencies and could sit their final exams twice a year.[13] Because European physicians had been interned, there was an acute shortage of medical personnel. The importation of pharmaceutical products was disrupted, and existing stock was appropriated by the Japanese military. In August 1942, a small group of medical students travelled from Surabaya to Jakarta to meet with fellow students, Rasjid, and several senior physicians who had been associated with the now inoperative Batavia Medical School.[14] Pointing to the urgent need for physicians, they implored the military administration to re-establish medical education. In response, a preparatory committee consisting of former Indonesian instructors was established to develop a

---

[10] Mrázek, *Sjahrir*, 226.
[11] Kanahele, 'Japanese Occupation', 53.
[12] Mrázek, *Sjahrir*, 226–31.
[13] T. Karimoeddin, 'Pendidikan Dokter Jaman Pendudukan Jepang (Ika Dai Gaku)', in *125 Tahun Pendidikan Dokter di Indonesia 1851–1976*, ed. M. A. Hanafiah, Bahder Djohan, and Surono (Jakarta: FKUI, 1976), 26.
[14] Among the students from Surabaya were Soejono Martosewojo, Eri Soedewo, and Tilam Purwohusodo. From Jakarta, medical students Koestedjo, Kaligis, Ibrahim Irsan, Abdul Hadi, and Imam Soedjoedi participated. See Soejono Martosewojo, 'Risalah Pembentukan Djakarta Ika Dai Gaku', in *125 Tahun Pendidikan Dokter di Indonesia 1851–1976*, ed. M. A. Hanafiah, Bahder Djohan, and Surono (Jakarta: FKUI, 1976), 33–34; and Soejono Martosewojo, Eri Soedewo, Sarnanto, Taufik Abdullah, and Idris Siregar, *Mahasiswa '45, Prapatan 10: Pengabdiannya* (Bandung: Patma, 1984), 5–14. A slightly reorganised and extended version of this book appeared as: O. E. Engelen, Aboe Bakar Loebis, Abdullah Ciptoprawiro, Soejono Joedodibroto, Oetarjo, and Idris Siregar, *Lahirnya Satu Bangsa dan Negara* (Jakarta: Universitas Indonesia, 1997).

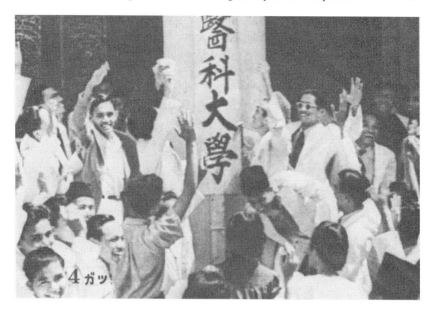

Figure 7.1 The opening of the Jakarta Ika Daigaku, 29 April 1943. *Djawa Baroe* 1 (15 December 1943), 19. Courtesy of the NIOD Institute for War, Holocaust, and Genocide Studies, Amsterdam

truncated, practical curriculum, forming a course of study one year shorter.[15] On 29 April 1943, the birthday of Japan's emperor, the Jakarta Ika Daigaku [Japanese: Medical College] was opened with a grand ceremony, beginning with a deep bow in the direction of the Imperial Palace in Tokyo and the raising of the Japanese flag. Enthusiastic speeches followed, praising the benevolence of Japan (Figure 7.1).

The Japanese military administration appointed several instructors of the former Batavia Medical School and the Surabaya Medical College as professors at the Ika Daigaku. All belonged to the Indonesian medical elite, held Dutch medical degrees, and, except one, held doctorates in medical science. For the first time, Indonesia's medical elite was in charge of medical education and medical care. They included prodigious medical researcher Achmad Mochtar, who was appointed director of Jakarta's leading institute for medical

---

[15] Members of this committee were: Abdulrachman Saleh, Achmad Mochtar, Asikin Widjaja Kusumah, Soemitro, Zainal Abidin, Hajat Hidajat, and Mohamad Sjaaf (the last two had been associated with the NIAS and the Surabaya Civil Hospital). See Martosewojo, 'Risalah Ika Dai Gaku', 34.

research.[16] His colleague Asikin, an internist, had received advanced medical training at several German medical institutions.[17] Soemitro Hadibroto became professor in ophthalmology.[18] Two had previously been associated with the NIAS: Mohamad Sjaaf, ophthalmologist, and Dajat Hidajat, paediatrician.[19] Their appointments enhanced and consolidated their professional standing. Professor Masamitsu Itagaki, a devout Christian and former dean of medicine at Kyushi Imperial University, Fukuoka, was appointed dean. Although he and a small number of other Japanese professors lectured in Japanese, Indonesian instructors taught in Malay. For the first time, medical students received instruction in Indonesia's national language. Two hundred ninety-one students enrolled – more than double the usual intake at the Dutch Medical School.

Like all organisations, the Association of Indonesian Physicians was disbanded in April 1942, although it informally continued its activities under the name Perkumpulan Tabib Indonesia (PERTABIN). The Association's new name used the word *tabib* – a physician or traditional Islamic healer – rather than the Dutch *dokter* [doctor or physician].[20] In August 1943, a preparatory meeting to resurrect the Association under the name Java Medical Service Association [Djawa Iji Hōkōkai] was held at the Ika Daigaku. After receiving guidance from Java's Supreme Military Commander, and the obligatory collective bow in the direction of the emperor's palace, Association president Rasjid thanked Satō for his trust in Indonesia's physicians and committed members to building the new Java within the Greater East Asia Co-Prosperity

---

[16] Achmad Mochtar graduated from the STOVIA in 1916; he received his medical degree at the University of Amsterdam in 1927 and his doctorate in medical science from the same university the same year. His thesis appeared as Achmad Mochtar, *Onderzoekingen omtrent Eenige Leptospiren-Stammen* (Amsterdam: Universiteitsboekhandel, 1927). In this thesis Mochtar disproved the widely held idea that leptospira causes yellow fever.

[17] Asikin's full name was Raden Djenal Asikin Widjaja Koesoema. He graduated from the STOVIA in 1914, received his medical degree at the University of Amsterdam in 1925, and earned his doctorate in medical science in 1940 from the Batavia Medical School. His dissertation appeared as Raden Djenal Asikin Widjaja Koesoemah, *Bijdrage tot de Kennis van de Bloedbilirubineverhoudingen bij Gezonden en Zieken in de Tropen* (Batavia: Kolff, 1932). Asikin was one of the students of Prof C. D. de Langen.

[18] Soemitro Hadibroto graduated from the STOVIA in 1915 and received his medical degree from the University of Amsterdam in 1930 and his doctorate in medical science from the Batavia Medical School in 1937. His dissertation appeared as Soemitro Hadibroto, *Het Trachoom op de Volksscholen te Batavia* (Batavia: Kolff, 1937).

[19] Sjaaf graduated from the STOVIA in 1913 and received his medical degree from the University of Amsterdam in 1922 and his doctorate in medical science from the same university in 1923. His dissertation appeared as Mohamad Sjaaf, *Vezelverloop in Netvlies en Oogzenuw* (Amsterdam: Buijten & Schipperheijn, 1923). Dajat Hidajat graduated from the STOVIA in 1916 and received his medical degree from the University of Amsterdam in 1927. He was employed at clinics in Utrecht, Leiden, Dusseldorf, Hamburg, Berlin, Vienna, and Munich before returning to the Indies.

[20] For the origin and meanings of the term *tabib*, see Jennifer Nourse, 'The Meaning of Dukun and Allure of Sufi Healers: How Persian Cosmopolitans Transformed Malay–Indonesian History', *Journal of Southeast Asian Studies* 44, no. 3 (2013), 400–22.

Sphere.[21] After several pompous speeches, the physicians present were invited to dinner, where they toasted the Japanese and vowed their support.[22] Two weeks later, the Java Medical Service Association was inaugurated at Jakarta's stately theatre with an audience of more than 240 physicians, dentists, pharmacists, Japanese military officials, and Indonesians holding positions in the advisory bodies established by the Japanese.[23] Solemnly, the audience pledged its allegiance to the Japanese emperor and swore to support Japan's war against European and American imperialism.[24] Professor Itagaki formally announced the demise of the pre-war Association and its replacement by a new, superior, and inclusive one.[25] In his speech, Sukarno highlighted the physicians' sacred obligations: 'Their work is *not only to treat the sick*, but also to look after and take care of the Indonesian people so that they become a very healthy and physically strong nation [*ra'jat sangat sehat dan koeat*].'[26] He urged attendees to dedicate themselves not only to their patients but 'to all layers of society'.[27]

Almost all members of the pre-war Association continued to be active.[28] T. Satō, the new director of the public health service, became the Association's advisor, with far-reaching control over its activities. R. Boentaran Martoatmodjo, who had not previously been an active member, became vice president. After graduating from the Batavia Medical College and working in various locations across the Indies, Boentaran obtained both a medical degree and a medical doctorate in the Netherlands.[29] In 1941, he became acting

---

[21] J. M. Gunseikan, 'Nasehat dan Petoendjoek', *Berita Ketabiban* 1, no. 1-2-3 (2604 [1944]), 5; 'Pelantikan dan Pendirian Badan Persiapan Djawa Izi Hookoo Kai', *Berita Ketabiban* 1, no. 1-2-3 (2606 [1944]), 6–7; Abdul Rasjid, 'Pedato dari Dr. Abdul Rasjid', *Berita Ketabiban* 1, no. 1-2-3 (2604 [1944]), 9–11. See also Abdul Rasjid, 'Samboetan Dokter-Dokter Indonesia: Terhadap Izi Hooko Kai', *Pembangoenan*, 13 August 1943, 2; Abdul Rasjid, 'Tabib Indonesia dan Pendirian Izi Hoko Kai', *Asia Raja*, 13 August 1943, 1.

[22] 'Pelantikan dan Pendirian', 8–9.

[23] 'Pemboekaan Pendirian "Izi Hookoo Kai" dengan Resmi pada Tanggal 30 VIII 2603', *Berita Ketabiban* 1, no. 1-2-3 (2604 [1944]), 17–18. For the constitution of the association, see *Djawa Izi Hookoo Kai, Osamu Serei No 28: Peratoeran Dasar, Peratoeran Khusus* (Jakarta: Gunseibanku, 2604 [1944]). See also 'Ichtiar oentoek Kesehatan Rakjat', *Tjahaja*, 26 August 1942, 2.

[24] 'Soerat Soempah', *Berita Ketabiban* 1, no. 1-2-3 (2604 [1944]), 25.

[25] Prof Itagaki, as quoted in 'Pemboekaan', *Berita Ketabiban* 1, no. 1-2-3 (2604 [1944]), 27.

[26] Soekarno, 'Pidato', *Berita Ketabiban* 1, no. 1-2-3 (2604 [1944]), 28. Emphasis in original.

[27] Soekarno, 'Pidato', 28.

[28] Leaders were Abdul Rasjid and R. Boentaran Martoatmodjo; administrators were Prof Achmad Mochtar and M. Sardjito aided by Bahder Djohan, Goedadi Wreksoatmodjo, M. Permadi, M. Soekarjo, M. Soetopo, R. Soeharto, Marzoeki, R. Sarwono Prawirohardjo, Aulia, Achmad Ramali, and R. M. H. Soetomo Tjokronegoro. Achmad Mochtar was the editor of *Berita Ketabiban*.

[29] Boentaran graduated from the STOVIA in 1918 and received his Dutch medical degree from the University of Leiden in 1930; a year later, he received his doctorate in medical science from the same university. His dissertation appeared as Boentaran Martoatmodjo, *Bijdrage tot de Studie van het 'Ultravirus Tuberculeux'* (Leiden: Boekhandel S. Garnade, 1931). See also R. Boentaran Martoatmodjo, 'Enkele Opmerkingen over de Bestrijding der Tuberculose als Volksziekte', in *Jubileumnummer 1911–1936* (Batavia: Kolff, 1937), 79–94.

director of Semarang's Central Civil Hospital and joined an underground organisation making preparations for the Japanese annexation. Boentaran also became head of the Semarang division of the Organisation to Aid the Victims of War [Penolong Korban Perang] (PEKOPE), a Java-wide organisation which attempted to undermine Dutch defences. When the Japanese arrived, Boentaran transformed this organisation into the local Committee for Indonesian Independence [Komite Indonesia Merdeka] to welcome the victors. The Semarang Committee coordinated the activities of all branches in Central Java until it was outlawed by the Japanese military administration.[30] Boentaran then became director of Semarang's main hospital and its public health service. In August 1943, both Rasjid and Boentaran were appointed to the Central Advisory Council, a new quasi-parliamentary body replacing the Volksraad. At the same time, the Indonesian Language Committee [Komite Bahasa Indonesia] was created to provide a platform for Indonesian intellectuals to develop a uniform Indonesian technical, scientific, and medical vocabulary.[31] Its physician members aimed to develop Malay medical terms to replace the Dutch and Latin medical vocabulary.[32]

The journal of the revived Association, named *Medical Reports* [*Berita Ketabiban*], was awash with pro-Japanese rhetoric. It heralded the central role of Indonesian physicians in building the new Java.[33] In an editorial, Rasjid urged all health professionals to cooperate, regardless of speciality, ethnic background, or religion, to realise 'final victory, which will create new conditions in East Asia for prosperity and well-being under the gallant leadership of Dai Nippon'.[34] The notion of pure science disregarding the needs of society, he wrote, 'has expired and is no longer useful'.[35] Physicians should eagerly accept their responsibilities, so that medicine could serve the common good instead of suffering from 'division and competition', as had been the case under the Dutch.[36] After 350 years of colonisation, Rasjid argued, there were a mere 600 physicians in the archipelago, and they were divided between European and

---

[30] Elly Touwen-Bouwsma, 'The Indonesian Nationalists and the Japanese "Liberation" of Indonesia: Visions and Reactions', *Journal of Southeast Asian Studies* 27, no. 1 (1996), 5, 7, 12.

[31] Kanahele, 'Japanese Occupation', 68.

[32] The result of the work of this committee, which continued after the Japanese surrender, was published as Ahmad Ramali and K. St. Pamoentjak, *Kamus Kedoktoran: Arti dan Keterangan Istilah* (Djakarta: Djambatan, 1953).

[33] Mas Sardjito, who was at the time associated with the Central Hospital at Semarang, had commenced publishing a medical journal with the name *Medical Reports* [*Medische Berichten*] in 1936. Rasjid announced that both *Medische Berichten* and the VIG magazine *Medisch Tribune* were subsumed in *Berita Ketabiban*. See Abdul Rasjid, 'Kata Pengantar', *Berita Ketabiban* 1, no. 1-2-3 (2604 [1944]), 2–4.

[34] Rasjid, 'Kata Pengantar', 3. His speech on the occasion of the induction of the preparatory commission for the establishment of a new physicians' association contained the same rhetoric and explicit allegiance to Japan. See Rasjid, 'Kata Pengantar', 9–11.

[35] Rasjid, 'Kata Pengantar', 3.

[36] Rasjid, 'Kata Pengantar', 4.

indigenous factions.[37] Medicine had served only the Dutch, with negligible benefit for Indonesians.

Boentaran's political career thrived. He was appointed vice chair of the Central Advisory Council and of several subcommittees. In September 1943, the Japanese military administration sent him and twenty others to Japan.[38] At the second meeting of the Java Medical Service Association, held in November 1943, again in Jakarta's theatre, Boentaran enthusiastically related his observations on Japan's health system. He emphasised the beneficial effects of sanitation and other public health measures, the quality of medical education, the great number of Japanese physicians, and the proliferation of neighbourhood clinics. Neighbourhood associations actively participated in health campaigns which reached the whole population. Boentaran exhorted Indonesian physicians to follow the Japanese example, so that medicine might strengthen the nation's physique.[39] He saw great potential for health initiatives: maternal and child health clinics, dietetic research, establishing norms for adequate nutrition, instigating health and exercise programs in all schools, supporting eugenics, conducting medical checks before marriage, providing adequate health care to all citizens, ameliorating poor living conditions, screening for tuberculosis, and undertaking public health education and preventative measures to eradicate contagious disease.[40] Although they were familiar with these ideas, Boentaran's forceful presentation impressed the audience. Afterwards, other speakers enthusiastically praised Japan's medical infrastructure and endorsed Boentaran's initiatives. Raden Soeharto, Sukarno's personal physician, called for greater public health education efforts and mobile medical response teams to fight epidemics.[41]

Boentaran's presentation inspired several additional proposals. One speaker suggested establishing a nutrition committee tasked with formulating minimal dietary requirements.[42] Another one extolled the importance of exercise and praised the physical education programs the Japanese had established in all

---

[37] Abdul Rasjid, 'Tabib Indonesia dan Pendirian *Izi Hookoo Kai*', *Berita Ketabiban* 1, no. 1-2-3 (2604 [1944]), 61.

[38] See Kanahele, 'Japanese Occupation', 105–07.

[39] Boentaran, quoted in 'Persidangan Oemoem Izi Hookoo Kai', *Berita Ketabiban* 1, no. 1-2-3 (2604 [1944]), 46.

[40] Boentaran's colleague Hendarmin emphasised, in an article in *Berita Ketabiban*, the importance of exercise and sports, which were advocated by the Japanese. See Hendarmin, 'Mempertegoeh Djasmani', *Berita Ketabiban* 1, no. 1-2-3 (2604 [1944]), 58–59.

[41] R. Soeharto, 'Kewadjiban Tabib dizaman Pembangoenan', *Berita Ketabiban* 1, no. 1-2-3 (2604 [1944]), 64–66. Raden Soeharto graduated from the Batavia Medical School in 1935. In 1941, he became Sukarno's personal physician as well as his personal assistant and remained in this position until his retirement. In 1946, he was appointed as treasurer of the Ministry of Defence. See R. Soeharto, *Saksi Sejarah Mengikuti Perjuangan Dwitunggal* (Jakarta: Gunung Agung, 1982).

[42] 'Bantoean Djawa Izi Hookoo Kai kepada "Komisi Makanan Dimasa Perang" dan kepada "Komisi Jamoe-Jamoe"', *Berita Ketabiban* 1, no. 4-5-6 (2604 [1944]), 10–12.

schools.[43] The neighbourhood associations established to promote enthusiasm for the empire and the Greater East Asia Co-Prosperity Sphere, argued another speaker, could also conduct public health education. Erecting neighbourhood clinics would make medical care available to all. Several physicians present volunteered their services.[44] The Japanese had declared three days of every month to be health days [*hari kesehatan rakyat*], devoted to intensive forms of public health education and street cleaning.[45] The meeting's overall message was clear: 'We must let go of … ways of working inherited from the days of the past [so that] we can contribute to the formation of a strong and healthy fatherland [*tanah air yang kuat dan sehat*].'[46]

Still another voice at the meeting pointed to the urgent need for further investigation into the efficacy of indigenous herbal medicine.[47] The Committee on Indigenous Medicine, established in 1941, was still functioning. Because European and North American pharmaceutical products could no longer be imported, Indonesian physicians were actively looking for substitutes. Sections of widely used herbal medicine manuals were reprinted and newspapers enthusiastically reported on the ways in which herbal medicines could fortify the new nation.[48] Raden Mochtar published a booklet with herbal prescriptions. Latin phrases and weight measures traditionally used by physicians gave the booklet a medical imprimatur. It also carried a strong political message: in

---

[43] Hendarmin, 'Mempertegoeh Djasmani', 58–59.

[44] 'Tonari-Gumi dan Kesehatan', *Berita Ketabiban* 1, no. 4-5-6 (2604 [1944]) 15–16.

[45] MSh., 'Menjehatkan Bangsa', *Berita Ketabiban* 1, no. 1-2-3 (2604 [1944]), 59–60. See also Boentaran Martoatmodjo, 'Pemadangan Singkat Perihal Kesehatan dan Makanan Rakjat dll.', *Berita Ketabiban* 1, no. 4-5-6 (2604 [1944]), 43–44.

[46] 'Tonari-Gumi dan Kesehatan', 17–18.

[47] T. Satō, 'Menjehatkan Rochani dan Djasmani Pendoedoek', *Berita Ketabiban* 1, no. 1-2-3 (2604 [1944]), 56; 'Bantoean Djawa Izi Hookoo Kai', 10–12.

[48] Some of these small volumes referred to a manual on herbal medicine that had appeared in 1885: Njonja W. van Blokland, *Doekoen Djawa: Oetawa Kitab dari Roepa-Roepa Obat njang Terpake di Tanah Djawa* (Batavia: Van Dorp, 1885); this book contained 351 pages. An extract in Javanese script was published in 1899 as Van Bloklan, *Ratjikan Obat Djawa I* (Soerakarta: Albert Rusche & Company, 1898). This version contained only thirty-five pages but was most likely part of a series. The publications during the Japanese occupation were most likely derived from this source. During the Japanese occupation, other versions appeared: Van Bloklan, *Ratjikan Djampi Djawi, Ingkang Winados, Karanganipoen Njonjah van Bloklan Ing Betawi; Kawedalaken denging Wirjapanitra, Solo* (Solo: Sadoe Boedi, 1942) (this book appeared in Javanese using Latin script); and Van Bloklan, *Serat Primbon Oesada, Van Bloklan; Kadjawekaken Mawi Askara Latyn dening Wirjapanitra*, 2nd print edn (Solo: Sadoe-Boedi, 2602 [1942]). The following manual was published as well: *Beberapa Toemboeh-Toemboehan Obat jang Berfaedah jang Terdapat di Djawa* (Djakarta: Djawa Gunseikanbu Naimubu Eiseikyoku, 1945). Another booklet on *jamu* published during the Japanese occupation was Isis Prawiranegara, *Oebar Kampoeng* (Djakarta: Djawa Goenseibankoe [Bale Poetaka], 2603 [1943]). For newspaper coverage, see 'Oesaha Membikin Obat2 Baroe di Djawa', *Sinar Baroe*, 27 April 1944, 3; '"Djamoe Indonesia' Memasoeki Zaman Baroe', *Kita-Sumatora-Sinbun: Soerat Kabar Harian*, 15 May 1944, 1; F. H. Dj., 'Obat Indonesia', *Sinar Baroe*, 19 May 1944, 3.

Dutch colonial times, medicine had primarily catered to Europeans, with expensive imported chemical and synthetic drugs.[49] Under Japanese guidance, a new type of medical care had been inaugurated. R. Mochtar urged Indonesians to embrace their own medical heritage, which provided affordable and effective treatments. Medicinal gardens should be established everywhere in a patriotic effort to supply the nation with medications. With alternatives no longer available, physicians turned to herbal medications out of necessity.[50]

Discontent among Medical Students

The reopening of the medical school had been contingent upon finding dormitory facilities for its students, and the premises of the Dutch Public Health Service at Prapatan 10 were refurbished for this purpose.[51] Benedict Anderson's arguments about the central role of educational institutions and associated dormitories during the Dutch colonial era apply with even greater force to the Japanese period. Anderson has argued that the 'utopian, voluntarist, and transcendent elements of traditional Javanese thought found their most ardent adherents' among these students.[52] Dormitories became focal points of political discussion and agitation against the Japanese. After the declaration of independence, they became centres where students organised resistance against the Allied forces and support to fledgling Indonesian state institutions. At that time, Anderson argues, the 'key institutional bases for the metropolitan undergrounds were *asrama*, or dormitories, for various types of *pemuda* [youth]'.[53]

The students who lived at the Prapatan 10 dormitory came from privileged, westernised households. Many only learned to speak Indonesian after the Japanese annexation.[54] Sjahrir's ideas were influential amongst these students, who praised science and democracy, were disinterested in traditional culture,

---

[49] Raden Mochtar, *Obat Obat dari Bahan-Bahan Negeri Sendiri* (Djakarta: Balai Poestaka, 1945), 9–10. For an extensive commentary on this publication, see Eric Andrew Stein, 'Vital Times: Power, Public Health, and Memory in Rural Java' (PhD, University of Michigan, 2005), 188–93.

[50] In *Berita Ketabiban*, one article on herbal medications for diabetes appeared, and one on experimentation with a raw food diet, following the experimental approach of a Japanese physician. A. Ramali, 'Pengobatan Penjakit Diabetes Mellitus dengan Obat Rempah-Rempah', *Berita Ketabiban* 1, no. 1-2-3 (2604 [1944]), 90–98; Aulia, 'Beberapa Pikiran tentang Terapi atau Pengobatan dengan Makanan Mentah', *Berita Ketabiban* 1, no. 1-2-3 (2604 [1944]), 68–77.

[51] In the Netherlands, in the Dutch East Indies, and in Indonesia today, the house number follows the street name rather than preceding it, as is common in English-speaking countries.

[52] Benedict R. O'G. Anderson, *Java in a Time of Revolution: Occupation and Resistance, 1944–1946*, Equinox Classic Indonesian Books (Jakarta: Equinox, 2006 [1972]), 9.

[53] Anderson, *Java in a Time of Revolution*, 39.

[54] J. D. Legge, *Intellectuals and Nationalism in Indonesia: A Study of the Following Recruited by Sutan Sjahrir in Occupied Jakarta* (Jakarta: Equinox, 2010 [1988]), 73.

and were opposed to the hierarchical organisation of traditional society.[55] Few had been politically active before the Japanese invasion, although some had participated in discussion groups devoted to philosophy and politics.[56] At Menteng 32, a ten-minute walk from Prapatan 10, several pre-war student associations had established a dormitory for students unable to return home. In August 1942, it was forced to relocate to Cikini 71.[57] Across the road, at Menteng 31, the Japanese Department of Propaganda established a dormitory for Indonesia's New Generation [Angkatan Baru Indonesia], where they trained as leaders of youth propaganda movements. It mainly housed students of the now-defunct Law School, who tended to be more radical than the medical students. Most had been politically active before the war. In October 1944, the Japanese Navy established a fourth dormitory, the Asrama Free Indonesia [Asrama Indonesia Merdeka], to train a cadre of Indonesian officials who would be ready to occupy administrative positions after independence was granted.[58] Indonesian nationalist leaders provided training and instruction at each dormitory, and preached nationalism. Disaffection with the Japanese administration increased steadily across all dormitories.

After the institutions of higher learning were closed, students remained in their dormitories with little to do. They were unable to go home and soon exhausted their financial resources. The Japanese military administration enticed them to become advocates of the Greater East Asia Co-Prosperity Sphere by employing them in their propaganda organisations. Sukarno, Hatta, and other nationalists who led these organisations interspersed their own nationalist ideologies through the formal training. After the imposition of curfews, students could discuss intellectual and political issues without Japanese interference. Some later reminisced: 'Because the Japanese could only see from the outside, they thought that we were adhering to their regulations ... They never guessed that the students inside the dormitory were being galvanised for the sake of Indonesia's national struggle.'[59] Unfortunately, the numerous memoirs written by the residents of the various dormitories do not mention when and why their enthusiasm for the Japanese cause gave way to resistance, probably because the authors did not care to elaborate on the former. Notwithstanding this, the dormitories established by the Japanese became sites of anti-Japanese ferment.

---

[55] Anderson, *Java in a Time of Revolution*, 40.

[56] R. Koestedjo, *Inilah Jalan Hikupku* (Jakarta: Rosda Jayaputra, 1996), 21–31.

[57] For a history of this dormitory, see H. N. Irna and Hadi Soewito, eds., *BAPERPI: Badan Perwakilan Peladjar-Peladjar Indonesia, Cikini 71* (Jakarta: Yayasan Tjikini 71, 1990), and Koestedjo, *Inilah Jalan Hikupku*, 33–37.

[58] Anderson, *Java in a Time of Revolution*, 44. This *asrama* was located at Kebon Sirih 80.

[59] Martosewojo et al., *Mahasiswa '45, Prapatan 10*, 11.

In October 1943, a dramatic incident took place at the Ika Daigaku. When Itagaki, the dean of medicine, ordered all junior students to shave their heads in accordance with Japanese military custom, several objected because this contravened Javanese cultural sensitivities.[60] A few days later, several Japanese soldiers, armed with bayonetted rifles, entered the lecture hall and forcefully shaved the heads of all students. This heavy-handed action came as a complete surprise as the Japanese had thus far treated medical students as a privileged elite. Several outraged students called for a student strike; from then on, no one attended lectures. The Indonesian professors were upset and feared that the students' action might lead to the closure of the medical school. They tried to convince the students to discontinue their protests. Sukarno and Hatta also met a group of medical students at the Cikini dormitory but were unable to dissuade them from striking. Two days later, the Kenpeitai arrested a number of student leaders.[61]

The student leaders were released after several days, but tensions increased dramatically two months later after a Japanese instructor slapped a medical student during a training exercise.[62] The Kenpeitai promptly arrested nineteen students – some were imprisoned for as long as two months.[63] The Ika Daigaku expelled eight students and suspended several others. Three expelled students, Soedjatmoko, Soedarpo, and Soebadio, visited Sukarno and criticised his pro-Japanese stance.[64] Sukarno later reflected:

The medical students had given me much difficulty. Many were Sjahrir's pupils. The prime result of his so-called underground work was that he'd inspired a small band of impatient, dissatisfied young men who nearly succeeded in getting themselves killed … It was Sukarno who pleaded they were just youngsters, not political brains, and it was Sukarno who freed them.[65]

---

[60] The well-known head-shaving incident at the Ika Daigaku is related in several sources. See, for example, Karimoeddin, 'Pendidikan Dokter Jaman Pendudukan Jepang (Ika Dai Gaku)', 28–30; Irna and Soewito, *BAPERPI Cikini 71*, 11–12; Martosewojo et al., *Mahasiswa '45, Prapatan 10*, 26–31; Margono Djojohadikusumo, *Herinneringen uit 3 Tijdperken: Een Geschreven Familie-Overlevering* (Jakarta: Indira, 1970), 148–50; M. Nursam, *Pergumulan Seorang Intelektual: Biografi Soedjatmoko* (Jakarta: Gramedia, 2002), 33–37; Rosihan Anwar, *Against the Currents: A Biography of Soedarpo Sastrosatomo* (Jakarta: Pustaka Sinar Harapan, 2003), 80–84; Mrázek, *Sjahrir*, 229; Legge, *Intellectuals and Nationalism*, 86–88; Ethan Mark, 'Appealing to Asia: Nation, Culture, and the Problem of Imperial Modernity in Japanese-Occupied Java, 1942–1945' (PhD thesis, Columbia University, 2003), 537–40.

[61] Among these students were Soebianto Djojohadikoesoemo, Soedarpo, Soedjatmoko, Daan Jahja, Eri Soedewo, Moeharto, Sanjoto, Soeroto Koento, and Oetario.

[62] Martosewojo et al., *Mahasiswa '45, Prapatan 10*, 32–37.

[63] Nursam, *Biografi Soedjatmoko*, 35.

[64] Anwar, *Biography of Soedarpo*, 83–84; Nursam, *Biografi Soedjatmoko*, 36–38; Mrázek, *Sjahrir*, 243.

[65] It is not unusual for Indonesians to refer to themselves using their own name. Soekarno, *Sukarno: An Autobiography as Told to Cindy Adams* (Indianapolis, IN: Bobbs-Merrill, 1965), 194.

After their acrimonious discussion, the three left Jakarta. The heavy-handed Japanese response left the remaining students hostile. The protests by the medical students later acquired symbolic significance as some of the first acts of resistance against the Japanese. The conflict at the Ika Daigaku also showed that Indonesia's elite physicians preferred a different course of action than the medical students. This indicated a broader generational conflict between Indonesia's older politicians, who sought to advance Indonesia's independence by collaborating with the Japanese, and various youth groups, who became increasingly hostile towards the Japanese and were not afraid of confrontation.

Health Conditions during the Japanese Period

In March 1944, the Japanese established the Java Service Association [Djawa Hōkōkai] to realise the 'divine mission of the Greater East Asia Holy War' by uniting all of Java's administrative structures and functional groups. The new association reached into every village in Java through its neighbourhood branches.[66] Affiliated with it was the Pioneer Corps [Barisan Pelopor], a paramilitary youth organisation established to build support for the Japanese cause and to strengthen the island's defences. The Corps was led by a physician named Moewardi, who had previously established various Indonesian scouting organisations.[67] It inadvertently brought student leaders in contact with disaffected youth all over Java and Madura.

Despite their impressive medical ideals, the Japanese accomplished little in Indonesia. As their military losses mounted, they committed ever greater resources to the war effort. Conditions on the archipelago deteriorated quickly. Indies physicians could not help but notice that the health of Indonesians was rapidly declining. As leading Indonesian physicians were appearing in theatrical displays staged by the Japanese, and professing their medical ideals, the Indonesian people suffered from poverty, malnutrition, infectious diseases, lack of effective medications, and the complete collapse of health care facilities. The prevalence of smallpox rose after vaccination programs were discontinued. During 1944, forced rice levies led to severe shortages and widespread malnourishment; the incidence of kwashiorkor (a severe form of malnutrition) and beriberi rose dramatically.[68] A drought led to widespread crop

---

[66] Kanahele, 'Japanese Occupation', 142. For the Djawa Hōkōkai, see Anderson, *Java in a Time of Revolution*, 27–34; Kanahele, 'Japanese Occupation', 138, 142–46, 154, 170, 177.

[67] See, for example, Moewardi, 'Kepandoean dalam Jong-Java', in *Gedenkboek Jong Java 1915 – 7 Maart – 1930: Kitab Peringatan Jong-Java* (Jakatera: Pedoman Besar Jong-Java, 1930), 141–80; Kanahele, 'Japanese Occupation', 166; Anderson, *Java in a Time of Revolution*, 30.

[68] About the food policies of the Japanese, in particular rice, see Paul Kratoska, *Food Supplies and the Japanese Occupation in South-East Asia* (New York: St. Martins, 1998).

failures. By early 1945, dead bodies were a common sight on Java's streets.[69] Since cotton had not been imported for years, clothing was scarce, and people dressed in jute bags or remained naked. 'Towards the end of the occupation', writes historian Shigeru Sato, 'Indonesia was on the verge of an economic catastrophe'.[70] In his novel *The Fugitive*, Pramoedya Ananta Toer described this time:

When you go to the city you see children sprawled lifeless at the side of the road. In front of the market and the stores, down beneath the bridge, on top of garbage heaps and in the gutters there are corpses. Nothing but corpses. The place is filled with the dead – children and the old people … In all my life this is the first time I've seen anything like it. Corpses. Wherever you go, unattended corpses.[71]

The archipelago also suffered a demographic calamity. Villages were left depleted after able-bodied workers were forcibly recruited to work on war projects. More than 300,000 left; less than half returned. Their state of health was appalling and mortality rates were high.[72] The few Indonesian physicians tasked with their care could do little to alleviate their suffering.

The war decisively disrupted quinine production. Before World War II, quinine was one of the few medications produced with biological materials (the bark of the cinchona tree) from the archipelago; during the Dutch colonial era, the Netherlands controlled more than 90 per cent of the world's supply.[73] The supply of cinchona had frequently caused friction between the Dutch colonial administration, Japan, and several other nations. Before the outbreak of hostilities, the Japanese had attempted to become self-sufficient with respect to quinine by establishing plantations on Taiwan.[74] They failed. When Germany

---

[69] Shigeru Sato, 'Forced Labourers and Their Resistance in Java under Japanese Military Rule, 1942–1945', in *Resisting Bondage in Indian Ocean Africa and Asia*, ed. Edward A. Alpers, Gwyn Campbell, and Michael Salman (New York: Routledge, 2007), 82–95; Shigeru Sato, '"Economic Soldiers" in Java: Indonesian Laborers Mobilized for Agricultural Projects', in *Asian Labor in the Wartime Japanese Empire: Unknown Histories*, ed. Paul H. Kratoska (Singapore: Singapore University Press, 2006), 130–31.

[70] Shigeru Sato, 'Indonesia 1939–1942: Prelude to the Japanese Occupation', *Journal of Southeast Asian Studies* 37, no. 2 (2006), 246.

[71] Pramoedya Ananta Toer, *The Fugitive* (Harmondsworth: Penguin, 1990), 33, as quoted by Sato, '"Economic Soldiers" in Java', 131.

[72] Sato, 'Forced Labourers'; Sato, '"Economic Soldiers" in Java'; Henk Hovinga, 'End of a Forgotten Drama: The Reception and Repatriation of *Rōmusha* after the Japanese Capitulation', in *Asian Labor in the Wartime Japanese Empire: Unknown Histories*, ed. Paul H. Kratoska (Singapore: Singapore University Press, 2006), 197–212; Remco Raben, 'Indonesian *Rōmusha* and Coolies under Naval Administration: The Eastern Archipelago, 1942–45', in *Asian Labor in the Wartime Japanese Empire: Unknown Histories*, ed. Paul H. Kratoska (Singapore: Singapore University Press, 2006), 197–212.

[73] Norman Taylor, *Cinchona in Java: The Story of Quinine* (New York: Greenberg, 1945).

[74] See Timothy Yang, 'Selling an Imperial Dream: Japanese Pharmaceuticals, National Power, and the Science of Quinine Self-Sufficiency', *East Asian Science, Technology, and Medicine* 6 (2012), 101–25.

occupied the Netherlands in 1940, it quickly seized the Dutch quinine production facilities. After the Japanese annexed the archipelago, the chemicals needed to produce quinine from cinchona could no longer be imported and production levels plummeted. All quinine stores were diverted to the Japanese military. The prevalence of malaria among Indonesians rose sharply, with many affected patients dying.[75] There were also global effects, felt most acutely by the American Expeditionary Force in the Pacific theatre of operations. American pharmaceutical companies produced Atabrine as an alternative, but this medication had undesirable side effects. By 1944, synthetic quinine and a variety of anti-malarial medications were produced by American pharmaceutical companies to support the war effort.[76]

Indonesian physicians openly discussed Java's disastrous state of health. In Semarang and surrounding areas, Boentaran reported, significant increases in malaria, dysentery, yaws, pneumonia, and other communicable diseases could be observed. Widespread malnutrition had decreased the population's resistance against disease, and he now regularly saw cases of kwashiorkor, which had been rare during Dutch colonial times. Mortality rates surpassed birth rates.[77] Urban populations had grown because hungry people migrated from the countryside. Achmad Mochtar warned that the prevalence of dysentery was rising.[78] In an investigation on malaria in Bogor and its surrounds, S. B. Zahar reported that a particularly virulent strain had claimed a high number of victims and that the disease had become endemic, rather than seasonal. He also noted widespread malnutrition and the increased prevalence of skin diseases, typhoid fever, and other contagious diseases.[79] Indonesian physicians avoided blaming the Japanese for these health concerns, referring tactfully instead to the extraordinary conditions of wartime. They continued to hail Japanese initiatives that would soon alleviate these conditions.

In December 1944, Boentaran was appointed advisor [*sanyo*] to the Health Bureau, and member of the Council of Political Advisors [Sanyo Kaigi or Dewan Sanyo], consisting of de facto department heads. Their council remained in session when the Central Advisory Council was adjourned. He also joined a subcommittee investigating problems related to rice distribution. Its report did not mince words.[80] It echoed Boentaran's earlier conclusions and demonstrated

---

[75] Sato, 'Prelude to the Japanese Occupation', 232.
[76] Vassiliki Betty Smocovitis, 'Desperately Seeking Quinine', *American Chemical Society* 6, no. 5 (2003), 57–58.
[77] Martoatmodjo, 'Pemadangan Singkat', 43–52.
[78] Achmad Mochtar, 'Dysenterie di Djawa', *Berita Ketabiban* 1, no. 1-2-3 (2604 [1944]), 38–43.
[79] S. B. Zahar, 'Pemeriksaan tentang Sakit Malaria dalam Bogor-Si dan Desa-Desa Sekitarnya', *Berita Ketabiban* 1, no. 4-5-6 (2604 [1944]), 19–27.
[80] The first half of this report has been presented in Benedict R. O'G. Anderson, 'The Problem of Rice: Stenographic Notes on the Fourth Session of the Sanyo Kaigi, January 8, 2605, 10.00

that the health of the Indonesian people had suffered dramatically, resistance to disease had declined sharply, and the death rate had surpassed the birth rate:

Every doctor whose opinion we asked acknowledged that malnutrition has caused a serious decline in the people's health, as well as in their ability to work and strength to resist disease. The deteriorating health of the people has been further accelerated by the shortage of medicines to prevent and cure disease, by the shortage of adequate clothing, and by the returning *romusha*, who usually bring back to their native villages all kinds of infections, particularly malaria and skin diseases.[81]

Referring to the health of the Indonesian population and to widespread pilfering and corruption in the rice distribution system, one Council member exclaimed: 'It is obvious that our society is suffering from an extremely grave illness.'[82] It became increasingly difficult for Indies physicians to hide their disillusionment with the Japanese – to ignore the fact that the grave illness was Japanese 'prosperity'.

Towards the Declaration of Indonesian Independence

In mid-1944, Japan's Supreme Command finally acknowledged that Japan was losing the war and that it required the full support of Indonesia's population to defend the archipelago. In January 1943, the Japanese had granted independence to Burma and to the Philippines, and Indonesian nationalists were deeply disappointed that no preparations whatsoever had been made for Indonesian independence. The popularity of the Japanese administration reached its nadir in 1944, and it responded with dramatic propaganda initiatives. In a speech to the Diet (the Japanese Imperial Parliament) on 7 September 1944, the newly appointed premier Koiso Kuniaki promised independence to Indonesia at an indeterminate point in the future. Indonesians were now permitted to discuss independence, raise the red-and-white flag, and sing *Indonesia Raya*, the Indonesian national anthem, in public. The Indonesians expressed their gratitude in numerous carefully staged celebrations.[83] It still took some time before any concrete steps towards independence were announced.

On 1 March 1945, the Japanese military administration announced the establishment of the Committee for the Investigation of Indonesian Independence.[84]

A.M.', *Indonesia*, no. 2 (1966), 77–123. The subcommittee on the problem of rice was chaired by Oto Iskandardinata.

[81] Anderson, 'The Problem of Rice', 92–93. At the time, venereal diseases were included among the skin diseases. The report referred to yaws and syphilis.

[82] Anderson, 'The Problem of Rice', 110.

[83] Kanahele, 'Japanese Occupation', 161–65.

[84] Benedict R. O'G. Anderson, *Some Aspects of Indonesian Politics under the Japanese Occupation, 1944–1945* (Ithaca, NY: Cornell University, Department of Far Eastern Studies, 1961), 16–17.

Two months later, on 29 April, the emperor's birthday, its composition was revealed. Solo's former court physician Dr Kandjeng Raden Toemenggoeng Radjiman Wediodiningrat (known as Radjiman when he addressed the first congress of Boedi Oetomo in 1908), representing the sultanates of Java's cultural heartland, was appointed chairman. Deliberations began at the end of May with a three-day meeting in the Volksraad building. On the first of June, Sukarno gave his famous speech on the five foundational principles of the future Indonesian state, now referred to as the *Pancasila*.[85] In the meantime, Indonesian students travelled all over Java as representatives of the various Japanese propaganda organisations. They expressed themselves with increasing vehemence and became a voice to be reckoned with, both by the Japanese military administration and by older Indonesian nationalists. On 7 June 1945, for example, several medical students organised a meeting at the Jakarta zoo to which all of Jakarta's high school students were invited.[86] Speakers defiantly declared that Indonesia's new generation was prepared to force independence through armed struggle, regardless of the sacrifices this would require. Speakers urged all youth to undertake military training. In July, several inhabitants of Prapatan 10 commenced military training with the Japanese youth military corps, the Defenders of the Homeland [Pembela Tanah Air] (PETA).[87]

On 17 July, the Japanese Imperial General Headquarters decreed that Indonesia should be granted independence as soon as possible.[88] On 6 August, the American Expeditionary Forces destroyed Hiroshima with a nuclear bomb. The following day, the Japanese command in Vietnam announced the establishment of the Committee for the Preparation of Indonesian Independence [Panitia Persiapan Kemerdekaan Indonesia] (PPKI). On 8 August, one hour before midnight, the Soviet Union declared war on Japan and invaded Japanese-occupied Manchuria. The next day, Sukarno, Hatta, and Radjiman flew to Saigon via Singapore to meet with Marshal Hisaichi Terauchi, head of Japan's Southern Area Command. On the day of their flight, a plutonium bomb destroyed Nagasaki. On 11 August, a ceremony was held in Terauchi's villa at Dalat, Vietnam, to inaugurate Sukarno and Hatta as the chairman and vice chairman of the Preparatory Committee. On 13 August, they flew back to Singapore, where Mohamad Amir and two other Sumatran representatives joined them to fly to Jakarta. Two days later, Japan capitulated. On the morning

---

[85] Soekarno, *Lahirnja Pantjasila: Filsafah Indonesia Tertjakup dalam Pantjasila* (Bandung: Duar-r, 1961).

[86] Mien Soedarpo, *Reminiscenses of the Past*, 2nd edn, 2 vols. (Jakarta: PT Ngrumat Bondo Utomo, 2005), vol. 1, 64; Martosewojo et al., *Mahasiswa '45, Prapatan 10*, 50–52; Anderson, *Java in a Time of Revolution*, 54–55.

[87] Soedarpo, *Reminiscenses of the Past*, vol. 1, 46, 65.

[88] For a detailed overview of these developments, see Anderson, *Java in a Time of Revolution*, 61–84.

of 17 August, Sukarno declared Indonesia's independence on the front steps of his house.[89] At the same time, a group of medical students at Prapatan 10 conducted a parallel ceremony, in case of misadventure.[90] That evening, Sukarno's voice, reading the declaration of independence, was broadcast through a radio transmitter that had been secreted by Abdulrahman Saleh, a lecturer at the Ika Daigaku. Indonesia's leaders had declared independence, but it would take another four and a half years of military conflict with the Dutch before sovereignty was formally transferred on 27 December 1949.

Conclusion

After Japan's annexation of the archipelago, health and medicine became more politicised than they had ever been. In the rhetoric of the new colonial forces, both health and medicine were essential to building a physically and spiritually strong nation able to resist the relentless attacks by imperialist forces. Japanese propaganda declared that in the Greater East Asia Co-Prosperity Sphere, medicine would realise its full potential because it was no longer limited by Western colonialism and capitalism.[91] Eric Stein has argued that the Japanese urged Indonesian physicians to re-envision their role in building their society.[92] Indonesian physicians working for the Japanese military administration were no doubt motivated by a mix of genuine enthusiasm, opportunism, and suppressed rage. It is not unlikely that, initially, most were enthusiastic about Japanese initiatives, particularly the reopening of the medical school. The Japanese interest in the archipelago's cultural heritage, their curiosity about *adat*, and the valorisation of Asian spirituality mirrored the interests of Indonesian nationalists.[93]

In the official, three-volume, government-issued history of health and medicine in Indonesia, only 6 of 433 pages are devoted to the Japanese occupation. The main conclusion is terse:

With regard to this short period there is not much to tell about the development of health; the narratives of various health figures provide similar accounts of events, which

---

[89] For a more detailed description of the events around the Indonesian declaration of independence, see Anderson, *Java in a Time of Revolution*, 61–84; Martosewojo et al., *Mahasiswa '45, Prapatan 10*, 57–88.

[90] Martosewojo et al., *Mahasiswa '45, Prapatan 10*, 86.

[91] See, for example, 'Mobilizasi Dokter', *Asia Raya*, 4 August 2603 [1943], as quoted in *Berita Ketabiban* 1, no. 1-2-3 (2604 [1944]), 67.

[92] Stein, 'Vital Times', 183–91. See also Eric Andrew Stein, 'Hygiene and Decolonization: The Rockefeller Foundation and Indonesian Nationalism, 1933–1958', in *Science, Public Health, and the State in Modern Asia*, ed. Liping Bu, Darwin H. Stapleton, and Ka-Che Yip (New York, 2012), 56–59.

[93] For common themes in Japanese and Indonesian thought and the initial enthusiasm of some Indonesians about the Japanese occupation, see Mark, '"Asia's" Transwar Lineage', 461–93.

essentially suggests a scaling down of health services due to lack of infrastructure and the worsening of public health due to lack of food.[94]

This official account emphasises disease, hunger, and starvation. The pioneering role of the Ika Daigaku in teaching in Indonesian is mentioned 'besides the absolutely miserable health problems [everywhere]'.[95] The chapter closes grimly, detailing the arrest and torture of several physicians and the execution of Achmad Mochtar, the most prolific Indonesian medical researcher, to divert attention from Japanese errors in the production of tetanus vaccines, which killed up to 1,000 forced labourers.[96]

Indonesian historians have given scant attention to the Japanese annexation and often treat it as a precursor to the Indonesian revolution.[97] Most accounts juxtapose the enthusiastic welcome of the Japanese with the universal hatred they came to inspire later on, omitting all intervening events. These accounts sidestep a number of uncomfortable questions that arise from discussions of warfare, annexation, and liberation: Who collaborated with the Japanese military administration, for what reason, to what extent, and to what end? Were the physicians appointed by the Japanese to teach at the Ika Daigaku enamoured of Japan's ideals, opportunists eager to enhance their professional status, Indonesian medical nationalists, or simply physicians deeply committed to their patients, practising medicine in whatever capacity they could? Did Indies physicians embrace the Japanese vision of liberating medicine, or were they simply being pragmatic? When and why did the enthusiasm of Indonesia's youth for Nippon's cause diminish, and morph into opposition? These questions are not addressed by Indonesia's official history of health and medicine or by the post-war autobiographies written by participants, which tend to emphasise the suffering experienced by all Indonesians and their strong, but necessarily covert, commitment to the cause of independence.[98] In addition,

---

[94] *Sejarah Kesehatan Nasional Indonesia*, 3 vols. (Jakarta: Departement Kesehatan RI, 2009), vol. 1, 71.

[95] *Sejarah Kesehatan Nasional Indonesia*, vol. 1, 72.

[96] *Sejarah Kesehatan Nasional Indonesia*, vol. 1, 74–75. For the circumstances leading up to Mochtar's execution, see Mohammad Ali Hanafiah, *Drama Kedokteran Terbesar* (Jakarta: Yayasan Gedung-gedung Bersejarah Jakarta, 1976); Richard Stone, 'Righting a 65-Year-Old Wrong', *Science* 329 (2 July 2010), 30–31; J. Kevin Baird and Sangkot Marzuki, *War Crimes in Japan-Occupied Indonesia: A Case of Murder by Medicine* (Washington, DC: Potomac Books, 2015).

[97] See Katherine E. McGregor, *History in Uniform: Military Ideology and the Construction of Indonesia's Past* (Singapore: National University of Singapore Press, 2007). In their emphasis on the Indonesian revolution, both Benedict R. O'G. Anderson and McTurnan Kahin underemphasise the continuities in Indonesian society between 1930 and 1955.

[98] In his analysis of the collection of autobiographical interviews deposited at the Indonesian National Archives, Ethan Mark emphasised the same points. See Ethan Mark, 'Suharto's New Order Remembers Japan's New Order: Oral Accounts from Indonesia', in *Representing the Japanese Occupation of Indonesia: Personal Testimonies and Public Images in Indonesia, Japan, and the Netherlands*, ed. Remco Raben (Zwolle: Waanders, 1999), 72–84.

they emphasise protest and resistance while glossing over the various ways in which Indonesians collaborated with the Japanese occupying forces.

There are several strategic reasons why autobiographical, biographical, and historical accounts written after 1950 avoid issues related to collaboration, commitment, and resistance. In independent Indonesia, past affinity with the Japanese, or the Dutch before them, could cause considerable damage to both individual and institutional reputations. During the Suharto era, accounts of the Japanese annexation and the Indonesian revolution became increasingly predictable, bolstering specific political causes.[99] Instead of detailing how individuals dealt with conflicting loyalties or challenging situations, most present a simplified, teleological narrative culminating in the declaration of independence. Even modest acts of resistance, including the student strike at the medical school, have been commemorated, because of the political legitimacy they conferred upon participating individuals and the medical profession as a whole. The student strike also reinforced the politically useful image of the brutality of the Japanese. The activities of the Java Medical Service Association and the enthusiastic reception of Japanese medical ideas by Indies physicians have, on the contrary, completely disappeared from historical accounts. Abdul Rasjid has been written out of Indonesian history. External histories rarely mention him. Because of the selective memory of most participants reinforced by historical accounts, the initial enthusiasm of Indies physicians for Japanese initiatives remains hidden from view. The most detailed accounts of the Ika Daigaku and the activities of medical students who lived at Prapatan 10 are found in publications by a small group of that dormitory's alumni. These accounts appeared during Suharto's New Order and should be viewed as attempts to enhance the reputation of the Indonesian medical profession by associating it with the Indonesian revolution.[100]

The different trajectories of Indonesia's small medical elite, its large body of Indies physicians, and its medical students in response to the presence of Japanese physicians and their medical ideals had profound consequences for the Indonesian medical profession. The medical elite cemented its dominant position over Indonesia's medical institutions when it took up the top positions in the archipelago's medical institutions vacated by its counterpart. The composition of this elite changed little before, during, or after the Japanese annexation.[101] The historical record does not make clear whether it collaborated with

[99] McGregor, *History in Uniform*.

[100] The most prominent accounts are Martosewojo et al., *Mahasiswa '45, Prapatan 10*; Engelen et al., *Lahirnya Satu Bangsa dan Negara*.

[101] With respect to medicine, the elite continuity thesis, as proposed by Alfred W. McCoy, applies. See Alfred W. McCoy, 'Introduction', in *Southeast Asia under Japanese Occupation* (New Haven, CT: Yale University Southeast Asia Studies, 1980), 1–13 and Peter Post and Elly Touwen-Bouwsma, 'Introduction', in *Japan, Indonesia, and the War: Myths and Realities* (Leiden: KITLV Press, 1997), 4–5.

the Japanese out of opportunism or because of conviction. Indies physicians tended to embrace Japanese medical ideals enthusiastically, which symbolically increased their social and political significance. Medical students, however, aligned not with the other segments of their profession but with various groups of disaffected youths, becoming increasingly hostile to the Japanese. As a consequence of these three divergent trajectories, Indonesia's medical elite was superbly placed to shape and control Indonesia's medical institutions after independence, while the group of Indies physicians, the Association of Indonesian Physicians, and Abdul Rasjid were discredited. Because they came to oppose the Japanese, medical students had placed themselves in an ideal position to build their post-war careers – they found themselves on the right side of history. They became leaders within Indonesia's post-war medical profession, in politics, in business, and in the military.

8   Medical Heroism and the Indonesian Revolution

On 17 August 1945, Sukarno and Mohammad Hatta proclaimed Indonesia's independence at a modest ceremony in front of Sukarno's house, close to the medical school and the University Hospital, formerly the Central Civil Hospital. After Japan's surrender two days earlier, the Allied forces had commanded the Japanese military administration to maintain peace and order until they were able to bring sufficient military personnel to take control. British forces began arriving in late September and commenced repatriating Japanese soldiers and European civilians, many of whom had been living in Japanese internment camps. The Dutch government refused to recognise Indonesia's independence, which would mean relinquishing its former colonies. Dutch bureaucrats tasked with re-establishing pre-war administrative institutions, now named the Netherlands Indies Civil Administration (NICA), followed closely on the heels of the British forces. Dutch troops soon joined them. When their number increased, tensions rose in Jakarta, on Java, and across the rest of the archipelago, and armed confrontations between Dutch military units and Indonesian militias multiplied. In 1947 and 1948, the Dutch launched two neo-colonial military campaigns, which led to outright warfare.[1] The Indonesian revolution was a lengthy and remarkably violent conflict, with numerous civilian casualties from interethnic strife among Indonesians as well as systematic

---

[1] There are several excellent studies on the Indonesian revolution. See, for example, George McTurnan Kahin, *Nationalism and Revolution in Indonesia* (Ithaca, NY: Cornell University Press, 1952); Anthony Reid, *The Indonesian National Revolution, 1945–1950* (Melbourne: Longman, 1974); Robert Cribb, *Gangsters and Revolutionaries: The Jakarta People's Militia and the Indonesian Revolution, 1945–1949* (Sydney: Allen & Unwin, 1991); and Benedict R. O'G. Anderson, *Java in a Time of Revolution: Occupation and Resistance, 1944–1946* (Jakarta: Equinox, 2006 [1972]), which covers the first eighteen months. Recent studies from the Netherlands have provided nuanced perspectives as well: J. J. P. de Jong, *Avondschot: Hoe Nederland Zich Terugtrok uit zijn Aziatisch Imperium* (Amsterdam: Boom, 2011); Ad van Liempt, *Nederland Valt Aan: Op Weg naar Oorlog met Indonesië, 1947* (Amsterdam: Balans, 2012); and J. J. A. van Doorn and W. J. Hendrix, *Ontsporing van Geweld: Het Nederlands–Indonesisch Conflict* (Zutphen: Walburg, 2012); J. J. P. de Jong, *De Terugtocht: Nederland en de Dekolonisatie van Indonesië* (Amsterdam: Boom, 2015).

violence by Dutch military forces, including summary executions.[2] It would be more than four years of conflict, extensive negotiations, official agreements, and truces announced and broken before the Netherlands transferred sovereignty to Indonesia on 27 December 1949. Indonesians across the archipelago celebrated exuberantly.

Although most Indonesians were united in their hatred of the Dutch, they had many different visions of the archipelago's future. Several politically inclined physicians participated in these debates, promoting different scenarios. Indonesia's medical profession suffered during the revolution years as an unprecedented number of alternate career paths became available to medical students and young physicians, and talent dispersed. Because of their linguistic skills and educational credentials, they were well qualified for positions in the administrative institutions of the new state. Some became military officers; others became politicians, bureaucrats, ambassadors, or businessmen. Those who remained physicians served in the armed forces or joined the Indonesian Red Cross to provide medical care near the battlefields, which enhanced their post-war reputations. Most members of Indonesia's small medical elite declared their support for the Republic of Indonesia. In January 1946, the instructors at the former Ika Daigaku moved to Yogyakarta, the heartland of the Indonesian Republic, to continue medical teaching under demanding and often dangerous conditions. When medical instruction ceased after the second Dutch military offensive, the medical students joined the dispersed guerrilla forces in the mountains. In the Dutch East Indies, several of their nationalist predecessors had stepped beyond the confines of medicine by engaging in journalism, politics, and other activities supporting the nationalist movement. These young physicians and medical students, in contrast, were able to further the cause of independence by following the calling of their profession. Their work reinforced the strong association between physicians and Indonesian nationalism.

The Declaration of Independence, Dutch Neo-Colonialism, and the Indonesian Revolution

In the first few weeks after the proclamation of independence, Indonesians worked frenetically to establish their new state with functioning government

---

[2] The use of systematic violence against Indonesian civilians by the Dutch military has only recently become a topic of discussion in the Netherlands. See Gert Oostindie, *Soldaat in Indonesië, 1945–1950* (Amsterdam: Prometheus, 2015) and Rémy Limpach, *De Brandende Kampongs van Generaal Spoor* (Amsterdam: Boom, 2016). For a general discussion on the violence that characterised the Indonesian revolution, see Bart Luttikhuis and A. Dirk Moses, eds., *Colonial Counterinsurgency and Mass Violence: The Dutch Empire in Indonesia* (London: Routledge, 2014).

institutions. A mere two hours after the proclamation ceremony, key nationalist leaders met to discuss the Indonesian constitution, the creation of a parliament, and the transfer of power from the Japanese military administration. That night, students painted slogans on buildings all over Jakarta announcing Indonesia's independence. The following day, the group of nationalists met again and elected Sukarno and Hatta as president and vice president of the Republic of Indonesia. The following weeks were filled with meetings, some of which were held at Prapatan 10.[3] The Central Indonesian National Committee [Komite Nasional Indonesia Pusat] (KNIP), a preliminary parliament, was established on 27 August 1945, followed by the first cabinet, which was appointed by Sukarno on 4 September. It closely resembled the board of advisors to the Japanese military administration to safeguard administrative continuity; Boentaran Martoatmodjo became the first minister of health.[4] Although the previous decade had witnessed vast political change, many bureaucratic functionaries continued to hold their positions. At the same time, it was important for the Republic of Indonesia to dissociate itself from the institutions established by the Japanese to demonstrate its legitimacy.

Two days after the declaration of independence, the Indonesian instructors at the Jakarta Ika Daigaku established the Indonesian Institute of Higher Education [Balai Perguruan Tinggi Republik Indonesia].[5] Sarwono Prawirohardjo, who had been associate professor of obstetrics and gynaecology and the assistant of Dean Masamitsu Itagaki, was appointed president of the Institute and dean of medicine.[6] In September, militant youth groups forcibly took possession of Jakarta's railway stations, tram system, radio station, and government institutions. The 'Beast Squad [Pasoekan Dadjal]', a militia drawn from the medical students at Prapatan 10, had launched this campaign by taking possession of the buildings of the medical school on 29

---

[3] Soejono Martosewojo, Eri Soedewo, Sarnanto, Taufik Abdullah, and Idris Siregar, *Mahasiswa '45, Prapatan 10: Pengabdiannya* (Bandung: Patma, 1984), 88–90.

[4] Benedict R. O'G. Anderson, *Java in a Time of Revolution: Occupation and Resistance, 1944–1946*, Equinox Classic Indonesian Books (Jakarta: Equinox, 2006 [1972]), 110–24.

[5] S. Somadikarta, Tri Wahyuning M. Irsyam, and Boen S. Oemarjati, *Tahun Emas Universitas Indonesia*, 3 vols., vol. 1: *Dari Balai ke Universitas* (Jakarta: Penerbit Universitas Indonesia, 2000), 11–25, 32–33. For an overview of academic initiatives during the Indonesian struggle for independence, see R. Thomas Murray, *A Chronicle of Indonesian Higher Education: The First Half Century, 1920–1970* (Singapore: Chopmen, 1973), 40–86; Sartono Kartodirdjo, Marwati Djoened Poesponegoro, and Nugroho Notosusanto, *Zaman Jepang dan Zaman Republik Indonesia, 1942–1998*, vol. 6, *Sejarah Nasional Indonesia* (Jakarta: Balai Pustaka, 2008), 285–89.

[6] For a biography, see Asvi Warman Adam, *Sarwono Prawirohardjo: Pembangun Institusi Ilmu Pengetahuan di Indonesia* (Jakarta: Lembaga Ilmu Pengetahuan Indonesia, 2009). For his activities as a member of Young Java, see Sarwono Prawirohardjo, 'Nasib Studiefonds Kita Dikemoedian Hari', in *Gedenkboek Jong Java 1915 – 7 Maart – 1930: Kitab Peringatan Jong-Java* (Jakatera: Pedoman Besar Jong-Java, 1930), 183–205.

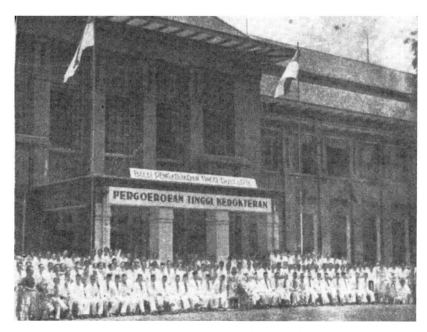

Figure 8.1 The Pergoeroean Tinggi Kedoktoran, Balai Pergoeroean Tinggi Republik Indonesia. Opening day. The walls of the building were covered with dark paint to camouflage the building from the air. Figure appeared in *Berita Film Indonesia*. Figure courtesy of Christopher Woodrich.

August. The next day, Itagaki officially handed the reigns of the institution to Sarwono.[7] The instructors at the Ika Daigaku were appointed to positions at the Indonesian Medical School [Pergoeroean Tinggi Kedokteran], and teaching commenced that afternoon (Figure 8.1). The Indonesian Red Cross [Palang Merah Indonesia] was founded on 7 September and organised several mobile medical teams. Bahder Djohan became secretary.[8] The Indonesian Medical School quickly graduated forty-five physicians, all of whom were exempted from taking their final exams because their services were urgently needed.

During the months immediately following the declaration of independence, all individuals who were willing and able worked to organise the institutions of the new state. Within days of the declaration, the provisional government asked Eri Soedewo, one of the leaders of Prapatan 10, to assist with

---

[7] Martosewojo et al., *Mahasiswa '45, Prapatan 10*, 127–28.
[8] Martosewojo et al., *Mahasiswa '45, Prapatan 10*, 120–24; Bahder Johan, *Bahder Johan: Pengabdi Kemanusian* (Jakarta: Gunung Agung, 1980), 85–100.

the organisation of the Indonesian armed forces.[9] Several medical students and young physicians who had received military training from the Japanese signed up as military officers. They set up a military training camp just outside Jakarta. Others became staff members of ministries and governmental institutions; their linguistic capacities were highly valued. Still others worked as journalists for newspapers and government-issued magazines. Because of these unprecedented opportunities, the urgent need for services, and their patriotism, many medical students opted for non-medical careers. Studying medicine had inspired them to embrace nation-building ideals; with the conditions that prevailed immediately after independence, they were able to participate in building a new nation, but it meant leaving medicine behind. Many eagerly embraced these opportunities, which helped fuel the revolution but depleted the medical profession.

On 25 August Soedewo and Chaerul Saleh, one of the radical student leaders at the Menteng 31 dormitory, debated the role of Indonesia's youth movements. Saleh had advocated military confrontation with the Japanese and replacing Indonesia's senior leadership, which was tarnished by its collaboration with the Japanese. Soedewo disagreed. Attacking the Japanese would be suicidal, he argued, and all youth groups should support Sukarno, Hatta, and the preliminary governmental structures that had been established thus far. Unable to resolve their differences, Saleh's associates left Prapatan 10, moved to Menteng 31, and called themselves the Young Indonesian Generation [Angkatan Pemuda Indonesia] (API [*api* = fire]).[10] Inspired by Sutan Sjahrir, medical students continued their participation in building state institutions. At the same time, an increasing number of militant youth groups started to prepare for armed conflict. The students at Menteng 31 were their leaders.

Several weeks passed before the British established a meaningful presence in Jakarta. Since the Indonesian archipelago had been transferred from General MacArthur's Southwest Pacific Area to Lord Mountbatten's British Southeast Asia Command only a few weeks before Japan capitulated, Mountbatten's staff had not been able to draw up detailed management plans.[11] His troops were already overextended, and the addition of the enormous area of the archipelago presented serious challenges. The British quickly realised that the new

---

[9] After several years serving in the military, Brigadier-General Soedewo resumed his medical training and specialised in surgery. From 1966 to 1972, he was president of Airlangga University. After that, he served as Indonesia's ambassador to Sweden. A biography of Eri Soedewo was written by his wife: Mang Eri Soedewo, *A Freedom Fighter: My Life with Eri-San* (Jakarta: Kata Hasta Pustaka, 2008).

[10] Cribb, *Gangsters and Revolutionaries*, 59; Martosewojo et al., *Mahasiswa '45, Prapatan 10*, 106–07; Anderson, *Java in a Time of Revolution*, 117–24.

[11] Richard McMillan, *The British Occupation of Indonesia, 1945–1946: Britain, the Netherlands and the Indonesian Revolution* (New York: Routledge, 2005), 2.

Republic had the population's support. Since their primary responsibilities were to repatriate Japanese soldiers and Dutch citizens, they decided to interfere as little as possible in local affairs. To the dismay of the Dutch, they negotiated with the Republican government to achieve their aims, thereby legitimising it. Nevertheless, tensions increased after Dutch soldiers started arriving. Jakarta's streets were unsafe while groups of former Dutch internees and armed bands of Indo-Europeans and Ambonese soldiers frequently clashed with Indonesian gangs and militias.[12] In early November, after a high British military official was shot under ambiguous circumstances in Surabaya, the British launched a major military offensive against Indonesian nationalists. Dentist Moestopo led the hastily organised Indonesian forces, assisted by several former students of the Surabaya Medical College.[13] On 4 January 1946, after the Allied military forces tightened their grip on Jakarta, the Republican government relocated to Yogyakarta.

On 21 January 1946, the Netherlands Indies Civil Administration established the Emergency University with psychiatrist P. M. van Wulfften Palthe as president.[14] Its Faculty of Medicine commenced teaching at the Cikini Hospital close to the Indonesian Medical School; sixty-three Dutch, sixty-three Chinese, and two Indonesian students enrolled.[15] In October 1946, C. D. de Langen succeeded van Wulfften Palthe. To his regret, he was unable to re-establish contact with his former students and accomplished little during his presidency. In March 1947, the Emergency University was renamed the University of Indonesia. In December, it opened a second Faculty of Medicine in the buildings of the former Surabaya Medical College.[16]

Medical education at the institutions associated with the Republic of Indonesia continued in various locations. In Jakarta, Sarwono Prawirohardjo led local endeavours. After Sardjito moved the Pasteur Institute from Bandung to Klaten, Central Java, in March 1946, he provided preclinical teaching at the local hospital.[17] At the same time, Asikin established clinical training in Surakarta. Before leaving Jakarta, Indonesian physicians had smuggled

[12] Anderson, *Java in a Time of Revolution*, 125–66.
[13] Suhario 'Kecik' Padmodiwiryo, *Student Soldiers: A Memoir of the Battle That Sparked Indonesia's National Revolution* (Jakarta: Yayasan Pustaka Obor Indonesia, 2015).
[14] P. M. van Wulfften Palthe and P. A. Kerstens, *Opening Nood-Universiteit: Redevoeringen* (Groningen en Batavia: Wolters, 1946).
[15] Van Wulfften Palthe and Kerstens, *Opening Nood-Universiteit*, 7.
[16] For an overview of the activities of the University of Indonesia, see *Universiteit van Indonesië: Gids voor het Academiejaar 1949–1950* (Batavia: Landsdrukkerij, 1949).
[17] For overviews of medical teaching during the Indonesian struggle for independence, see Murray, *Chronicle of Indonesian Higher Education*; *The Medical Faculty, Its Allied Departments and Its Relation to the National University of Indonesia: A Brief Report Prepared by the Ministry of Health, Republic of Indonesia* (Yogyakarta: Ministry of Health, RI, 1950) (this text is most likely written by Sardjito); M. Sardjito, *The Development of the Universitas Gadjah Mada* (Yogyakarta: Universitas Gadjah Mada, 1955).

pharmaceuticals and medical equipment to Central Java. In September 1946, additional teaching facilities were established in Malang, under Sjaaf, with medical equipment from Surabaya. Medical students alternated between attending classes, participating in guerrilla warfare, and volunteering for the Indonesian Red Cross. In March 1946, the Dutch authorities took possession of the buildings of the Indonesian Faculty of Medicine and repurposed them for the Dutch Emergency University. Indonesian medical teaching continued at the hospital next door, now renamed University Hospital [Roemah Sakit Pergoeroean Tinggi].[18] In an arrangement that defies the imagination, the Dutch Faculty of Medicine and the remnant of its Indonesian counterpart were neighbours for the next two and a half years.

On 15 November 1946, representatives of the Netherlands and the Republic of Indonesia signed the Linggardjati agreement, a triumph for Sjahrir, the Republic's prime minister, who had tirelessly advocated diplomacy over armed conflict.[19] Mohammad Roem had led the negotiations for the Republic. Sjahrir, appointed because he had not taken a position in the Japanese military administration, had been prime minister of three cabinets since November 1945. His success caused considerable resentment among the youth militias advocating armed struggle. According to the terms of the agreement, the Netherlands recognised Republican rule over most of Java and Sumatra and incorporated the Republic into a future federal state. The Dutch occupation forces subsequently established a number of puppet states to counterbalance the Republic's influence. Because the agreement was unpopular in both Indonesia and the Netherlands, however, armed conflict resumed.

In December 1946, the Dutch military administration established the State of East Indonesia [Negara Indonesia Timur]. It encompassed all islands east of Java and Kalimantan, including Sulawesi, the Moluccas, Bali, West Timor, and the Lesser Sunda Islands. This new state covered a vast area and a multitude of ethnic groups, and lacked any obvious *raison d'être*. In 1946, Minahasan ophthalmologist S. J. Warouw, the second chairman of Young Minahasa, became one of the main advocates for a federal Indonesian state with close ties to the Netherlands.[20] He had previously gained some administrative experience after he was elected to Makassar's city council in the late 1930s. In an elaborate manifesto, he argued that a federal state was needed because of the great diversity of ethnic groups in Indonesia. He made his point using various psychological, philosophical, historical, sociological, and theological arguments.

[18] 'Geneeskundige Hoogeschool', *Het Dagblad*, 21 March 1946, 1. See also P. M. van Wulfften Palthe, 'Het Ontstaan der Nooduniversiteit van Nederlandsch-Indië', *Nederlands Tijdschrift voor Geneeskunde* 90, no. 26 (29 June 1946), 748–50.

[19] Rushdy Hoesein, *Terobosan Sukarno dalam Perundingan Linggardjati* (Jakarta: Kompas, 2010).

[20] S. J. Warouw, *Indonesië in Rijksverband* (N.p.: Author, 1946).

Warouw became the minister of health in the State of East Indonesia when it was created, and for the final three months of 1947, he was acting prime minister, but achieved little.[21] In 1949, Warouw advocated independence for the Minahasa, hoping – to no avail – to influence the final negotiations between the Dutch and the Indonesians.[22] After independence, he returned to his medical career. He was involved in establishing the Faculty of Medicine at the University of Makassar and in 1964 became the first president of the Indonesian Christian University Tomohon, just outside Manado.

Dutch Physicians on the Indonesian Revolution

Several Dutch physicians participated in debates on the future of the archipelago. P. M. van Wulfften Palthe, whose militant attitude had hardened during the Japanese occupation, was strongly opposed to the Indonesian Republic. In late 1945, he formulated a psychoanalytic interpretation of the Indonesian struggle for independence, but the Dutch military authorities soon silenced him.[23] In his analysis, van Wulfften Palthe synthesised the views of colonial psychiatrists on the inherently primitive, emotional, and childish nature of the Indonesian mind with psychoanalytic insights and a rather dated form of crowd psychology. He suggested that the Indonesian hatred for the Japanese had been transferred to the Dutch after Japan's capitulation, which had come about without any effort or struggle.[24] Because these residual feelings of hatred found no outlet, they intensified. As a consequence, he argued, Indonesians had collectively regressed to a primitive, highly emotional state which would inevitably explode in a collective form of amok, with violent outbursts erroneously directed towards the Dutch.[25] Indonesian militias consisting of bandits, Japanese-trained soldiers, unkempt youth, and even a few Indonesian intellectuals, all

---

[21] See Ide Anak Agung Gde Agung, *From the Formation of the State of East Indonesia Towards the Establishment of the United States of Indonesia* (Jakarta: Yayasan Obor Indonesia, 1996), 144, 312–31.

[22] S. J. Warouw, *Minahassa Strijdt voor Zelfbeschikkingsrecht en Vrijheid* (The Hague: Komite Ketatanegaraan Minahassa, 1949).

[23] P. M. van Wulfften Palthe, 'Ingezonden: Psychological Aspects of the Indonesian Problem', *Nederlands Tijdschrift voor Geneeskunde* 93, no. 49 (3 December 1949), 4118–19. See also files in the Dutch National Archives, The Hague, Collection 190 J. W. Meyer Ranneft, 1910–1968, access number 2.21.121, file number 486, 'Beschouwingen over de Indonesische Kwestie'.

[24] v. W. P. [P. M. van Wulfften Palthe], 'Haatgevoelens', *Het Dagblad*, 22 January 1946, 1. For an extensive analysis of van Wulfften Palthe's psychoanalytic interpretation of the Indonesian revolution, see Hans Pols, 'The Totem Vanishes, the Hordes Revolt: A Psychoanalytic Interpretation of the Indonesian Struggle for Independence', in *Globalizing the Unconscious: Psychoanalysis, Colonial Trauma, Sovereignties*, ed. Warwick H. Anderson, Deborah Jenson, and Richard Keller (Durham, NC: Duke University Press, 2011), 141–65.

[25] P. M. van Wulfften Palthe, 'Psychologische Beschouwing omtrent den Huidigen Toestand op Java', *Nederlands Tijdschrift voor Geneeskunde* 90, no. 18 (4 May 1946), 426.

in a trance-like state, gave irrational impulses free rein, leading to the formation of uncontrollable, hyper-aggressive mobs. Only decisive military action – prohibiting all meetings, dispersing all groups, and disarming gangs – could keep these primitive impulses at bay and prevent further violent eruptions; negotiation and rational discussion would be counterproductive. It is doubtful whether Indonesian intellectuals were aware of van Wulfften Palthe's imaginative fusion of reactionary political ideas and psychoanalytic thinking. His theories illustrate merely the chasm between the warring camps.[26]

Van Wulfften Palthe's views were not remarkable among Dutch physicians. Near the end of the first military incursion, the Dutch Ministry of Overseas Territories (formerly the Ministry of Colonies) received a request to send out physicians to Indonesia. In October 1947, physician E. Kits van Waveren, the founder and chair of the Medical Coordination Committee, established by the Royal Dutch Association of Physicians to coordinate medical assistance in Indonesia, travelled to the archipelago to ascertain the need for medical manpower. In his report, he contrasted the hospitals run by the Dutch ('clean … excellently organised … packed with patients') and those run by Indonesians in areas recently conquered by the Dutch military forces ('gross neglect, disorganisation, and mismanagement … dirty … almost empty').[27] The report lacked critical contextual information: the Republican hospitals visited by Kits van Waveren were located in areas the Dutch had blockaded for more than two years, preventing access to medical equipment, medicines, food, and basic necessities. The area had subsequently been devastated by the Dutch 'liberation'. It was no surprise that conditions in these hospitals were sub-optimal. Nevertheless, Dutch physicians interviewed by Kits van Waveren attributed these conditions to the character deficits of their Indonesian colleagues:

They lack the initiative, originality, motivation, and the creative higher (and scientific) mental powers and organisational capacities of Westerners … [Indonesian] physicians and students do not think independently to a sufficient degree, they are good learners and at times very good at memorising, but are often helpless when they encounter situations and problems of which the solution has not been taught.[28]

Their Indonesian colleagues, explained the Dutch physicians, excelled in routine tasks but lacked initiative. They tended towards indolence and superstition, and practiced medicine without compassion. Kits van Waveren had interviewed Indonesian physicians at the Jakarta University Hospital but did not allow their

---

[26] Van Wulfften Palthe could publish an English translation of his ideas only at the end of 1949, when he no longer was a civil servant of the Netherlands Indies Civil Administration. See P. M. van Wulfften Palthe, *Psychological Aspects of the Indonesian Problem* (Leiden: Brill, 1949).

[27] E. Kits van Waveren, 'De Artsenpositie in Indonesië', *Nederlands Tijdschrift voor Geneeskunde* 91 (1947), 3437.

[28] Kits van Waveren, 'De Artsenpositie in Indonesië', 3438.

views to influence his report. He noted that Indonesian physicians supported the Republic but did not elaborate further.[29]

Kits van Waveren's report caused a stir in Dutch medical circles. Within a week, he was forced to resign as chair of the Medical Coordination Commission. The board of the Dutch Association of Tropical Medicine condemned his report because of his derogatory comments about Indonesian physicians. Even van Wulfften Palthe criticised the report, emphasising that health conditions in Indonesia would improve only when Indonesian and Dutch physicians cooperated.[30] The president of the Dutch University of Indonesia, physician C. Bonne, also protested.[31] Kits van Waveren's ideas reflected Dutch propaganda, which emphasised Dutch largesse in the provision of medical care to Indonesians while highlighting the poverty and substandard medical care in areas controlled by the Republicans. More importantly, he had failed to accept Indonesian physicians as colleagues and legitimate interlocutors.

Taking Sides: Indonesian Physicians during the Revolution

In colonial times, Indies physicians were cosmopolitan in orientation and articulated hybrid identities containing both Dutch and Indonesian elements. Indonesia's medical elite had enjoyed advanced medical training in the Netherlands and were consequently much closer to the colonial European social sphere. The Indonesian revolution required both groups to take sides. Several Indonesian physicians had chosen to live in the Netherlands before the Japanese annexation or soon after the declaration of independence. Others favoured a federal Indonesian state, which would, in their opinion, safeguard ethnic and religious diversity. Still others vied unreservedly for the Republic. Tracing their decisions and choices, made before, during, and after the Indonesian revolution, sheds light on the way they envisaged their own future and that of the archipelago.

Some members of the Indonesian medical elite felt an affinity for the Dutch and moved to the Netherlands upon retirement. In 1933, Javanese physician Mas Soewarno, the first secretary of Boedi Oetomo and an instructor in ophthalmology at the Surabaya Medical College, moved to the Netherlands with his Dutch wife, a gynaecologist, and their son, in the hope that the Dutch climate would have a beneficial effect on his tuberculosis. At the end of 1945, he briefly returned to the archipelago to treat the eye diseases of former Dutch

---

[29] Kits van Waveren, 'De Artsenpositie in Indonesië', 3435.

[30] 'Ingezonden: De Artsenpositie in Indonesië, II', *Nederlands Tijdschrift voor Geneeskunde* 91, no. 52 (27 December 1947), 3756; P. M. van Wulfften Palthe, 'Ingezonden: De Artsenpositie in Indonesië', *Nederlands Tijdschrift voor Geneeskunde* 92, no. 2 (10 January 1947), 122.

[31] C. Bonne, 'Uitzending van Artsen uit Nederland', *Medisch Maandblad* 2, no. 17 (1947), 336.

internees.[32] Christian Moluccan physician H. D. J. Apituley, who had been a stridently pro-Dutch Indonesian member of the Volksraad from 1927 to 1934, retired to the Netherlands in 1935. Psychiatrist Ronald Tumbelaka, a Minahasan Christian who had served as inspector of institutions for the insane for the Indies Public Health Service, moved to the Netherlands in 1938 to take up a position at a Dutch mental hospital. He returned to Indonesia in September 1945 to assist in the reorganisation of health services in those parts of Java under Dutch control but soon realised that Indonesia's independence was inevitable. He was kidnapped and murdered when he returned from a visit to the Buitenzorg mental hospital in August 1946, probably by a militant Indonesian militia who thought that he sympathised with the Dutch.[33]

The first generation of Indies physicians was modernist, advocating closer ties between the Netherlands and the Dutch East Indies. Christian Ambonese physician W. K. Tehupeiory, the founder of the Association of Indies Physicians, had been a prominent physician in private practice during the Dutch colonial era. He never abandoned his political allegiance to the Netherlands and continued to display a portrait of Queen Wilhelmina in his living room during the Japanese period. Probably because of his popularity and his poor state of health (he had suffered a series of minor strokes), the Japanese military administration did not intervene.[34] After 1945, Tehupeiory's brother-in-law, the Christian Ambonese psychiatrist and nationalist J. A. Latumeten, cautiously re-established contact with him, fully aware that associating with individuals holding pro-Dutch sympathies was not without risk. Tehupeiory died of a stroke in November 1946. At his funeral, representatives of the Dutch occupying forces and the Indonesian Republic gave speeches. Among them were Latumeten, the (Dutch) interim mayor of Jakarta, the Christian Ambonese physician Johannes Leimena, Professor C. D. de Langen, Abdul Rasjid representing the resurrected Association of Indonesian Physicians, and several representatives of Protestant and Maluku associations.[35] Warring sides found common cause. After the first Dutch military campaign, such a gathering was unimaginable.

In the first months of 1946, Latumeten had been appointed professor of psychiatry at the Indonesian Medical School and inspector of mental hospitals

---

[32] Mas Soewarno, 'Iets over Kampogen', *Nederlands Tijdschrift voor Geneeskunde* 90 (14 January 1946), 213–16.

[33] Herman Keppy, 'Beschaamt de Minahassa Niet', in *Pendek: Korte Verhalen over Indische Levens* (Amsterdam: West, 2013), 75–80.

[34] Letter, J. A. Latumeten to Annie Tehupeiory, 21 July 1946. Archive Willem Karel Tehupeiory, inventory number 6, International Institute of Social History, Amsterdam.

[35] 'Dr. Tehupeiory', *Het Dagblad*, 1 November 1946, 1. For a historical novel on the life of W. K. Tehupeiory based on extensive archival research, see Herman Keppy, *Tussen Ambon en Amsterdam* (Amsterdam: Conserve, 2004).

at the Indonesian Ministry of Health. Unlike Tehupeiory, he had long favoured independence. Despite his outspoken political ideas (he had been one of the main organisers of the physicians' strike in 1919), he received a fellowship for advanced medical training in the Netherlands, where he lived from 1922 to 1925.[36] He was active in the increasingly radical Perhimpunan Indonesia and orchestrated a response to the views of Dutch colonial psychiatrists on the nature of the Indonesian mind. After he returned to the Indies, Latumeten ceased participating in political activities and focused on medicine. He held appointments at several mental hospitals before he became the first superintendent of the new Sabang mental hospital in 1927. In 1936, he was appointed superintendent at the Lawang mental hospital, where he remained during the Japanese period. In May 1945 he was arrested by the kenpeitai, and nearly died of starvation in prison. He was released after Japan's capitulation but was in very poor health. A militant youth group promptly banned him from the asylum since, as a Christian Moluccan physician who had held respectable positions in the colonial era, he was viewed with automatic suspicion. The youngsters were almost certainly not aware of his nationalist ideals and earlier activities.[37] Latumeten never fully recovered, and died in Jakarta in 1948.

Mohammad Amir had been politically active for most of his life. During his time at the Batavia Medical College he was the main ideologue of Young Sumatra and served as its second chairman. After graduating in 1923, he moved to the Netherlands with a bursary from the Dutch Theosophical Association for advanced medical training, specialising in psychiatry. He married a Dutch woman and was active in the Perhimpunan Indonesia but withdrew after the Theosophists threatened to discontinue his bursary.[38] Amir published widely in Theosophical journals and in Indonesian newspapers, and co-founded the weekly cultural magazine *Observation* [*Penindjauan*] in 1934.[39] The same

---

[36] Latumeten received his Dutch medical degree in 1924 and his doctorate in medicine in 1925 with the dissertation Jonas Andreas Latumeten, *Over de Kernen van den Nervus Oculomotorius* (Utrecht: Den Boer, 1924).

[37] Letter, J. A. Latumeten to Maartje Johanna (Annie) Tehupeiory-Ommering (Tehupeiory's estranged wife), 21 July 1946.

[38] Amir was awarded a Dutch medical degree in 1926 at the University of Amsterdam and received his doctorate in medical science in 1928 at the University of Utrecht with a dissertation on a gynaecological topic: Mohamad Amir, *Bijdrage tot de Kliniek en Therapie der Deflexieliggingen* (Utrecht: Smits, 1928). For a biography of Amir, see Wisnu Subagyo, *Dr. Mohamad Amir: Karya dan Pengabdiannya* (Jakarta: Departemen Pendidikan dan Kebudayaan, Direktorat Sejarah dan Nilai Tradisional, Proyek Inventarisasi dan dokumentasi Sejarah Nasional, 1986).

[39] Amir's co-editor of *Penindjauan* was G. S. S. J. Ratulangi. About this cultural weekly see Andrew Goss, *The Floracrats: State-Sponsored Science and the Failure of the Enlightenment in Indonesia* (Madison: University of Wisconsin Press, 2011), 110–11. Amir frequently wrote for the Theosophical journal *The Pioneer* [*De Pionier*]. For a collection of Amir's political and

year, he became the first director of the psychiatric clinic in Medan, the thriving urban centre of the Deli plantation area. He left in 1937 to become the private physician to the sultan of Langkat, a man with strong hypochondriacal beliefs who lived in constant fear of being poisoned. Before the Japanese annexation, Amir was known as a Western-educated intellectual who hoped that Indonesians would retain their cultural heritage while appropriating the fruits of Western science and medicine. After the Japanese annexation, he focused on his medical practice and secretly aided interned Dutch citizens. In 1943, after several minor strokes, he became decidedly pro-Japanese, and was appointed to the Sumatran equivalent of Java's Advisory Council.[40] The head of Sumatra's Japanese military administration requested that he join Sukarno, Hatta, and Radjiman on their flight to Jakarta after they returned from Saigon to discuss Indonesia's independence.[41]

Amir was present at the declaration of independence on 17 August 1945, and was appointed minister in Sukarno's first cabinet and vice governor of Sumatra. He was instructed to spread news of Indonesia's independence in Sumatra and to establish Indonesian government institutions there. Without the support of a local militia, however, Amir's position in Medan was weak. When British troops landed in October 1945 with Dutch officials in tow, the situation quickly deteriorated. Because of their ability to grant land tenancy rights to the Deli plantations, the sultanates in Deli had become extremely wealthy, which fostered resentment among the rest of the population. The sultanates supported the Allies and fully expected the return of pre-war conditions, but in February 1946, during Sumatra's social revolution, most sultans were murdered together with their families.[42] Young revolutionaries grew suspicious of Amir because of his European lifestyle and his Dutch medical training. After several failed assassination attempts, Amir and his family fled to a British evacuation camp and were transported to the Netherlands. He returned to Sulawesi to work as a physician, regretting that he could no longer take part in the revolution. He only remained there for a short time, however; after a second series of strokes, he was transported to the Netherlands, where he died in hospital on 29 December

---

cultural writings, see M. Amir, *Boenga Rampai: Himpoenan Karangan jang Terbit Diantara Tahoen 1923 dan 1939* (Medan: Centrale Courant en Boekhandel, 1940).

[40] See 'De Rol door Dr Amir Gespeeld in de Sociale Revolutie ter S. O. K.', NIOD Institute for War, Holocaust, and Genocide Studies Archives, Access number 400, file 2131. See also 'Notes Made by Dr. Amir Concerning the Indonesian Revolution, 1946', NIOD Archives, Access number 400, file 4739.

[41] The other representatives were T. M. Hassan, who was appointed governor of Sumatra, and Abdul Abbas.

[42] Anthony Reid, *The Blood of the People: Revolution and the End of Traditional Rule in Northern Sumatra* (New York: Oxford University Press, 1979). Reid mentions Amir several times, on pp. 123, 144, 148, 152, 218, 224–25, 234, and 244.

1949, without regaining consciousness. Two days prior, the Netherlands had transferred sovereignty to the Republic of Indonesia.[43]

Physicians joined opposing factions during the Indonesian revolution. After Amir's departure, the situation in Sumatra became increasingly chaotic, with various militias fighting against the Allies and, at times, each other. One group, the Fifth Militia [Pasukan V], was organised by Mangaradja Soangkoepon, Abdul Rasjid's father. Although it aimed to bring stability to the area, it was seen by other militias as assisting the Dutch.[44] It was at one point led by the Christian Toba-Batak physician F. J. Nainggolan, whose family had been murdered by a rival militia.[45] In December 1947, the State of East Sumatra [Negara Sumatera Timur] was founded as a Dutch puppet state. Tengkeu Mansoer, a member of the family of the sultan of Asahan and, previously, the first president of Young Sumatra, became head of state.[46] Nainggolan became health minister. In July 1948, the Dutch military administration established the Assembly for Federal Consultation with the aim of creating a federal United States of Indonesia. By that time, the Dutch had created fifteen separate puppet states, but with little success, since the majority of the representatives of these states came to sympathise with the Republic. Mansoer and Nainggolan resumed their medical careers after independence.

The Dutch Military Campaigns, 1947–1948

On 21 July 1947, the Dutch military forces commenced their first incursion, 'Operation Product', into Republican territory, to capture economically productive areas on Java and the east coast of Sumatra. The Dutch occupation to this point had been very costly, since the territory under Dutch control was small and economically insignificant. The recently established United Nations condemned the Dutch offensive. Sjahrir, then representing the Republic at the United Nations, proposed possible solutions to the conflict, and the Security Council established the Committee of Good Offices to assist the parties to

---

[43] Interview of the author with Anton Amir, Mohammad Amir's son. Middelburg, The Netherlands, 24 September 2013. Anneke Amir (Mohammad Amir's daughter), Dagboek 1943–1946, in possession of the Amir family.

[44] Reid, *Blood of the People*, 164.

[45] Nainggolan had graduated from the STOVIA in 1918. Novelist Beb Vuyk has written a literary rendition of the biography of Dr Nainggolan; see Beb Vuyk, 'De Laatste Waardigheid', in *Verzameld Werk* (Amsterdam: Querido, 1972), 446–61. In Vuyk's rendition, Dr Nambela represents Dr Nainggolan.

[46] Dr Tengkeu Mansoer was a nephew of the sultan of Asahan. He graduated from the STOVIA in 1920 and received his Dutch medical degree from the University of Leiden, where he specialised in surgery, in 1926. He received his doctorate in medical science from the same university in 1928. He married a Dutch woman. His dissertation appeared as Tengkoe Mansoer, *De Lachgasnarcose in de Heelkunde* (Leiden: Patria, 1928).

arrive at a peaceful solution. The Dutch offensive ceased on 5 August 1947, after the conquest of most of Java and the plantation area around Medan, East Sumatra. Conditions within the Republic rapidly deteriorated, and at least 6 million refugees flocked to the small Republican area which was effectively blockaded by the Dutch. Food and other essentials became scarce.

After the Dutch military incursion, medical teaching in Malang ceased and students and instructors moved to Klaten, taking whatever medical equipment they could. Klaten, Surakarta, and Yogyakarta were now close to the fighting lines. When they were not receiving instruction or working, medical students served at the front lines as members of the Indonesian Red Cross or as soldiers.[47] The Indonesian military forces engaged in guerrilla warfare while medical students and physicians provided medical care to battle casualties under trying conditions. Members of the Indonesian medical elite actively supported the Indonesian revolution, which elevated their already stellar pre-war reputations. In Jakarta, the position of Indonesian physicians and medical students deteriorated. On 24 August 1948, the Dutch military occupied Jakarta's University Hospital, which had been the last institution in Jakarta under Republican control.[48] Physicians removed whatever medical supplies and equipment they could to the nearby home of Bahder Djohan. When Dutch soldiers arrived, all 1,200 hospital employees walked out in an act of collective defiance. Medical instruction continued at the homes of radiologist W. Z. Johannes, Bahder Djohan, psychiatrist Slamet Imam Santoso, and Sarwono Prawirohardjo.[49]

The second Dutch military offensive, which aimed to overthrow the Republican government in Yogyakarta, commenced on 19 December 1948. With both international opinion and sentiment in the archipelago increasingly favouring the Republic, the Dutch thought that a decisive military victory was the only viable option.[50] The Dutch occupied Yogyakarta within a day and arrested Sukarno, Hatta, and most Indonesian government ministers. Sukarno, Hatta, and Sjahrir were exiled to Bangka island, off the coast of East Sumatra.

---

[47] For an overview of the organisation of medical care by the Republic and the logistical challenges it faced, see B. Bouman, *Ieder voor Zich en de Republiek voor Ons Allen: De Logistiek Achter de Indonesische Revolutie, 1945–1950* (Amsterdam: Boom, 2006), 49–50, 153–59, 170–74, 183–84, 219–23, 314–19, 375–76.

[48] 'C. B. Z. op Salemba Overgenomen', *Het Dagblad*, 24 August 1948, 1. See also Robert Cribb, 'The Nationalist World of Occupied Jakarta, 1946–1949', in *From Batavia to Jakarta: Indonesia's Capital 1930s to 1980s*, ed. Susan Abeyasekere (Melbourne: Monash University, 1985), 97.

[49] For biographies of W. Z. Johannes, a Christian physician from the island of Rote near Timor, see Zaidir Djalal, *Prof. Dr. W. Z. Yohannes* (Jakarta: Mutiara, 1978); and M. Soenjata Kardarmadja, *Prof. Dr. Wilhelmus Zakarias Johannes* (Jakarta: Departemen Pendidikan dan Kebudayaan, 1985).

[50] Julius Pour, *Doorstoot naar Djokja: Pertikaian Pemimpin Sipil-Militer* (Jakarta: Kompas, 2009).

The United Nations was outraged; its Committee of Good Offices had been ignored. The second offensive ended on 5 January 1949 after a forthright Security Council condemnation. The United States suspended its Marshall Aid to the Netherlands because the Dutch had spent these funds on its military forces fighting in Indonesia rather than on national reconstruction (the United States had effectively bankrolled both military offensives). A week later, the Security Council demanded the immediate release of the Republican cabinet and the establishment of an interim government. The Dutch government finally accepted that it had no option but to relinquish all claims to its former colonies. From August to November 1949, details of the transfer of sovereignty were negotiated in the Netherlands.

Because all medical teaching in Central Java had ceased, many physicians and medical students joined the guerrilla forces in the mountains surrounding Yogyakarta. On 7 May 1949, after a truce, medical education resumed in Yogyakarta. Hamengkubuwono IX, the city's sultan, made the residences of the crown prince available. Sardjito, who led the establishment of the new centre for medical education, described how the new premises were modified: 'The carriage house is transformed into a polyclinic, the guard house into a laboratory for bacteriology, the servants' room into a laboratory for chemistry, the ceremonial reception halls are used for lectures halls, and so on.'[51] The situation was less than ideal: there was limited medical equipment, medications were scarce, and the facilities were unsuitable. The Dutch blockade of Central Java had led to severe shortages of virtually everything. Sardjito related how medical equipment was smuggled from Klaten to Yogyakarta:

Students, employers and staff alike must turn smuggler, and carefully tend their fine instruments in their disguised packages along atrociously bad back roads which could be negotiated only on bicycle or on foot. The difficulties encountered during the removal can be realized if one imagines that the main road between Jogjakarta and Klaten – a distance of 20 miles – was wrecked by Indonesian guerrillas. Bridges were destroyed, tank traps blocked the road. Besides, Dutch troops and air forces controlled the countryside.[52]

Several other facilities for higher education were also transferred to Yogyakarta. On 19 December 1949, exactly one year after the start of the second Dutch offensive, the University of Gadjah Mada was established.[53] Sardjito was appointed president (a position he occupied until 1961) and dean of medicine. Yogyakarta's sultan donated a large plot of land just outside the city to the university, and a new campus was built over the following decades.

---

[51] Sardjito, *Development UGM*, 8.
[52] Sardjito, *Development UGM*, 7–8.
[53] Sutaryo, *Sejarah Fakultas Kedoktoran UGM – Rumah Sakit UGM/RSUP Dr. Sardjito* (Yogyakarta: Puspagama, 2016), 27–84.

Today, the university hospital is named after Sardjito. On 27 December 1949, the Netherlands formally transferred sovereignty to the Federal Republic of Indonesia [Republic Indonesia Serikat]. Indonesian independence had finally been recognised. On 17 August 1950, Indonesia's Independence Day, the fifteen federal states established by the Dutch became part of the unitary Republic of Indonesia.

The Dispersal of Medical Talent during the Indonesian Revolution

After Indonesia's declaration of independence, many medical students and young physicians became military officers, journalists, politicians, businessmen, or government officials. Several were involved in establishing the administrative institutions of the new state, writing and disseminating information for the outside world, and representing the Republic in international political bodies. Their association with the nascent Indonesian military led to many joining its ranks. When the military came to play an increasingly significant role in running the Indonesian economy, several physicians became businessmen. The involvement of so many young physicians and medical students in building the new nation led to a depletion of the medical profession.

The careers of several medical students at the former Ika Daigaku illustrate the highly fluid situation following the declaration of independence. Soedjatmoko, famous for his intellectual and philosophical interests, was born in a privileged Javanese family in January 1922. His father, K. W. T. Saleh Mangoendiningrat, was court physician to Solo's Sunan and had advocated research into traditional herbal medications during the second congress of the Association of Indonesian Physicians. Soedjatmoko strongly objected to the feudal orientation of Javanese society and refused to use his aristocratic title.[54] In 1940, after enrolling at the Batavia Medical School, he became a voracious reader and was active in several student associations and moderate nationalist youth groups. Like several of his fellow students, Soedjatmoko was concerned about Japan's fascist regime. Throughout the Japanese period, he was close to Sutan Sjahrir, and married Sjahrir's sister in 1951. The 1943 hair-cutting incident at the Ika Daigaku strengthened Soedjatmoko's anti-Japanese attitude, and he and Soedarpo were the leaders of the ensuing protests. After Soedjatmoko was imprisoned by the kenpeitai for four weeks and expelled from medical

---

[54] For Soedjatmoko's biography, see M. Nursam, *Pergumulan Seorang Intelektual: Biografi Soedjatmoko* (Jakarta: Gramedia, 2002). For a biography of Mohamad Saleh Mangoendiningrat, Soedjatmoko's father, see M. Nursam, *Prof. Dr. Dr. Moh. Saleh Mangundiningrat: Potret Cendekiawan Jawa* (Jakarta: SUN, 2006). Both biographies were commissioned by the family and written by the same author.

school, he became highly critical of Sukarno, Hatta, and other Indonesian political leaders for their collaboration with the Japanese. Upon his release from prison, Soedjatmoko returned to his family in Solo, dejected, and assisted his father in his medical practice.

When Soedjatmoko heard of the declaration of independence, he returned to Jakarta and was hired, along with his friend Soedarpo, by the Department of Propaganda in the government of Prime Minister Sutan Sjahrir. They worked for the English-language publication *The Voice of Indonesia* and the Dutch-language journal *Insight* [*Inzicht*], the main competitor of *Outlook* [*Uitzicht*], published by the Dutch Information Service. Their aim was to inform foreign journalists about the state of affairs in Indonesia. Unofficially, they became multilingual government employees who maintained contact with several ministers and appeared at key diplomatic and political discussions. In 1947, Sjahrir sent Soedjatmoko to New York to lead the diplomatic campaign for the Republic's international recognition. In 1951, Soedjatmoko returned to Indonesia and was elected to parliament as a representative of Sjahrir's socialist party in 1955. After Sukarno banned the party in 1958, Soedjatmoko spent two years as a guest lecturer at Cornell University.[55] When Suharto became president, Soedjatmoko served as Indonesia's representative at the United Nations and as ambassador to the United States. He also became a member of several international think tanks, joined the Club of Rome, and was elected to the board of trustees of the Ford Foundation. In 1980, he became the president of the United Nations University in Tokyo.[56] After Soedjatmoko's death, his wife published a collection of his most influential essays on humanism and cosmopolitanism.[57]

Until 1952, Soedjatmoko's close friend Soedarpo followed a very similar career trajectory.[58] After his expulsion from the Ika Daigaku, Soedarpo left

---

[55] During his stay at Cornell University, Soedjatmoko published an edited book: Soedjatmoko, *An Introduction to Indonesian Historiography* (Ithaca, NY: Cornell University Press, 1965). From this time also comes Soedjatmoko, *Southeast Asia Today and Tomorrow* (Honolulu, HI: East-West Center Press, 1969).

[56] Soedjatmoko published several more essays and books. See Soedjatmoko, *Development and Freedom* (New Delhi: Centre for Policy Research, 1980) and Soedjatmoko, *The Primacy of Freedom in Development* (Lanham, MD: University Press of America, 1985).

[57] Kathleen Newland and Kamala Chandrakirana Soedjatmoko, eds., *Transforming Humanity: The Visionary Writings of Soedjatmoko* (West Hartford, CT: Kumarian Press, 1994). The United Nations University also published a tribute: Soedjatmoko, Selo Soemardjan, and Kenneth W. Thompson, *Culture, Development, and Democracy: The Role of the Intellectual, a Tribute to Soedjatmoko* (Tokyo: United Nations University Press, 1994). See also Soedjatmoko, *Asia di Mata Soedjatmoko* (Jakarta: Kompas, 2010) and Soedjatmoko, *Menjadi Bangsa terdidik Menurut Soedjatmoko* (Jakarta: Kompas, 2010).

[58] For Soedarpo's biography, see Rosihan Anwar, *Against the Currents: A Biography of Soedarpo Sastrosatomo* (Jakarta: Pustaka Sinar Harapan, 2003). See also the memoirs of his wife: Mien Soedarpo, *Reminiscenses of the Past*, 2nd edn, 2 vols. (Jakarta: Ngrumat Bondo Utomo, 2005).

Batavia to live with his older brother, physician Sapoean, and assisted him in his medical practice. He too returned to Jakarta after the declaration of independence and was soon dispatched by the medical students living at Prapatan 10 to travel around Java discussing future political initiatives with local leaders. After his return to Jakarta, he joined Soedjatmoko at the Department of Propaganda. In May 1948, Soedarpo became a member of the Indonesian delegation to the United Nations and helped to establish Indonesia's consular offices in New York. After two years working at the Indonesian embassy in Washington, DC, he decided to leave government service and became a businessman. In the 1950s, the Indonesian government passed laws that required all international shipping lines to open locally owned offices. Soedarpo took advantage of this opportunity and established local companies to run these offices, benefitting from generous government subsidies. After the nationalisation of all Dutch-owned businesses in 1958, Soedarpo built a large shipping company.[59] He also started several other businesses and amassed a large fortune.

Ibnu Sutowo also started his business career during the Indonesian revolution. His main accomplishment was turning state oil company Pertamina into a highly profitable enterprise, before he brought it to the brink of collapse through precarious investments, financial mismanagement, nepotism, and corruption.[60] In 1940, Sutowo graduated from the Surabaya Medical College and was placed in southern Sumatra. During the Indonesian revolution he joined the Indonesian military and rose quickly through the ranks. In 1945 he was asked to oversee the redevelopment of South Sumatra's oil fields. The Indonesian military had a major role in the reorganisation and steering of major industries; in 1957, all oil production in Indonesia was nationalised and Lieutenant-General Sutowo was put in charge of the national oil company, Pertamina. In November 1963, Sutowo, still managing Pertamina, was appointed as the minister for oil and natural gas. In 1970, Pertamina had debts totalling more than $10 billion, around 30 per cent of Indonesia's gross domestic product, creating severe financial problems for the country. Sutowo was nevertheless honourably dismissed from his position and cleared of all corruption charges. He retained his enormous wealth and continued to run more than thirty companies.

---

[59] The Dutch shipping company was called the Royal Package Shipping Company [Koninklijke Paketvaart Maatschappij] (KPM); Soedarpo's company was called National Indonesian Shipping [Pelayaran Nasional Indonesia] (PELNI), and it still operates most major lines in Indonesia today.

[60] Several biographies have been written about Ibnu Sutowo. See Mara Karma, *Ibnu Sutowo Mengemban Misi Revolusi: Sebagai Dokter, Tentara, Pejuang Minyak Bumi* (Jakarta: Pustaka Sinar Harapan, 2001) and Ramadhan, *Ibnu Sutowo: Saatnya Saya Bercerita!* (Jakarta: National Press Club, 2008). See also Hamish McDonald, *Suharto's Indonesia* (Melbourne: Fontana, 1980), 143–65.

A number of physicians acquired legendary reputations during the Indonesian revolution. Physiologist Abdulrahman Saleh had been the very popular secretary of the Ika Daigaku, a radio pioneer, and an airplane enthusiast. He was killed on 29 July 1947 when the Dutch armed forces shot down his plane as he was about to land near Yogyakarta. It was stocked with medicines acquired in Singapore. Adnan Kapau Gani is another legendary physician. Before the Japanese annexation, he had starred in two popular movies.[61] During the revolution, his career developed rapidly, as physician, military officer, and then politician. He became known as a master smuggler, conveying weapons and military supplies past the Dutch blockade and into the Republic. He sold Sumatra's oil and agricultural products such as rubber and coffee on the international market to obtain hard currency to finance the military resistance against the Dutch. Physician Satrio enlisted as a military officer in 1946 and was placed in Banten, West Java. Because the Indonesian Red Cross was severely under-resourced in the region, medical practitioners had to improvise. To inoculate the local population against smallpox, Satrio injected four buffaloes with two smuggled ampoules containing cowpox. The serum derived from these animals enabled him to inoculate 240,000 people.[62] In 1957, Major-General Satrio became a professor of medicine at the University of Indonesia; from 1959 to 1966 he served as the minister of health and from 1970 to 1982 as the president of the Indonesian Red Cross.[63]

Conclusion

During the Dutch colonial period, several Indonesian physicians were noted for their engagement in political affairs, their participation in the nationalist movement, and their journalistic work. In 1948, Sukarno and Hatta honoured these physicians by declaring 20 May, the day Boedi Oetomo was founded, a national holiday – National Awakening Day [Hari Kebangkitan Nasional].[64] By equating the founding of Boedi Oetomo with the origins of the Indonesian nationalist movement, the new leaders of the Republic buttressed their ideal of a secular state, undercut the historical significance of the Islamic Union,

[61] Ruben Nalenan and Iskandar Gani, *Dr. A. K. Gani: Pejuang Berwawasan Sipil dan Militer* (Jakarta: Yayasan Indonesianologi, 1990) and Rosihan Anwar, 'Dimensi Pendidikan Kedoktoran: Kepemimpinan, Humanisme, Kejuangan', in *Sejarah Kecil: Petite Histoire Indonesia* (Jakarta: Kompas, 2009), 6–8.

[62] Matia Madjiah, *Kisah Seorang Dokter Gerilya: Dalam Revolusi Kemerdekaan di Banten* (Jakarta: Sinar Harapan, 1986), 201–11.

[63] Satrio, *Perjuangan dan Pengabdian: Mosaik Kenangan Prof. Dr. Satrio, 1916–1986* (Jakarta: Arsip Nasional, Republik Indonesia, 1986).

[64] The link between 20 May 1908, the date Boedi Oetomo was founded, and 17 August 1945, the declaration of Indonesian independence, was explicitly made in Ki Hadjar Dewantara and Wurjaningrat, *20 Mei Pelopor 17 Augustus* (Bandung: Djapenpro Djabar, 1950).

and attempted to sideline various Islam-based political parties that envisaged Indonesia as an Islamic nation. The historical significance of Boedi Oetomo had earlier been enhanced by the publication of a volume commemorating the tenth anniversary of its founding, written by a group of Indies students in the Netherlands including Goenawan Mangoenkoesoemo and Soewardi Soerjaningrat.[65] The essays written for this anniversary volume were far more radical than the politics advocated by its founders. Boedi Oetomo became more important over time because several nationalists saw it as a precursor for their preferred model of nation-building. However it was later inflected, the founding of Boedi Oetomo represented a clear moment of political engagement by physicians and medical students during the first part of the twentieth century.

The diversity of political opinion among Indonesian physicians became clear once again during the Indonesian revolution. Physicians opposing the Republican cause or favouring federalism occupied various political positions. Because of the severe shortage of physicians after 1950, most of them returned to their medical careers without suffering any ill consequences. Their political careers, however, were over. Indies physicians who had embraced Japanese medical visions were discredited after Japan's capitulation. They too returned to their medical careers, politically jaded. Indonesia's small medical elite fared much better. During the Japanese period, it remained focused on medicine. During the revolution, it maintained medical education and continued to provide medical services under difficult conditions. When the government of the Republic moved to Java's heartland, most elite physicians followed and continued their work there. The eagerness of medical students and their teachers to support the Republican troops when the battle moved to Central Java earned them the respect of Indonesian freedom fighters, and this was the foundation for their later reputations as nationalists. Following independence, this medical elite played leading roles in the development of Indonesia's medical infrastructure. They staffed the Ministry of Health, hospitals, clinics, and the newly established medical schools. Under the Dutch colonial administration, the highly vocal and politically active Association of Indies Physicians kept health care and medical education on the political agenda, but was discredited after it embraced Japan's political cause during the occupation. After 1950, Indonesia's apolitical medical elite became known for its patriotism, and reaped the associated benefits, consolidating its position in Indonesia's universities and government bureaucracies.

---

[65] Sosro Kartono, Noto Soeroto, and Soewardi Soeryaningrat, eds., *Soembangsih: Gedenkboek Boedi Oetomo, 1908–1918* (Amsterdam: Tijdschrift Nederlandsch Indië Oud & Nieuw, 1918).

9   Medicine in Independent Indonesia: National Physicians and International Health

On 27 December 1949, during a formal ceremony at Amsterdam's Royal Palace, Dutch Prime Minister Willem Drees, Queen Juliana, and Indonesian Prime Minister and Vice President Mohamad Hatta signed the Act that transferred sovereignty over the Dutch East Indies to the United States of Indonesia. At the same time, the sultan of Yogyakarta and the High Representative of the (Dutch) Crown for the Dutch East Indies signed similar documents at the latter's palace bordering Jakarta's large central square, now known as Freedom Square [Medan Merdeka]. Soldiers lowered the Dutch flag and raised the Indonesian one. The next day, tens of thousands of jubilant Indonesians celebrated their country's hard-won independence and welcomed Sukarno, the first president of independent Indonesia, to the newly named Freedom Palace [Istana Merdeka]. Despite the ecstatic atmosphere and the exuberance of the crowd, Indonesia's leaders knew they faced daunting tasks. Indonesia was a fractured nation without a functioning state apparatus. Its economy and infrastructure had been devastated by eight years of war. The heroes of the revolution now faced the task of rebuilding the country and transforming the legacies of Dutch and Japanese colonialism into state institutions that could serve the new nation.

The health of Indonesians had suffered tremendously. Large parts of the population were malnourished, smallpox had broken out again, and malaria, tuberculosis, trachoma, typhoid fever, leprosy, and yaws were rampant. Only a few health care institutions were still functioning, and the number of physicians and health care professionals was a fraction of what was needed. Addressing the nation's health problems required rebuilding and expanding health care facilities, educating large numbers of physicians and paramedical personnel, implementing public health measures, and organising extensive health education campaigns. Indonesian medical doctors had previously been *nationalist* physicians; they were now *national* physicians, medical doctors working in the state's health care institutions. The first step in decolonising medicine was to take control of health care institutions, medical schools, and the government health administration. Indonesia's physicians then shaped Indonesia's health care, combining elements from two different models: the metropolitan model of Europe and North America, which emphasised specialisation, hospital-based care, and medical technology; and a rival model emphasising social medicine, sanitary and public health measures, and public health education.

Never fond of political engagement during the Dutch and Japanese colonial periods, Indonesia's medical elite became resolutely apolitical in independent Indonesia. During Sukarno's rule, they successfully inured themselves against national politics while maintaining their professional autonomy. Their association with the international medical community proved beneficial. To meet the demands of Suharto's dictatorial state, they had to relinquish all political involvement. Indonesia's national physicians found that even though their social position improved in the years following independence, the political engagement that had once distinguished their profession completely disappeared. Despite the strong political participation of nationalist physicians in the colonial era, and notwithstanding the growing body of well-trained national physicians following independence, medicine and health care have never been political priorities in independent Indonesia. Indonesia has lagged in a number of health indicators, and continues to lag, in comparison to its immediate neighbours in Southeast Asia.[1] The ideals of Indonesia's nationalist and national physicians still await realisation.

Health in Sukarno's Indonesia: Plans and Ambitions

Indonesians faced enormous challenges in building a functioning state in the midst of several separatist movements and armed insurrections threatening the new nation. Although opposition to Dutch and Japanese colonialism had created a semblance of national unity, this crumbled soon after the transfer of sovereignty. In January 1950, Dutch military officer Raymond Westerling, already notorious for his part in civilian massacres in south Sulawesi in 1947, unsuccessfully organised a coup. A few months later a group of Christian Moluccan men recently discharged from the disbanded colonial army proclaimed the independent Republic of South Maluku; order was restored by the Indonesian army later that year, but sporadic fighting continued for more than a decade. Darul Islam, led by former NIAS student S. M. Kartosoewirjo, embarked on a campaign of guerrilla fighting on Java and Sulawesi with the aim of establishing an Islamic state ruled by sharia law.[2] The 1958 uprising of

---

[1] Susan Abeyasekere poses the same question by contrasting elite versus egalitarian health policies, and by analysing the positions of Indonesian nationalists in the Volksraad on health care policy. See Susan Abeyasekere, 'Health as a Nationalist Issue in Colonial Indonesia', in *Nineteenth and Twentieth Century Indonesia: Essays in Honour of Professor J. D. Legge*, ed. David P. Chandler and M. C. Ricklefs (Melbourne: Monash University Press, 1986), 1–14. According to Abeyasekere, Indonesian nationalists hardly ever advocated egalitarian health policies, but she mentions Abdul Rasjid as a notable exception.

[2] For Westerling and the Republic of the South Moluccas, see, for example, George McTurnan Kahin, *Nationalism and Revolution in Indonesia* (Ithaca, NY: Cornell University Press, 1952),

the self-declared Revolutionary Government of the Republic of Indonesia in Sumatra led to the abrogation of democracy and the inauguration of Sukarno's Guided Democracy.[3] From its inception, the new country experienced continuous political instability, internal conflict, and external pressures to such an extent that governments rarely held power more than a year. Since political parties doubled as patronage networks, there was high personnel turnover in state institutions whenever government changed hands.[4] Lastly, the newly independent nation was plagued by severe economic problems. After eight years of war, Indonesia's economy barely functioned and most of its infrastructure had been destroyed. Hyper-inflation was a regular threat, and the life of ordinary Indonesians grew increasingly difficult.

In late 1949, the University of Gadjah Mada was established in Yogyakarta.[5] The following year, officials inaugurated the University of Indonesia [Universitas Indonesia], which incorporated all departments of the Dutch University of Indonesia as well as those of the Institute of Higher Education of the Republic of Indonesia. In 1950 the Surabaya Medical School, which had been revived in 1948 by the Dutch occupying forces, was transferred to the University of Indonesia, and in 1954 it became part of the newly established University of Airlangga.[6] Establishing educational institutions became a key priority for Indonesian politicians, who saw their importance for the country's economic development. The number of such institutions grew exponentially in the 1950s, mainly to meet the manpower needs of Indonesia's enlarged administration. Bahder Djohan, who served as the minister of education and culture in 1950–51 and 1952–53, helped formulate a nationalistic educational program

---

453–61. A small number of Moluccan ex-soldiers and their families were transferred to the Netherlands by the Dutch government with the promise they could return to Indonesia after the Dutch government had made arrangements for them; this never happened. The great majority stayed in Indonesia; the soldiers among them became members of the Indonesian armed forces. For a history of the Republic of the South Moluccas, see Fridus Steijlen, *RMS, van Ideaal tot Symbool: Moluks Nationalisme in Nederland, 1951–1994* (Amsterdam: Spinhuis, 1996). For a biography of Kartosoewirjo, see Chiara Formichi, *Islam and the Making of the Nation: Kartosuwiryo and Political Islam in Twentieth-Century Indonesia* (Leiden: KITLV Press, 2012).

[3] For biographies of Sukarno, see Bob Heering, *Soekarno: Founding Father of Indonesia, 1901–1945* (Leiden: KITLV Press, 2002); J. D. Legge, *Sukarno: A Political Biography* (London: Allan Lane, 1972).

[4] See Herbert Feith, *The Decline of Constitutional Democracy in Indonesia* (Jakarta: Equinox, 2007 [1962]). See also Herbert Feith and Lance Castles, eds., *Indonesian Political Thinking, 1945–1965* (Jakarta: Equinox, 2007 [1970]) and Jemma Purdey, *From Vienna to Yogyakarta: The Life of Herb Feith* (Sydney: University of New South Wales Press, 2011), 148–206.

[5] Sutaryo, *Sejarah Fakultas Kedokteran UGM – Rumah Sakit UGM/RSUP Dr. Sardjito* (Yogyakarta: Puspagama, 2016), 32.

[6] Sandiantoro, *Jejak Jiwa, di Listasan Zaman (1913–2013): Mengenang yang Silam, Meretas Masa Depan* (Surabaya: Peringatan 1 Abad Pendidikan Dokter di Surabaya, 2013), 67–81.

which enlisted institutions of higher education to further the nation's development. The program aimed to reduce illiteracy, improve access to primary education, and graduate large numbers of teachers. The Indonesian language was promoted by prohibiting the use of Dutch in higher education – English was tolerated.[7] Universities were directed to hire Indonesian rather than foreign staff, adopt a practical orientation in both teaching and research, and maintain a harmonious relationship with the state.[8] With the departure of most Dutch instructors in 1950, however, the universities faced severe staff shortages. The Faculty of Medicine at the University of Indonesia was an exception.[9] During the 1950s, several new universities were founded, and most had Faculties of Medicine. The graduates of the oldest three Faculties were appointed to the new ones, while a number of professors travelled between cities to teach at several universities.

In September 1950, nearly 100 Indonesian physicians met in Jakarta to establish the Indonesian Medical Association [Ikatan Dokter Indonesia] (IDI). Rasjid's Association of Indonesian Physicians had been discredited because of its collaboration with the Japanese and so they opted not to revive it. The new association's first president was Sarwono Prawirohardjo, professor of gynaecology at the University of Indonesia. The association's aims echoed those of its predecessor: 'raising the level of health of the people; striving for fundamental rights of man in obtaining physical and mental health, according to the principle of social justice; raising the level of medical and related sciences; and striving for an appropriate position for its members'.[10] Full membership was reserved for Indonesians; others could become associate members. Several

[7] For Bahder Djohan's autobiography, see *Bahder Johan: Pengabdi Kemanusian* (Jakarta: Gunung Agung, 1980). For the changing role of scientific research and university teaching in Indonesia after 1950, see also Adam Messer, 'Effects of the Indonesian National Revolution and Transfer of Power on the Scientific Establishment', *Indonesia*, no. 58 (1994), 41–68.

[8] For an overview of science in independent Indonesia and how it operated under the constraints of increasing state control, see Andrew Goss, *The Floracrats: State-Sponsored Science and the Failure of the Enlightenment in Indonesia* (Madison: University of Wisconsin Press, 2011), 141–69. For general overviews, see William K. Cummings and Salman Kasenda, 'The Origin of Modern Indonesian Higher Education', in *From Dependence to Autonomy: The Development of Asian Universities*, ed. Philip G. Altbach and Viswanathan Selvaratnam (Dordrecht: Kluwer, 1989), 143–66; R. M. Koentjaraningrat and H. W. Bachtiar, 'Higher Education in the Social Sciences in Indonesia', in *The Social Sciences in Indonesia*, ed. R. M. Koentjaraningrat (Jakarta: LIPI, 1975), 1–42; and Bachtiar Rifai and Koesnadi Hardjasoemantri, *Perguruan Tinggi di Indonesia* (Jakarta: Departemen Perguruan Tinggi dan Ilmu Pengetahuan, 1965). See also R. Thomas Murray, *A Chronicle of Indonesian Higher Education: The First Half Century, 1920–1970* (Singapore: Chopmen, 1973), 43–52, 87–122.

[9] Messer, 'Effects of the Indonesian National Revolution', 47.

[10] 'Announcement [of the Founding of Ikatan Dokter Indonesia]', *OSR News* 2, no. 11 (1950), 141. For the Ikatan Dokter Indonesia, see Vivek Neelakantan, *Science, Public Health and Nation-Building in Soekarno-Era Indonesia* (Newcastle upon Tyne: Cambridge Scholars, 2017), 189–91.

young physicians who had fought the Dutch became board members and served on various committees. The association's headquarters were in Jakarta, in close proximity to the Ministry of Health, other government institutions, and the Republic's leading medical school.

Indonesians hoped to rebuild the country and to enjoy increasing prosperity. Reiterating views on progress and development [*kemajuan*] that had been articulated from the 1880s onward, Indonesians again appropriated Western ideas of development, now primarily in the field of economics [*pembangunan*].[11] They looked for international assistance, and both the United States and the Soviet Union stepped up their foreign assistance programs during the Cold War, seeking to win hearts and minds in the newly decolonised nations. Indonesia's development program bore an uncanny resemblance to the one proposed during the Dutch colonial era, as both viewed the country's traditional and backward population as the main obstacle to development.[12] Anthropologist Tania Murry Li has highlighted how both development regimes assumed that administrators and foreign experts were superior.[13] Education and training therefore continued to be high priorities; American ambassador to Indonesia from 1958 to 1965 Howard Jones characterised them as the most important tools in the 'struggle

---

[11] On Indonesian ideas of development, in particular during the Suharto era, see Ariel Heryanto, *Language of Development and Development of Language: The Case of Indonesia* (Canberra: Australian National University, Research School of Pacific and Asian Studies, 1995). Also see Theodore Friend, *Indonesian Destinies* (Cambridge, MA: Belknap Press of Harvard University Press, 2003). For post-war ideas on development, which were articulated in the United States and disseminated through international organisations such as the United Nations and the World Health Organization, see Arturo Escobar, *Encountering Development: The Making and Unmaking of the Third World*, 2nd edn (Princeton, NJ: Princeton University Press, 2012 [1995]). See also Michael E. Latham, *Modernization as Ideology: American Social Science and 'Nation Building' in the Kennedy Era* (Durham: University of North Carolina Press, 2000); *The Right Kind of Revolution: Modernization, Development, and U.S. Foreign Policy from the Cold War to the Present* (Ithaca, NY: Cornell University Press, 2010).

[12] Suzanne Moon, *Technology and Technical Idealism: A History of Development in the Netherlands East Indies* (Leiden: CNWS, 2007).

[13] Tania Murray Li, *The Will to Improve: Governmentality, Development, and the Practice of Politics* (Durham, NC: Duke University Press, 2007), 31–60. Anderson highlights the similarities between the Ethical Policy and Suharto's development regime: Benedict R. O'G. Anderson, 'Old State, New Society: Indonesia's New Order in Comparative Historical Perspective', in *Language and Power: Exploring Political Cultures in Indonesia* (Jakarta: Equinox, 2006 [1983]), 96–99, 109–19. For general critiques on development policies, see Escobar, *Encountering Development*; James C. Scott, *Seeing Like a State: How Certain Schemes to Improve the Human Condition Have Failed* (New Haven, CT: Yale University Press, 1998); and James Ferguson, *The Anti-Politics Machine: Development, Depoliticization, and Bureaucratic Power in Lesotho* (Minneapolis: University of Minnesota Press, 1994). For an excellent historiographical overview of critiques of development, see Christopher Shepherd, *Development and the Environment Politics Unmasked: Authority, Participation and Equity in East Timor* (New York: Routledge, 2013), 21–29. For a critique of recent development programs in Indonesia, see Anna Lowenhaupt Tsing, *Friction: An Ethnography of Global Connection* (Princeton, NJ: Princeton University Press, 2005).

for the Indonesian mind'.[14] Like the Dutch colonial administrators before, the new regime also celebrated Indonesia's National Awakening, which called for development through education, and with the assistance of science, technology, and medicine.[15]

Sukarno eagerly accepted international assistance but refused to surrender Indonesia's hard-won sovereignty. Opposing the United States in its insistence on free trade, the abolition of tariffs, and free reign for American corporations, Sukarno aimed to make Indonesia self-sufficient, particularly with respect to food.[16] He sought to avoid becoming overly dependent on one donor country, playing the major powers against each other. In April 1955, Indonesia hosted the first Asian-African Conference in Bandung, which later inspired the formation of an alliance between several recently decolonised nations which together hoped to form a third, independent voice in international affairs.[17] During the late 1950s Sukarno gradually turned away from the United States and towards China and the Soviet Union (Figure 9.1). When the tension with the United States came to a head, Sukarno bluntly told the Americans: 'Go to hell with your aid.' At that moment, Indonesia's economy had collapsed, hyper-inflation had made its monetary reserves worthless, democracy had been abrogated, and Indonesia had withdrawn from the United Nations and the International Monetary Fund.

During Sukarno's rule, the Indonesian medical profession compensated for the state's weakness and shortage of funds with its idealism and nationalist conviction. Although Indonesia's physicians were acutely aware that they needed outside expertise and funding, they accepted it with ambivalence. To build a health infrastructure, Indonesia received assistance from the World Health Organization (WHO), the United Nations Children's Fund (UNICEF), the United States Agency for International Development (USAID), and various other international organisations. Early in 1950, officials from the US Technical Cooperation Administration Mission arrived in Jakarta, with health and medicine significant parts of their brief. In 1953, a team of physicians from the World Health Organization travelled around the country giving lectures and holding discussions with local physicians.[18] One of these physicians reported

---

[14] Quoted by Suzanne Moon, 'Takeoff or Self-Sufficiency: Ideologies of Development in Indonesia, 1957–1961', *Technology and Culture* 39, no. 2 (1998), 203.

[15] Ariel Heryanto, 'Questioning the Relevance of National Awakening Today', *Jakarta Post*, 21 May 2008.

[16] Bradley R. Simpson, *Economists with Guns: Authoritarian Development and U.S.–Indonesian Relations, 1960–1968* (Stanford, CA: Stanford University Press, 2008), 13–36.

[17] For the 1955 Bandung conference, see See Seng Tan and Amitav Acharya, eds., *Bandung Revisited: The Legacy of the 1955 Asian-African Conference for International Order* (Singapore: NUS Press, 2008) and Christopher J. Lee, *Making a World after Empire: The Bandung Moment and Its Political Afterlives* (Athens: Ohio University Press, 2010).

[18] *Lectures of the World Health Organization Visiting Team of Medical Scientists to Indonesia* (Djakarta: Ikatan Dokter Indonesia, 1953).

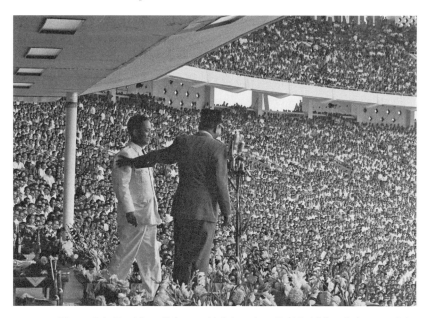

Figure 9.1 President Sukarno (right) praises D. N. Aidit, chairman of the Indonesian Communist Party (PKI), during a rally at Jakarta's Merdeka Sports Stadium on 23 May 1965, marking the anniversary of the PKI. © AP Photo

that the 'spread of medical men and of hospital provision is very thin indeed and it will be many years before funds and manpower can meet the needs of the population for public health and medical care by international standards'.[19] The challenges faced by the Ministry of Health were so enormous, indeed, that they could only be met by '"supermen"'. Its officials were also doubly burdened, with an 'immense and excessive amount of paper work'.[20] Later that year, the WHO invited Indonesian Minister of Health Johannes Leimena to visit Norway, Britain, Yugoslavia, Egypt, India, and Malaya to study the organisation of public health. Afterwards, Leimena presented his plans for Indonesia at the second meeting of the Expert Committee on Public Health Administration at the WHO's Geneva headquarters.[21]

---

[19] Alan C. Stevenson, 'WHO Visiting Team of Medical Scientists to Indonesia 1953: Report on Public Health Administration in Indonesia' (1953), 3. Typescript, National Library of Medicine, National Institutes of Health, Bethesda, MD.

[20] Stevenson, 'WHO Visiting Team of Medical Scientists', 2, 48.

[21] J. Leimena, *Some Aspects of Health Protection to Local Areas in Indonesia* (Djakarta: Ministry of Health, 1953).

Both Indonesian and visiting physicians were aware of the country's enormous health challenges. E. Ross Jenney, chief of the US Technical Cooperation Administration Mission to Indonesia and head of its Public Health Division from 1950 to 1953, reported as follows: 'Public health problems are widespread and profound, complicated by great distances, poor communications, illiteracy, and poverty … The exasperating contrast between what is and what could be – the obvious unreasonableness of it – places a tremendous burden of proof upon all the precepts of planning for human welfare.'[22] Jenney's deputy surveyed health conditions in various areas on Java, concluding:

The poverty and disease existing among the population of this rich agricultural area … appear representative of much of rural Java. Despite the seeming agricultural prosperity of [this area], nutritional deficiencies are almost universal. Superimposed upon poverty and malnutrition are diseases induced by poor housing, lack of sanitation, overcrowding, and lack of education. Families are unable to work because of debility and sickness; thus they are caught in the vicious cycle of illness and poverty.[23]

Almost all physicians were engaged in patient care, the deputy continued, and 90 per cent of the Ministry of Health budget was spent on curative care and administration; the small remainder was left to promote public health.[24] Ameliorating health conditions would require drastic changes.

Indonesia faced a severe shortage of physicians and paramedical personnel in addressing the enormous medical needs of the country. Almost all European physicians had left and a great number of medical students and young physicians had opted out of medicine to pursue careers as politicians, government officials, businessmen, and military officers. In 1950, Indonesia had around 1,200 physicians, or 1 per 75,000 inhabitants.[25] More than 20 per cent resided in Jakarta and most of the remainder in other urban areas, so the majority of Indonesians in rural areas had no access to medical care. Several strategies were implemented to rectify the shortage. With international assistance, the Ministry of Health sent several promising medical students and leading physicians abroad to receive advanced medical training and to inspect successful health programs.[26] After their return, they became instructors at the country's faculties of medicine. In 1949, pathologist and cancer specialist

[22] E. Ross Jenney, 'Public Health in Indonesia', *Public Health Reports* 68, no. 4 (1953), 414–15; see also E. Ross Jenney, 'Technical Assistance for Public Health in the Republic of Indonesia', *Public Health Reports* 68, no. 7 (1953), 707–13.
[23] Warren A. Ketterer, 'Village Polyclinics in Middle Java', *Public Health Reports* 68, no. 6 (1953), 561.
[24] Ketterer, 'Village Polyclinics', 561.
[25] J. Leimena, *The Upbuilding of Public Health in Indonesia* (Djakarta: Pertjetakan Negara, 1952), 13, 12. This book was a translation of J. Leimena, *Membangun Kesehatan Rakjat* (Djakarta: Noordhoff-Kolff, 1952).
[26] Jenney, 'Technical Assistance', 707–13.

R. M. Sutomo Tjokronegoro from the University of Indonesia embarked on the first of many international trips to establish contacts with medical schools abroad and to organise opportunities for advanced training for Indonesian medical students.[27] In 1951, he approached the dean of medicine at the University of California Medical Center in San Francisco proposing to form an affiliation between both institutions. The result was a far-reaching restructuring of medical education in Indonesia.[28]

In the 1950s, Indonesia's universities adhered to the academic model introduced by the former Batavia Medical School, which emphasised free study according to a self-directed schedule. Graduating physicians were highly qualified but, because of the high dropout rate, few in number. Following its affiliation with the University of California, the Faculty of Medicine at the University of Indonesia implemented the American guided model, and began admitting students in cohorts and holding mandatory exams throughout the year. Practical demonstrations and laboratory work alternated with compulsory lectures. In addition, formal selection procedures were introduced to manage the burgeoning interest in medical education. The number of graduating physicians increased markedly after 1960, when the first cohort trained under the new model received their diplomas.[29] The affiliation with the University of California Medical Center also included advanced medical training for more than 100 Indonesian academic physicians at American universities, and visits of around thirty American medical educators to Indonesia. When the model of guided study proved successful, the University of Indonesia implemented it

---

[27] R. M. Sutomo Tjokronegoro graduated from the Batavia Medical School in 1937. He was appointed assistant instructor in pathology and forensic medicine the same year. In 1942, he became the acting editor of the *Medical Journal of the Dutch Indies*. He served as assistant professor of pathology at the Jakarta *Ika Daigaku* and became professor at the Faculty of Medicine at the University of Indonesia in 1950. For a biography, see Mardanas Safwan, *Riwajat Hidup dan Pengabdian Prof. Dr. Sutomo Cokronegoro* (Jakarta: Lembaga Sejarah dan Antropologi, 1972).

[28] Francis Scott Smyth, 'Health and Medicine in Indonesia', *Journal of Medical Education* 38, no. 8 (1963): 693–96; Bruce L. Smith, *Indonesian-American Cooperation in Higher Education* (East Lansing: Institute of Research on Overseas Programs, Michigan State University, 1960); John S. Wellington, 'Indonesian Physicians Studying Abroad,' *Journal of Medical Education* 43 (1968), 1183–91; John S. Wellington, 'Medical Science and Technology,' in *Indonesia: Resources and Their Technological Development*, ed. Howard M. Beers (Lexington: University Press of Kentucky, 1970), 165–73; Soedjono Djoened Poesponegoro, *Laporan Perkembangan Pendidikan Dokter pada Fakultas Kedokteran Universitas Indonesia Djakarta/Report on the Development of Medical Education at the School of Medicine, University of Indonesia, Djakarta* (Jakarta: FKUI, 1960); Anne M. Schmidt, 'History of the University of California School of Medicine Affiliation with Medical Faculty of Universities at Djakarta and Surabaja (University of California-San Francisco, 1976)', in *Projects in Medical Education: Indonesia Papers 1951–1966*, UCSF Archives. See also Neelakantan, *Science, Public Health*, 188–231.

[29] Schmidt, 'History University of California Medicine Affiliation'; Poesponegoro, *Laporan*. See also Francis Scott Smyth, 'University of California Medical Science Teaching in Indonesia', *Journal of Medical Education* 32, no. 5 (1957), 344–49.

across all faculties. The Faculties of Medicine at the University of Airlangga and the University of Gadjah Mada introduced similar reforms.[30]

While Indonesia's academic physicians were reforming the medical curriculum, staff members at the Ministry of Health debated health policy. Christian Moluccan physician Johannes Leimena was the minister of health from 1947 until 1953 and again from 1955 to 1959, and remained involved in health matters until 1966.[31] Leimena was motivated by his Christian beliefs and ideals of social justice. He saw Christianity and health as forces that could foster a world community, overcoming ethnic, religious, and political differences.[32] He welcomed the assistance of international health organisations and proposed a blueprint for the organisation of Indonesia's health care incorporating suggestions of the WHO's Expert Advisory Panel.[33] In 1952, Leimena presented the so-called Bandung plan, named after the city where it was first implemented.[34] It defined health care delivery at four levels, starting with hospital care in urban centres, auxiliary hospitals in several districts, polyclinics in sub-districts (Figure 9.2), and health posts in outer villages. Conditions that could not be treated in the health posts and polyclinics were referred to the auxiliary hospitals or to the main hospital. Leimena proposed to integrate public health initiatives, public health education, and curative care at all four levels. The same year, public health became a compulsory component of medical curricula. Physicians were also required to work in remote areas for a period of three years upon graduation in an attempt to spread medical care more evenly over the archipelago.[35] Physicians working for public hospitals, clinics, and universities were able to supplement their income in private practice during

---

[30] Neelakantan, *Science, Public Health*, 142–76.

[31] On Leimena see R. Z. Leirissa, *Kewarganegaraan yang Bertanggungjawab: Mengenang Dr. J. Leimena* (Jakarta: Gunung Mulia, 1995) and Victor Silean, Jerry Rudolf Sirait, Yanedi Jagau, Abraham Simatupang, Marojahan Doloksaribu, John Pieris, Nikson Gans Lalu, and Midian Saragi, *Dr. Johannes Leimena: Negarawan Sejati dan Politisi Berhati Nurani* (Jakarta: Gunung Mulia, 2007).

[32] See, for example, Johannes Leimena, 'World Health and World Community', *Ecumenical Review* 8, no. 4 (1956), 407–09. See also Jan Sihar Aritonang and Karel Adriaan Steenbrink, eds., *A History of Christianity in Indonesia* (Leiden: Brill, 2008).

[33] For the critique of colonial medicine by Indonesian physicians in the 1950s, see Murakami Saki, 'Call for Doctors!: Medical Provision and the State during Indonesian Decolonisation, 1930s–1950s', in *Cars, Conduits, and Kampongs: The Modernization of the Indonesian City, 1920–1960*, ed. Freek Colombijn and Joost Coté (Leiden: Brill, 2014), 37–39. For the involvement of the WHO Expert Advisory Panel, see Leimena, *Membangun Kesehatan Rakjat*, 4. This preface was omitted in the English translation. Leimena's coverage of Hydrick's Banyumas project takes five pages (out of fifty-three); there are several references to the Intergovernmental Conference on Far-Eastern Countries on Rural Medicine, held at Bandung in 1937.

[34] This plan was presented in Leimena, *Upbuilding of Public Health in Indonesia*, 26–43. The most extensive discussion of the Bandung plan can be found in Neelakantan, *Science, Public Health*, 67–91.

[35] For an overview of developments in public health in the 1950s, see Neelakantan, *Science, Public Health*, 29–66.

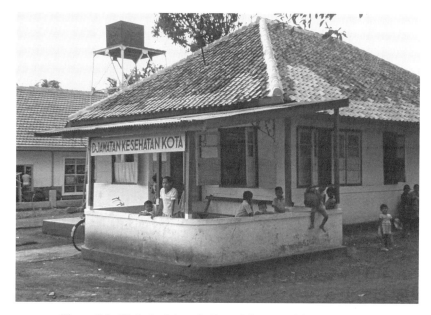

Figure 9.2 Clinic in Jakarta's Pasar Minggu neighbourhood, operated by the City Health Service, 1964. Reproduced with the permission of Robert T. Rubin, MD, PhD. © 2015 by Robert T. Rubin

the afternoon. Initially, this arrangement was suitable because the physicians building the nation's health infrastructure did not constitute an undue burden on the state. It became counterproductive later, since private practice was profitable only in the larger urban centres and physicians tended to concentrate there, making it almost impossible to staff rural health centres.

The greatest cause of ill health in Indonesia was malaria, which was a disease of special interest to the WHO. In 1953, an American physician called Indonesia 'one of the world's most malarious areas' and found that around 40 per cent of the population was affected.[36] In 1951, Indonesian physicians had implemented several pilot projects targeting the mosquitoes that transmitted malaria with a variety of control measures, including quinine distribution, swamp drainage, and DDT spraying, without results. In 1955, the WHO announced its Global Malaria Eradication Program, which relied almost exclusively on DDT spraying.[37] This program was typical of the vertical disease

[36] Warren A. Ketterer, 'Economic Benefits of Malaria Control in the Republic of Indonesia', *Public Health Reports* 68, no. 11 (1953), 1056.
[37] See Randall M. Packard, 'Malaria Dreams: Postwar Visions of Health and Development in the Third World', *Medical Anthropology* 17, no. 3 (1997), 279–96; Socrates Litsios, 'Malaria

eradication programs embraced by the WHO in the 1950s, which relied on technology-driven interventions targeting specific diseases, with little local participation or public health education. The malaria eradication program supported developmental initiatives which aimed to stimulate agriculture and foster a productive labour force. In 1958, the WHO commenced an ambitious nationwide anti-malaria campaign in Indonesia – the second largest in the world, after India.[38] It was highly successful until mosquitos developed resistance to DDT and various toxic effects of this chemical compound became manifest. Organisational and financial problems further contributed to the program's failure. Because of political upheaval and Sukarno's increasingly anti-American attitude during the early 1960s, American funding diminished markedly. The program was re-established in 1968 but again failed to eradicate malaria.

Indonesia's leading physicians deliberately chose to focus on building the nation's medical infrastructure and to refrain from involvement in party-based politics and other forms of political participation. They did so to safeguard medicine from politics, and their success is seen in the relative peace within the medical profession in a country increasingly torn by political conflict. As the 1950s progressed, however, Indonesia became progressively unstable and economic problems proliferated, which led to severe problems in running medical institutions.[39] In the early 1960s, Sukarno issued several stark ideological statements and decreed that schools and universities incorporate them in their curricula. Socialist and communist politicians incited student groups to hold demonstrations against allegedly counter-revolutionary professors and administrators who appeared to flout Sukarno's increasingly radical ideology.[40] Dr Soebandrio, the minister of foreign affairs and one of the last physicians-turned-politician argued that the Indonesian revolution was not yet finished, as Indonesians had merely replaced the Dutch in government and business, leaving an exploitative social structure in place. He therefore called for a social revolution to complete the national one.[41]

Control, the Cold War, and the Postwar Reorganization of International Assistance', *Medical Anthropology* 17, no. 3 (1997), 255–78. See also Randall M. Packard, *The Making of a Tropical Disease: A Short History of Malaria* (Baltimore, MD: Johns Hopkins University Press, 2007).

[38] Vivek Neelakantan, 'The Campaign against the Big Four Endemic Diseases and Indonesia's Engagement with the WHO during the Cold War 1950s', in *Public Health and National Reconstruction in Post-War Asia: International Influences, Local Transformations*, ed. Liping Bu and Ka-che Yip (London: Routledge, 2015), 161–63. Neelakantan, *Science, Public Health*, 92–141.

[39] An analysis is provided in the famous monography by Feith, *The Decline of Constitutional Democracy in Indonesia*.

[40] 'The Indonesian University Situation', *Minerva* 4, no. 3 (1966), 434–35.

[41] See, for example, Soebandrio, *Pangaruh Revolusi Indonesia Didunia* (Jakarta: Departemen Luar Negeri RI, 1962). In 1966, Soebandrio was sentenced to death; his sentence was commuted to life imprisonment. He was released from prison in 1995.

Activists also sought to ban Western books from university libraries, remove all neo-colonial and imperialist traces from curricula, and mandate compulsory lessons in Marxism. A mixture of hyper-inflation and various forms of political obstruction led to a decline in the quality of instruction. Laboratory equipment became scarce and could not be replaced. Because academic salaries stagnated, lecturers were forced to take additional jobs to make ends meet. By 1965, universities could no longer function, the economy had come to a standstill, and Sukarno's rule was all but untenable.[42] Indonesia found itself in a social, political, and economic crisis.

Health under Suharto: Building a National Health Infrastructure

The dramatic murder of six generals on 30 September 1965, allegedly by Communists, provided General Suharto with the opportunity to move to the centre of political life.[43] He insisted Sukarno give him emergency powers to stem the crisis.[44] Suharto immediately banned the Communist Party, and in subsequent months up to 1.5 million alleged Communists were murdered by militias and gangs with army support.[45] They also targeted Chinese Indonesians because of their perceived links with Communist China and their dominance in the economy. Indonesian students, encouraged by the armed forces, organised demonstrations around the building of Jakarta's Faculty of Medicine demanding the eradication of communism, the end of corruption, and lower prices for basic goods which rampant inflation had rendered unaffordable.[46]

---

[42] Mortimer Rex, *Indonesian Communism under Sukarno: Ideology and Politics, 1959–1965* (Ithaca, NY: Cornell University Press, 1974).

[43] John Hughes, *The End of Sukarno: A Coup That Misfired, a Purge That Ran Wild* (Singapore: Archipelago, 2002 [1967]); Robert Cribb, ed., *The Indonesian Killings of 1965–1966: Studies from Java and Bali* (Melbourne: Centre of Southeast Asian Studies, Monash University, 1990).

[44] For a biography of Suharto, see R. E. Elson, *Suharto: A Political Biography* (Cambridge: Cambridge University Press, 2001).

[45] John Roosa, *Pretext for Mass Murder: The September 30th Movement and Suharto's Coup d'Etat in Indonesia* (Madison: University of Wisconsin Press, 2006). Joshua Oppenheimer recently made two documentaries that attracted international attention to these events: Joshua Oppenheimer, *The Act of Killing* (Copenhagen: Final Cut for Real, 2012); Joshua Oppenheimer, *The Look of Silence* (Copenhagen: Final Cut for Real, 2014).

[46] For overviews of the student activism between 1965 and 1968, see Stephen A. Douglas, *Political Socialization and Student Activism in Indonesia* (Chicago: University of Illinois Press, 1970), 153–201; Murray, *Chronicle of Indonesian Higher Education*, 222–34; François Raillon, *Les Étudiants Indonésiens et L'ordre Nouveau: Politique et Idéologie du Mahasiswa Indonesia, 1966–1974* (Paris: Editions de la Maison des Sciences de l'Homme, 1984); Edward Aspinall, 'Indonesia: Moral Force Politics and the Struggle against Authoritarianism', in *Student Activism in Asia: Between Protest and Powerlessness*, ed. Meredith L. Weiss, Edward Aspinall, and Patricio M. Abinales (Minneapolis: University of Minnesota Press, 2012), 153–79; Doreen Lee, 'Images of Youth: On the Iconography of History and Protest in Indonesia', *History and Anthropology* 22, no. 3 (2011), 307–36. Firman Lubis describes his participation in these

Styling themselves after the youth militias that had played a central role in the Indonesian revolution, they called themselves the generation of 1966 [*Angkatan 66*].[47] Beset by student strikes and general political chaos, most universities closed for at least twelve months. During the next two and a half years, Suharto consolidated his power; he was declared Indonesia's president in 1968. The military dominated his strong and highly centralised government, which maintained stability for some three decades through the brutal repression of all dissent.

Suharto's resolute stance against communism gained him the trust of the United States, which was unsuccessfully fighting communism in Vietnam. Indonesia rejoined the United Nations, the World Bank, and the International Monetary Fund. After Suharto acceded to American demands to open its borders for American corporations, Indonesia received extravagant financial aid, development assistance, and generous debt rescheduling. In the 1970s, Indonesia attracted the second-highest distribution of foreign aid in the world. The economy grew significantly, inflation returned to normal levels, and standards of living improved noticeably. Suharto appointed a team of economists trained in the United States, dubbed the 'Berkeley mafia' or the 'Technocrats', to take charge of economic planning.[48] Large sectors of the economy were opened for foreign investment, and foreign capital streamed into the country. Suharto's Indonesia rejected non-alignment and firmly associated itself with the United States. Indonesia now followed American views on development and Suharto became known as Father Development [Bapak Pembangunan]. His reign was styled as the New Order [Orde Baru], and its blend of terror and economic development was a mixed blessing for the country.[49] Indonesians paid a high price for the rise in their standard of living, which was accompanied by massive corruption, intricate patronage networks, and random state-sanctioned violence.

The development programs implemented by the Suharto regime led to significant increases in income and prosperity. The average per capita income

---

demonstrations as a young medical student. See Firman Lubis, *Jakarta 1960-an: Kenangan Semasa Mahasiswa* (Jakarta: Masup, 2008), 227–67.

[47] For regular updates on the situation as it unfolded, see 'Politics in the World of Science and Learning: Indonesia', *Minerva* 4, no. 2 (1965), 302; 'The Indonesian University Situation', and 'Students' Role in Indonesian Political Changes', *Minerva* 4, no. 4 (1966), 584–85; 'Continuing Student Agitation in Indonesia', *Minerva* 5, no. 1 (1966), 116–23; 'Rampant Disorder: Indonesia', *Minerva* 5, no. 2 (1966), 300–01.

[48] Simpson, *Economists with Guns*.

[49] Heryanto, *Language of Development*. For overviews of the New Order, see Hal Hill, *Indonesia's New Order: The Dynamics of Socio-Economic Transformation* (Sydney: Allen & Unwin, 1994); Hamish McDonald, *Suharto's Indonesia* (Melbourne: Fontana, 1980). For American views on development, see Latham, *Modernization as Ideology* and *The Right Kind of Revolution*. The 'mixed blessing' characterisation has been provided by Adrian Vickers in his *A History of Modern Indonesia* (Cambridge: Cambridge University Press, 2005), 174–201.

increased from around US $50 in 1968 to US $1,125 in 1996. Between 1965 and 1998, life expectancy rose from 48.7 to 66.6 years; infant mortality declined from 131 to 44.7 per 1,000 births. During the same period, the number of physicians rose from 0.032 per 1,000 people (or 1 per 30,000) to 0.162 (1 physician per 6,000).[50] Leimena's vision of a national health care infrastructure built around community health centres was realised. Several new medical schools were founded, leading to a significant increase in the number of graduating physicians. Backed by a strong and highly centralised state, Indonesia's national physicians were able to considerably strengthen their position. At the same time, they had to give up any form of political involvement since the Suharto regime had fully depoliticised Indonesian society. The Indonesian medical profession therefore continued to focus on building the nation's health infrastructure and related professional matters. Under Sukarno, remaining aloof from politics was a strategic decision made to strengthen the medical profession and establish health care institutions. Under Suharto, it became a political necessity.

Christian Moluccan army physician Gerrit A. Siwabessy was the minister of health from 1966 to 1978.[51] When he took up his position he removed all employees suspected of holding communist sympathies and embarked on the delicate task of rebuilding Indonesia's relationship with the WHO and UNICEF.[52] At the 1968 National Health Conference he presented plans to provide health care through community health centres [*pusat kesehatan masyarakat; puskesmas*] (echoing Leimena's earlier proposals).[53] In rural areas, these clinics would cooperate with a variety of agricultural and economic development programs. Siwabessy amended his plans after consultation with the WHO and UNICEF; both organisations were contemplating ways of meeting the health care needs of the poor in developing nations.[54] His health plans were subsequently incorporated in Suharto's first Five Year Development

---

[50] These data are available through the World Bank. See www.worldbank.org, accessed on 30 November 2015.
[51] For Siwabessy's autobiography, see G. A. Siwabessy, *Upuleru: Memoar Dr. G. A. Siwabessy* (Jakarta: Gunung Agung, 1979). In Moluccan Malay, *Upuleru* means 'God' or 'Protector'; it was Siwabessy's nickname amongst the students living at Prapatan 10. For essays on Siwabessy's accomplishments, see Victor P. H. Nikijuluw and Erlita Rachman, eds., *Sang Upuleru: Mengenang 100 Tahun Prof. Dr. Gerrit Augustinus Siwabessy (1914–2014)* (Jakarta: Gramedia, 2014).
[52] Wasisto Broto, Thomas Suroso, Rushdy Hoesein, and Abdul Syukur, *Sejarah Pembangunan Kesehatan Indonesia 1973–2009* (Jakarta: Kementrian Kesehatan Republik Indonesia, 2009), 17–19.
[53] Linda Shields and Lucia Endang Hartati, 'Primary Care in Indonesia', *Journal of Child Health Care* 10, no. 1 (2006), 4–8.
[54] An exploration of alternative forms of health care is provided in Voyo Djukanovic and Edward P. Mach, eds., *Alternative Approaches to Meeting Basic Health Needs of Populations in Developing Countries* (Geneva: World Health Organization, 1975).

Plan [Repelita I, 1969–74]. Training facilities for physicians and auxiliary health personnel were expanded to staff the planned community centres. During the second Five Year Development Plan (1974–79), these centres were established all over the country.

In 1978, the International Conference on Primary Health Care was held at Alma Ata, Kazakhstan, USSR. After the WHO's malaria education campaign had failed, attendees proposed alternative strategies for promoting health amongst poor rural populations. These focused upon primary health clinics, public health initiatives, and public health education.[55] Participants agreed that technology-intensive, hospital-based medical care was not an efficient method of providing health care to rural populations; instead, they proposed 'horizontal' programs based on a greater number of clinics offering essential services. As well as providing immunisation, maternal and child health care, family planning, nutrition, and the treatment of the most common diseases in the region, the clinics were to deliver public health education. The conference's conclusions resembled those of the Inter-Governmental Conference of Far-Eastern Countries on Rural Hygiene held in Bandung in 1937.[56]

The Indonesian delegation to the Alma Ata conference reported on primary health care initiatives already undertaken in their country. Surveys conducted two years before the conference had demonstrated that primary health clinics had been established in more than 200 villages.[57] Between 1966 and 1974, for example, delegate Gunawan Nugroho and his wife, also a physician, had developed two innovative programs near Surakarta. In the process, they had observed widespread malnutrition. Rather than focusing on providing medical treatment, they introduced new rice strains and invited government officials to educate villagers on the use of fertilisers and modern agricultural methods. Nugroho then obtained a small loan to fund an irrigation dam. After a few years, he noted that malnutrition had disappeared and that infant mortality rates had declined, even though 'nothing particular had been done in … health care delivery.'[58] After villagers had collected funds by selling excess rice on the market, they embarked on a housing improvement program. In a

---

[55] Socrates Litsios, 'The Long and Difficult Road to Alma Ata: A Personal Reflection', *International Journal of Health Services* 32 (2002), 709–32; Socrates Litsios, 'The Christian Medical Commission and the Development of the World Health Organization's Primary Health Care Approach', *American Journal of Public Health* 94, no. 11 (2004), 1884–93; Marcos Cueto, 'The Origins of Primary Health Care and Selective Primary Health Care', *American Journal of Public Health* 94, no. 11 (2004), 1864–74.

[56] Litsios, 'The Long and Difficult Road to Alma Ata', 720.

[57] *Primary Health Care (Village Community Health Development) in Indonesia* (Jakarta: Ministry of Health, RI, 1978), 11. This was Indonesia's report to the Alma Ata conference.

[58] Gunawan Nugroho, 'A Community Development Approach to Raising Health Standards in Central Java, Indonesia', in *Health by the People*, ed. Kenneth W. Newell (Geneva: World Health Organization, 1975), 96.

second village, Nugroho successfully encouraged villagers to establish a goat cooperative and a modest health insurance scheme. He concluded on the basis of these experiences that health was of essential importance for community development, and that health conditions would improve only with full community participation. Agricultural development, community organisation, public health education, volunteer training, and the provision of basic health care must work in unison. The Nugrohos' health projects were among several community-based health projects that inspired the formulation of the primary health care approach by WHO officials that were discussed at the Alma Ata conference.[59]

Indonesia's community health centres did not quite meet expectations.[60] Physician Januar Achmad identified several problems.[61] Physicians lacked enthusiasm and worked in the community centres only during their three years of compulsory service to the government before promptly returning to the urban centres. Working in the community centres did nothing for their careers, and worse still, their time was consumed by cumbersome administrative work which left little time for medical care.[62] Most of the actual treatment was provided by nurses who had not been trained to do so.[63] Local governments viewed community health centres as a source of income, and appropriated more than 75 per cent of the profits they generated, which left other health initiatives unfunded. There was little time for public health education because of the heavy workload. The rigid programs of the Ministry of Health, finally, meant that health centres could not respond effectively to local needs, and while the program was formulated by the Ministry of Health, the clinics were established and operated by the Interior Ministry.[64] Health officials, then, had little control over the program as it unfolded.

[59] For descriptions, see Nugroho, 'Community Development Approach Central Java', 91–111; James C. McGilvray, *The Quest for Health and Wholeness* (Tübingen: German Institute for Medical Missions, 1981), 80–81. See also Arif Haliman and Glen Williams, 'Can People Move Bureaucratic Mountains?: Developing Primary Health Care in Rural Indonesia', *Social Science & Medicine* 17, no. 19 (1983), 1449–55. For a similar initiative, see L. Hendrate, 'A Model for Community Health Care in Rural Java', *Development Digest* 19, no. 1 (1981), 107–14. See also Litsios, 'Christian Medical Commission', 1888–89.

[60] Lorraine Corner and Y. Rahardjo, 'New Direction in Health Policy in Indonesia: The Need for a Demand-Oriented Perspective', in *Health and Development in Southeast Asia*, ed. Paul Cohen and John Purcal (Canberra: Australian Development Studies Network, Australian National University, 1995), 77.

[61] Januar Achmad, *Hollow Development: The Politics of Health in Soeharto's Indonesia* (Canberra: Australian National University, 1999).

[62] Achmad, *Hollow Development*, 95.

[63] Rosalia Sciortino, 'Rural Nurses and Doctors: The Discrepancy between Western Concepts and Javanese Practices', in *Health Care in Java: Past and Present*, ed. Peter Boomgaard, Rosalia Sciortino, and Ines Smyth (Leiden: KITLV Press, 1996), 111–28; Rosalia Sciortino, *Care-Takers of Cure: An Anthropological Study of Health Centre Nurses in Rural Central Java* (Yogyakarta: Gadjah Mada University Press, 1995).

[64] Paulus Hidayat Santosa, 'Participation from Below in Hierarchical Bureaucracies: The Unsolved Dilemma in Indonesian Primary Health Care', in *The Hidden Crisis in Development:*

The Suharto regime received major praise from international health organisations for implementing family planning programs to curb population growth.[65] Suharto and his technocrats became interested in population control when they courted Western powers and found that aid was contingent on the institutionalisation of such programs. The Ford Foundation had already enabled several Indonesian physicians to attend family planning meetings in other developing nations and had provided modest funds for earlier family planning initiatives. In December 1967, Suharto signed the World Leaders' Declaration on Population and was able to convince various Muslim political groups to endorse his plans. The following year, he founded the precursor to the National Family Planning Co-ordinating Board, which reported directly to him.[66] This organisation became known as Indonesia's most dynamic, most creative, and least bureaucratic government institution. The Board established hundreds of clinics throughout Indonesia with financial assistance from USAID and, later, from the United Nations Population Fund (UNPFA, which awarded Suharto its population award in 1989). It reached families everywhere, using the motto 'Two is enough [*dua anak cukup*].'[67] The Board employed physicians and nurses but relied also on large numbers of volunteers, particularly the leaders of the village organisations which had originally been established by the Japanese. Between 1965 and 1997, the reported fertility rate in Indonesia declined from 5.91 to 2.78 per woman, or about 53 per cent (Figure 9.3).[68]

Development Bureaucracies, ed. Philip Quarles van Ufford, Dirk Kruijt, and Theodore Downing (Tokyo: United Nations University, 1988), 211–22; see also Glen Williams and Satoto, 'Socio-Political Constraints on Primary Health Care: A Case Study from Java', *Development Dialogue* 1 (1980), 85–101.

[65] For a historical overview, see Terence H. Hull and Valerie J. Hull, 'From Family Planning to Reproductive Health Care: A Brief History', in *People, Population, and Policy in Indonesia*, ed. Terence H. Hull (Singapore: Equinox for ISEAS, 2005), 1–69. See also Donald P. Warwick, 'The Indonesian Family Planning Program: Government Influence and Client Choice', *Population and Development Review* 12, no. 3 (1986), 453–90. For an overview of the international population control initiative, see Matthew Connely, *Fatal Misconception: The Struggle to Control World Population* (Cambridge, MA: Belknap Press of Harvard University Press, 2008).

[66] Firman Lubis, 'History and Structure of the National Family Planning Program', in *Two Is Enough: Family Planning in Indonesia under the New Order, 1968–1998*, ed. Firman Lubis and Anke Niehof (Leiden: KITLV Press, 2003), 31–55; Terence H. Hull, 'The Political Framework for Family Planning in Indonesia: Three Decades of Development', in *Two Is Enough: Family Planning in Indonesia under the New Order, 1968–1998*, ed. Firman Lubis and Anke Niehof (Leiden: KITLV Press, 2003), 57–81.

[67] Firman Lubis and Anke Niehof, eds., *Two Is Enough: Family Planning in Indonesia under the New Order, 1968–1998* (Leiden: KITLV Press, 2003). Between 1970 and 1975, a pilot project was undertaken in the village of Serpong, west of Jakarta; see Anke Niehof and Firman Lubis, 'Family Planning in Practice: Cases from the Field', in *Two Is Enough: Family Planning in Indonesia under the New Order, 1968–1998*, ed. Firman Lubis and Anke Niehof (Leiden: KITLV Press, 2003), 121–30. For a personal account of this project, see Firman Lubis, *Jakarta 1970-An: Kenangan Sebagai Dosen* (Jakarta: Masup, 2010), 231–53.

[68] Lubis and Niehof, *Two Is Enough*, 1. See also Terence H. Hull, 'Fertility Decline in the New Order Period: The Evolution of Population Policy, 1965–90', in *Indonesia's New Order: The*

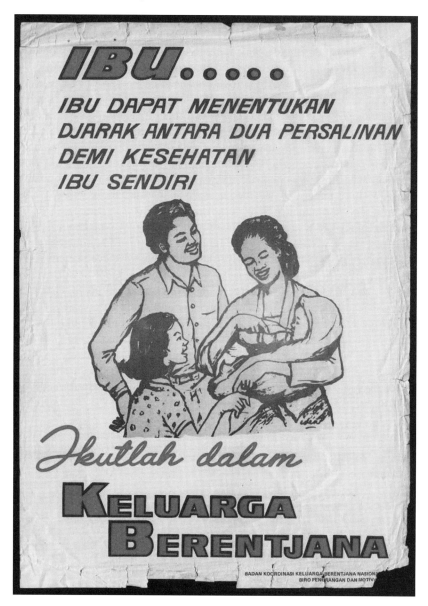

Figure 9.3 Poster advocating family planning, around 1970. The text reads: 'Mothers … you can choose the time between pregnancies for your own health. Follow family planning.' Author's collection

Although the Board established numerous clinics across the country, its members quickly realised that outreach programs would be needed in addition to clinic-based services. Rewards were offered to local bureaucrats according to the number of 'acceptors' in their villages and districts, and while these bureaucrats sometimes applied undue pressure on women to participate, the forceful methods employed in China and India were not replicated in Indonesia.[69] In flagrant disregard for privacy, some villages erected central noticeboards showing the types of birth control used in each household. Family planning services were limited to married couples to prevent antagonising religious associations. Noting the unusually high infant and maternal mortality rates in Indonesia, family planning advocates increasingly emphasised maternal and child health as well as reproductive choice. In response, health care was offered at monthly village meetings which were held in association with the community health centres. At these meetings [posyandu; pos pelayanan terpadu, integrated service post], nurses weighed children, provided advice to pregnant women, dispensed nutrition information, and administered vaccinations.[70] These health and family planning meetings were highly successful and demonstrated the importance of integrating family planning services within the health care system.

In 1958, the WHO endorsed the Global Strategy for the Eradication of Smallpox. At that time, Indonesia had the second highest incidence of smallpox in the world, after India. Although some vaccination campaigns had been run before 1965, they had failed in the absence of a comprehensive health care system. Indonesia's anti-smallpox campaigns were interrupted during political unrest and economic crises, but resumed in 1968 (Figure 9.4). 'Challenges included overcoming popular resistance to vaccination, circumventing the non-involvement of top provincial leaders, and navigating byzantine bureaucratic structures', writes historian of medicine Vivek Neelakantan.[71]

Dynamics of Socio-Economic Transformation, ed. Hal Hill (Sydney: Allen & Unwin, 1994), 123–45.

[69] Juliette Koning, 'Family Planning Acceptance in a Rural Central Javanese Village', in *Health Care in Java: Past and Present*, ed. Peter Boomgaard, Rosalia Sciortino, and Ines Smyth (Leiden: KITLV Press, 1996), 147–69; Kartono Mohamad, 'Family Planning', in *Indonesia in the Soeharto Years: Issues, Incidents and Images*, ed. John H. McGlynn, Oscar Motuloh, Suzanne Charlé, Jeffrey Hadler, Bambang Bujono, Margaret Glade Agusta, and Gedsiri Suhartono (Jakarta: Lontar, 2007), 132–34.

[70] Ayami Saito, 'The Development of *Posyandu*: Historical and Institutional Aspects', in *Critical and Radical Geographies of the Social, the Spatial and the Political*, ed. Toshio Mizuuchi (Osaka: Department of Geography, Osaka City University, 2006), 80–97. For an ethnographic project investigating how *posyandu* are run, see Nathalie Köllmann and Corrie van Veggel, 'Posyandu: Theory and Practice', in *Health Care in Java: Past and Present*, ed. Peter Boomgaard, Rosalia Sciortino, and Ines Smyth (Leiden: KITLV Press, 1996), 95–100.

[71] Vivek Neelakantan, 'Eradicating Smallpox in Indonesia: The Archipelagic Challenge', *Health and History* 12, no. 1 (2010), 62; Scott Naysmith, 'Disease Control in Democratic Indonesia',

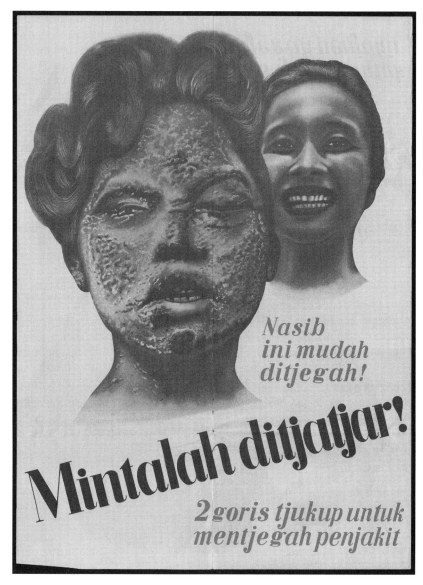

Figure 9.4 Poster for Indonesia's campaign for the eradication of smallpox, around 1970. The text reads: 'This fate is easily preventable: Ask to get vaccinated! Two scratches [the scar left by the two-pronged needle used in this campaign] are enough to prevent (this) disease.' Author's collection

Conditions paralleled those in India, where campaigns were successful when physicians, politicians, and local powerbrokers supported them, a sufficient number of vaccinators had been trained, and a basic health care infrastructure had been established.[72] In Indonesia, upper echelons of the government bureaucracy compelled lower-level civil servants to provide assistance. Citizens were vaccinated in systematic and efficient campaigns but received little information about the benefits of vaccination. Eradication efforts focused on vaccination, surveillance, and containment; affected individuals were isolated and quarantined to remove the possibility of contagion, sometimes by force. These campaigns were successful: the last case was reported in 1972, and in 1974, the country was declared smallpox-free.

In the 1990s, newspapers and magazines published commentaries relating to the detrimental effects of 'progress'. The lifestyle diseases and chronic degenerative conditions common in the West were becoming more prevalent amongst Indonesians. Anthropologist Stephen Ferzacca interprets these reports as indirect expressions of a deep dissatisfaction with the New Order regime under the guise of neutral, medical vocabulary, which provided an acceptable way of expressing political disaffection. Using a medical vocabulary to provide political commentaries was, argues Ferzacca, inspired by the political engagement of Indonesian physicians during the colonial era.[73] At this time, Suharto liberalised the banking system, leading to a proliferation of banks, not all of them with sound financial bases. Their vulnerability was exposed by the 1997 Asian financial crisis. The Indonesian rupiah lost 80 per cent of its value, a great number of businesses collapsed, and the economy shrank by 13 per cent. Unemployment rose dramatically, living standards declined, and the number of people living below the poverty line increased markedly.[74] The International Monetary Fund offered Indonesia large loans that were conditional upon severe austerity programs. Many people were furious about the economy's decline, leading to increasing public critique of the flagrant corruption in Suharto's circles. In 1998, students demonstrated on the streets of Jakarta, recalling

---

Inside Indonesia, no. 111 (2013), www.insideindonesia.org/disease-control-in-democratic-indonesia-2; accessed on 12 July 2015.

[72] See Sanjoy Bhattacharya, *Expunging Variola: The Control and Eradication of Smallpox in India, 1947–1977* (Hyderabad: Orient BlackSwan, 2006). See also Sanjoy Bhattacharya and Sharon Messenger, eds., *The Global Eradication of Smallpox* (Hyderabad: Orient BlackSwan, 2010). Bhattacharya has also analysed vaccination campaigns in colonial India; see Sanjoy Bhattacharya, Mark Harrison, and Michael Worboys, *Fractured States: Smallpox, Public Health and Vaccination Policy in British India, 1900–1947* (Hyderabad: Orient BlackSwan, 2005).

[73] Steven Ferzacca, 'Mediations of Health and the Development of a Nation: Late Suharto, Late Modernity', in *Liberalizing, Feminizing and Popularizing Health Communications in Asia*, ed. Liew Kai Khiun (Farnham, MA: Ashgate, 2012), 15–42.

[74] World Bank, 'The World Bank on the Social Impact of the Indonesian Crisis', *Population and Development Review* 24, no. 3 (1998), 664–66.

their central role in Sukarno's downfall. Anti-Chinese riots again broke out.[75] Suharto's position became untenable, and he resigned on 21 May.

Conclusion

Between 1950 and 1998, Indonesia's national physicians solidified their profession's social position. During the Sukarno era, physicians were committed to building a national health care system. They compensated for difficulties caused by the state's weakness and financial problems with their nationalist zeal. During the Suharto era, medical schools, hospitals, and community health clinics multiplied. Backed by a strong and centralised state, and supported by international health organisations, Indonesian physicians made decisive professional gains. Because they were not permitted to participate in politics, they focused on professional matters exclusively. Indonesia's national physicians developed a hybrid model of health care incorporating elements from two different models. Many followed European and North American approaches, which rewarded specialisation and working in technology-intensive, hospital-based settings. Some, however, were inspired by social medicine and public health, and aimed to realise medical ideals similar to those Indies physicians had advocated in the 1930s. Because working in community health centres lacked professional and financial incentives and therefore failed as viable career options for ambitious physicians, most opted for the first model.

After 1950, the two-tier colonial medical profession disappeared, so that Indonesian physicians no longer worked in the shadows of colleagues who had received Western education, held higher medical degrees, and earned more generous remunerations. Yet they continued to rely on outside expertise and assistance from first-world physicians, who continued to reinforce dependency in their Indonesian colleagues. No longer a subordinated elite in a colonial society, Indonesian doctors entered a global world in which they still occupied a subordinate position, even in health matters within their own country.

Despite the political engagement of Indies physicians during Dutch colonial times, and despite Abdul Rasjid's program of medical nationalism which inspired unprecedented enthusiasm and activity in the late 1930s, Indonesia's physicians have never succeeded in making health and medicine national priorities. A 2015 World Bank report highlights the continuing shortages of physicians and other health personnel, and unequal access to health care for low-income earners and inhabitants of specific regions and of all rural areas.

[75] Lee, 'Images of Youth'.

It concludes that Indonesia 'continues to suffer from serious challenges in the number and distribution, and in particular the quality, of its health workers'.[76] Before 2014, the country spent a mere 3.1 per cent of its GDP on health care, the lowest rate of ASEAN. Its infant mortality rates remain high (22.8 per 1,000 live births in 2015), as do maternal mortality rates (220 per 100,000 live births in 2010). In 2012, there were still only 0.2 physicians per 1,000 inhabitants.[77] Because physicians and other health personnel have to pay unofficial fees to attain employment in the still underfunded public system, access to health care for the poor continues to be adversely affected.[78] Those who can afford it prefer to travel to Singapore, Malaysia, Australia, or China for medical treatment because they believe that the medical care in these places is superior. Many think that foreign physicians' attitudes towards their patients are better. In 2007, more than 100,000 Indonesians travelled abroad for medical treatment; in 2014, this number had risen to 600,000.[79]

It might be possible to explain the relatively poor state of medical care in contemporary Indonesia by analysing the ambitions of the medical profession between 1925 and 1965. In colonial times, many Indies physicians were politically engaged and therefore familiar with the state's bureaucracies and political processes. During the 1920s, a small group of elite physicians emerged who chose medicine over political involvement. After 1945, the influence of the first group declined considerably, which left apolitical physicians in charge of building Indonesia's medical schools and health infrastructure. The aloofness of Indonesia's national physicians was reinforced by political factors. Indonesia consequently lacked physicians familiar with politics and government bureaucracies capable of eliciting political commitment to the nation's

---

[76] Claudia Rokx, John Giles, Elan Satriawan, Puti Marzoeki, Pandu Harimurti, and Elif Yavuz, *New Insights into the Provision of Health Services in Indonesia: A Health Workforce Study* (Washington, DC: World Bank, 2010), 3. See also A. Kurniati, E. Rosskam, M. M. Afzal, T. B. Suryowinoto, and A. G. Mukti, 'Strengthening Indonesia's Health Workforce through Partnerships', *Public Health* 129 (2015), 1138–49.

[77] Joint Committee on Reducing Maternal and Neonatal Mortality in Indonesia, *Reducing Maternal and Neonatal Mortality in Indonesia: Saving Lives, Saving the Future* (Washington, DC: National Academy of Sciences, 2013). See also Paul C. Webster, 'Indonesia Makes Maternal Health a National Priority', *The Lancet* 380 (8 December 2012), 1981–82; and Michael J. Dibley and Meiwita Budiharsana, 'Keeping Women and Babies Healthy within an Unequal System', *Inside Indonesia*, no. 119 (2015), www.insideindonesia.org/keeping-women-and-babies-healthy-within-an-unequal-system-2; accessed on 12 July 2015.

[78] Andrew Rosser, 'Realising Free Health Care for the Poor in Indonesia: The Politics of Illegal Fees', *Journal of Contemporary Asia* 42, no. 2 (2012), 255–75.

[79] Tommy Dharmawan, 'Indonesian Doctors' Attitude', *Jakarta Post*, 15 May 2010; Tommy Dharmawan, 'Are Indonesian Physicians Ready for ASEAN Economic Community?', *Jakarta Post*, 6 December 2014, 7. See also Catherine Smith, 'Traveling for a Cure', *Inside Indonesia*, no. 111 (2013), www.insideindonesia.org/traveling-for-a-cure-2; accessed on 12 July 2015; and 'Doctors Association Seeks to Boost Local Health Services by Awarding High-PR', *Jakarta Post*, 28 April 2009.

health. Instead of political engagement, Indonesia's physicians pursued professional incentives, which rewarded specialisation and technologically intensive hospital-based care. This left the nation's *puskesmas* as the least desirable option for a medical career. During colonial times, pursuing professional and social advancement was motivated by the emancipatory desire of gaining equality with European doctors, or the political motive of fighting discrimination on racial or ethnic grounds. After independence, these ideological motives no longer prevailed, which left only professional and personal advancement.

Conclusion: The Rise and Decline of the National Physician

A Dutch novel published just before the end of the Indonesian struggle for independence begins, enigmatically, with the statement 'Oeroeg was my friend.'[1] The novel, *Oeroeg*, follows the return to Indonesia of a young Dutch engineer with the hastily organised Dutch armed forces seeking to reclaim the former colonies. The narrator yearns to find his Indonesian childhood friend Oeroeg, and reflects upon their shared childhood in the mountainous area around Bandung where his father owned a tea plantation. Oeroeg's father was the plantation manager and reported to the father of the narrator, who was appalled to find that the two young boys had grown to be inseparable. The two continued their friendship after moving to Batavia to attend Dutch high schools. Once there, Oeroeg behaved like many young Indonesian high school students, dressing and acting as a European and speaking exclusively Dutch. He was reticent about his background as a native country boy.[2] After finishing school, he enrolled at the Surabaya Medical College. There he became more confident and mature, and committed himself to the Indonesian nationalist movement. To the reader, it is clear that Oeroeg's political sophistication far outstrips that of the narrator, who remains naïve about the nature of colonial life. Just before the narrator leaves the Indies, Oeroeg forcefully argues that Indonesians no longer need *wayang* puppets, *gamelan*, superstition, or indigenous healers. They require factories, warships, modern clinics, schools, and, above all, a say in their own affairs.[3]

---

[1] I follow the English translation: Hella S. Haasse, *The Black Lake* trans. Ina Rilke (London: Portobella, 2012 [1948]), 1. Haasse's novel first appeared, anonymously, in 1948, as a gift given by booksellers to customers during Dutch book week. It has since been reprinted more than fifty times in the Netherlands. Remarkably, the novel appeared before the second Dutch act of military aggression. Few commentators have speculated on the meaning of the Dutch title of the book. The name Oeroeg is not a common Sundanese (or even Indonesian) name. Striking is the first syllable, 'ur-', which means proto-, primitive, or original, but also superior or great. Spelling Oeroeg backwards (a practice not uncommon in the Dutch East Indies, as Dutchmen often gave their last name, spelled backwards, to their mixed-race children) results in *goeroe* [guru], Malay for teacher.

[2] Haasse, *The Black Lake*, 78.

[3] Haasse, *The Black Lake*, 103.

In the final pages of the novel, the narrator and Oeroeg are reunited as adults. They meet in the forest close to the headquarters of the former tea plantation. The demarcation line between the Dutch and Republican territories were not far away and there is frequent incidental fighting nearby. Oeroeg appears suddenly, now a military physician with the characteristic appearance of a young Indonesian freedom fighter – dishevelled, with long hair tied up with a cloth – and snarls at his former friend that he does not have any business in Indonesia and should return home. He warns him that he will shoot him if he does not leave. It is only at this point that the narrator realises that the chasm between their worlds has become unbridgeable. Oeroeg now represents, for the narrator, Indonesia's inescapable, unfathomable otherness, a trope normally used to describe traditional villagers, not physicians or freedom fighters. The Indonesian declaration of independence and the Dutch neo-colonial military offensive had turned these once inseparable friends into strangers.

Oeroeg's life trajectory was not exceptional for young Indonesian men who studied medicine in the Dutch East Indies. It resembled especially the lives of those students attending the Surabaya Medical College in the 1930s, at a time when the few Indonesian students at the elite Batavia Medical School were not particularly interested in politics.[4] During the colonial period, many Indonesian medical students identified with modern Western culture, disavowed their indigenous origins, and adopted the appearance, behaviour, and tastes of upper-middle-class Europeans. They viewed their medical training as a means of social advancement, and celebrated modern science, technology, and medicine as the most effective tools to improve the life of their fellow Indonesians. They styled themselves as future professionals, tasked with realising the promises of modern science. After completing their studies, however, many became aware of the ambiguous position they occupied in colonial society. Their professional aspirations were regularly encouraged, but their attainment was continuously deferred. The ambiguity in their social standing inspired many Indonesian physicians to engage in an endless and at times almost obsessive analysis of the position of their profession in colonial society. Some extended the analysis to colonial society itself, and this motivated them to engage in colonial politics.

In colonial times, Indonesian physicians participated in public debates by publishing articles in newspapers and magazines, joining political parties, organisations, and social movements, becoming members of city councils and the colonial parliament, strengthening the Indonesian medical profession, and advocating health policies. They were public intellectuals who interpreted

---

[4] Thus far, no commentator of Haasse's novel has commented on the political importance of the NIAS during the 1930s, when most students at the Batavia Medical School were no longer interested in politics, or the importance of physicians and medical students in the Indonesian nationalist movement.

colonial society according to medical and scientific hermeneutics.[5] After the introduction of the Ethical Policy, these physicians contributed to debates about the possibility and trajectory of modernisation in the Indies. They saw themselves, and were seen by their contemporaries, as especially qualified to analyse the colonial social body and its social evolution. Their dedication to health and medicine, their association with the cosmopolitan medical profession, and, in the 1930s, their participation in international health organisations, enabled them to transcend their positions as colonial subjects. They formulated alternative identities, criticised colonial arrangements, and fought with other Indonesians for independence. Warwick Anderson argues that 'the clinic and the laboratory should be added to those sites where the nation – any nation – may be imagined.'[6] After independence, these nationalist physicians became Indonesia's national physicians, building Indonesia's health care system in close association with the state. Because they no longer found themselves in an oppositional relation to the state and because of post-independence political realities, they relinquished their political engagement and focused on health and medicine exclusively.

One of the origin stories told about the Indonesian nation – the founding of Boedi Oetomo – was set in a medical college and featured physicians and medical students. It is not often that such characters figure in national origin narratives, and it is rare that the nationalist ideals of physicians have been acknowledged and commemorated by non-physicians. Focusing on the role of physicians in the Indonesian nationalist movement offers new directions for theories of nationalism, at least those that pertain to Southeast Asia. Apart from highlighting the role of trade, the printing press, religion, and education, most theorists have identified the ideas and activities of the educated indigenous middle class as pivotal in the interpretation of social conditions and the mobilisation of the masses against colonial regimes. Representatives of the middle class became aware of the social strictures placed upon them in colonial societies, and had the means to mount coherent critiques of these impediments. In many Southeast Asian countries, as elsewhere, these intellectuals were often physicians, and their nationalism was distinctly medical.[7] In most colonies, physicians were the only professionals who had received schooling

---

[5] I follow Warwick Anderson's analysis of the social ideas of Australian physicians who engage in 'midlevel, mundane theorizing that commonly occurs when one does science or practices medicine in a society a long way from Europe'. Warwick Anderson, *The Cultivation of Whiteness: Science, Health and Racial Destiny in Australia* (Melbourne: University of Melbourne Press, 2002), 3.

[6] Anderson, *Cultivation of Whiteness*, 2.

[7] Warwick Anderson and Hans Pols, 'Scientific Patriotism: Medical Science and National Self-Fashioning in Southeast Asia', *Comparative Studies in Society and History* 54, no. 1 (2012), 93–113.

in biology and physiology, and so were the only ones familiar with the powerful metaphors offered by these disciplines. Biological and physiological models helped physicians to see the diseased state of the colonial body and to identify obstacles to the evolution of indigenous society. As disciples of science, they had an unshakeable belief in progress. In this book, I have analysed the characteristics and various expressions of medical nationalism in the Dutch East Indies and Indonesia. Further analysis of medical nationalism is called for, focusing on physicians in other colonial contexts by investigating how their nationalism manifested itself under a range of political conditions. More work is needed, similarly, to explore the ways in which other professionals bound their identities to the developing nation, and how other scientific disciplines contributed to nationalistic formulations and political action.

During the past two centuries, both individual physicians and the medical profession as a whole have maintained a close, in places intimate, relationship with the state. In the nineteenth century both the French and German states were keenly interested in medicine because political leaders believed that national strength and military superiority were dependent upon the health of the population. In the 1880s, the figure of the national physician emerged in Germany with its system of state-employed physicians. National physicians may be defined as medical doctors employed by the state and working in state-run health institutions who were responsible for curative care and public health. These physicians developed strong national sensibilities and firm convictions about the central role of medicine and the medical profession in building and maintaining the health of the nation. During Dutch and Japanese colonial times, Indonesian physicians formulated nationalistic views in opposition to the colonial state. After independence, these nationalist physicians became 'normalised' as national medical doctors, and were placed in charge of building new medical schools, a health infrastructure, and a strong medical profession. During Sukarno's rule, Indonesian physicians astutely focused on health and sought to insulate their profession from political interference by withdrawing from political activity. Under Suharto, they built Indonesia's health infrastructure backed by a strong state, a raft of international health organisations, and ample funding, and their social position rose accordingly. The Suharto regime decisively depoliticised society, however, and physicians were therefore prohibited from engaging in political affairs. Unlike their colonial predecessors, Indonesia's national physicians were no longer public intellectuals or political agitators.

Indonesia's physicians opted for active political engagement under a specific set of circumstances. After the turn of the twentieth century, political commentary increasingly relied on biological and physiological metaphors, making Indies physicians unusually suitable to participate in political debates. The international belief in progress and development accorded educated individuals unusually important social positions. However, the two-tier medical system of the Dutch East Indies, which provided Indies physicians with second-rate medical degrees and access to inferior positions, motivated them to question colonial arrangements, first with respect to medicine and, second, with respect to colonial society as a whole. It was among this group of Indies physicians that political activists could be found. The small but growing Indonesian medical *elite*, which held European degrees and earned the same salaries as their European colleagues, instead focused on medical matters and remained aloof from political involvement. After Indonesian independence, the relatively large but now dwindling group of Indies physicians no longer played a significant role. Indonesia's medical elite, reacting to new political realities, continued to maintain its apolitical stance.

The Decline of Indonesia's National Physician

The decade following Suharto's resignation was characterised by far-reaching social and political change.[8] B. J. Habibie, Suharto's vice president, served as president from 1998 to 1999 and abolished media censorship, liberalised the press, scrapped laws limiting the activities of political organisations, and oversaw the organisation of national elections. He implemented the economic reforms stipulated by the International Monetary Fund, including the liberalisation of the economy and the privatisation of state enterprises. He also diminished the size of government bureaucracies and further opened the Indonesian economy by abolishing tariffs, state subsidies, and restrictive legislation. These measures exacerbated the economic crisis that had led to Suharto's resignation and further increased the number of Indonesians living in poverty. To stave off regional separatist movements and armed insurrections, Habibie initiated a far-reaching decentralisation plan, devolving authority and decision-making power to the regencies. The centralised administrative practices of the New Order were replaced by numerous regency-based programs – a mass of uncoordinated piecemeal initiatives. Local politicians took (and continue to take) advantage of decentralisation by establishing new regencies so that they could tap into large central subsidies. In creating local government institutions and hiring civil servants en masse, they built local patronage networks, entrenching their power.[9]

[8] See, for example, Edward Aspinall and Greg Fealy, *Local Power and Politics in Indonesia: Decentralisation & Democratisation* (Singapore: Institute of Southeast Asian Studies, 2003); and Mark Turner, Owen Podger, Maria Sumardjono, and Wayan K. Tirthaysa, *Decentralisation in Indonesia: Redesigning the State* (Canberra: Asia Pacific Press, 2003).

[9] Elizabeth Pisani, *Indonesia Etc.: Exploring the Improbable Nation* (London: Granta, 2014), 122–32.

These decentralisation policies overall were detrimental for Indonesia's state of health. Disparities between regions grew.[10] After 1998, all regencies were required to establish health departments and a large number of civil servants with minimal experience in health were appointed to them. Currently, the national Ministry of Health disburses health funding to the regencies but scarcely regulates how it is spent. A small amount is allocated to the provinces to oversee and inspect health programs, but few have the tools to do so and the allocation does not cover the costs.[11] Several national programs have been reduced or discontinued; disease surveillance systems have collapsed with regencies not passing information to the Ministry of Health or failing to collect it in the first place. Public health programs have declined. Regional disparities in health care provision are more pronounced than ever, with rural and poor areas disadvantaged by the concentration of physicians and other health personnel in urban areas. An increasing number of physicians exclusively work in city-based private practices.[12] The agile and highly effective family planning program has declined.[13] In the past fifteen years, facilities for monitoring the quality of medical education and education programs for paramedical personnel have been inadequate.

Despite the generally detrimental consequences of decentralisation for the provision of health care, it has become much easier to develop and implement initiatives at the regency and distict level to address local health issues. Feedback from patients in regional hospitals and community health centres has started to influence how health care is provided. Since 2006, local politicians have routinely included new health initiatives and health insurance schemes, for the poor or for all constituents, in their election campaigns; the number of these schemes has consequently multiplied.[14] Non-governmental organisations

---

[10] For an overview of conditions in 1990, see Broto Wasisto, 'Pembangunan Kesehatan di Indonesia: Masalah dan Prospeknya', *Prisma* 6 (1990), 36–53. For an overview of developments in Indonesia's universities after the fall of Suharto, see 'Indonesian Universities in Transition: Catching Up and Opening Up', *Bulletin of Indonesian Economic Studies* 48, no. 2 (2012), 229–51.

[11] Elizabeth Pisani, conversation with author, London, 5 October 2015.

[12] Country Office for Indonesia World Health Organization, *WHO Country Cooperation Strategy 2007–2012: Indonesia* (New Dehli: WHO Regional Office for South-East Asia, 2008). See also Peter Heywood and Nida P. Harahap, 'Health Facilities at the District Level in Indonesia', *Australia and New Zealand Health Policy* 6, no. 13 (2009), www.anzhealthpolicy.com/content/6/1/13; accessed on 30 July 2015; and Paul C. Webster, 'Indonesia: The Midwife and Maternal Mortality Miasma', *Canadian Medical Association Journal* 185, no. 2 (2013), E95–E96.

[13] Hari Fitri Putjuk, 'Indonesia's Family Planning Program: From Stagnation to Revitalization', *Devex International Development News* (25 September 2015), www.devex.com/news/indonesia sfamilyplanningprogramfromstagnationtorevitalization84387; accessed on 10 November 2015.

[14] Andrew Rosser and Ian Wilson, 'Democratic Decentralisation and Pro-Poor Policy Reform in Indonesia: The Politics of Health Insurance for the Poor in Jembrana and Tabanan', *Asian Journal of Social Science* 40 (2012), 608–34; Edward Aspinall and Eve Warburton, 'A Healthcare Revolution in the Regions', *Inside Indonesia*, no. 111 (2013), www.insideindonesia .org/a-healthcare-revolution-in-the-regions-2; accessed on 12 July 2015.

(NGOs) have undertaken a range of initiatives to address local health problems, often very effectively. Despite these promising developments, health care institutions have decreased in number and quality, and the health of Indonesians as a national population has declined. Because the formerly powerful and highly centralised Indonesian state has been replaced by a patchwork of little-coordinated regency governments, the social position of Indonesia's national physicians has eroded together with national health programs and institutions – they have become local doctors.

During the 1990s, global health, a new approach to the world's health challenges pioneered and promoted by the World Bank, came to dominate the agenda of international health organisations, muting the influence of the World Health Organization.[15] Global health tends to favour vertical programs, technological intervention, and pharmaceutical innovation, all built around specific diseases which are often infectious, threatening human life beyond any one country's borders, and which require a forceful and coordinated response exceeding the capacities of national governments. HIV/AIDS was the first condition to elicit a global response, followed by other conditions including severe acute respiratory syndrome (SARS), Ebola, and avian and swine influenza.[16] Emphasis often is placed on biosecurity and attempts to prevent infectious disease from spreading. Less attention is paid to horizontal initiatives such as long-term programs to strengthen national health services, primary health care, public health education, or the involvement of local communities in health initiatives. The social and economic roots of disease are largely ignored. Following the rise of neo-liberalism in the 1980s, global health programs have favoured public-private partnerships, NGOs, and private sector involvement, which came with an increased emphasis on financial accountability, cost-effectiveness, market-oriented policies, and, where possible, full privatisation. Neo-liberal theorists advocate a diminished role for central governments; the global health initiatives influenced by them hold national governments as secondary in the pursuit of health.

---

[15] Theodore M. Brown, Marcos Cueto, and Elizabeth Fee, 'The World Health Organization and the Transition from "International" to "Global" Public Health', *American Journal of Public Health* 96, no. 1 (2004), 62–72; Andrew Lakoff, 'Two Regimes of Global Health', *Humanity: An International Journal of Human Rights, Humanitarianism, and Development* 1, no. 1 (2010), 59–79; Paul Farmer, Jim Yong Kim, Arthur Kleinman, and Matthew Basilico, eds., *Reimagining Global Health: An Introduction* (Berkeley: California University Press, 2013). See also Vincanne Adams, 'Against Global Health: Arbitrating Science, Non-Science, and Nonsense through Health', in *Against Health: How Health Became the New Morality*, ed. J. M. Metzl and A. Kirkland (New York: New York University Press, 2010), 40–60.

[16] The HIV epidemic boosted a global approach to health and disease as coordinated and global reaction was required Allan M. Brandt, 'How AIDS Invented Global Health', *New England Journal of Medicine* 368, no. 23 (6 June 2013), 2149–52. For Indonesian health initiatives in response to AIDS, see Elizabeth Pisani, *The Wisdom of Whores: Bureaucrats, Brothels and the Business of AIDS* (New York: Norton, 2009).

While advocates of global health often celebrate the free, almost uninhibited flow of individuals, information, technologies, and medications around the world, critics point to the pronounced inequalities in access to information, medications, and financial resources that constrict this flow.[17] Some have criticised global health initiatives for neglecting primary health care institutions supporting disadvantaged populations in their preoccupation with biotechnological innovation, drug development, and biosecurity.[18] In many respects, global health reveals the legacy of colonial medicine, which often was characterised by disease-specific interventions and a focus on epidemics and a concern with population control.[19] Global health initiatives tend to focus on former tropical colonies, reinforcing the old and stale idea that dangerous epidemics originate in that region, amongst the unhygienic masses. For the physician and historian of medicine Jeremy Greene and his co-authors, 'the history of [colonial] tropical medicine helps explain why in rich countries the phrase "global health" connotes diseases of "elsewhere" – problems affecting an othered "them" rather than an inclusive "us".'[20] Current quarantine measures and the culling of livestock to prevent disease outbreaks, for example, affect poor people in developing nations far more than they affect wealthy nations. The project as a whole appears to promote the health of wealthy nations by taking a neo-colonial stance towards the rest of the world, which is characterised as the source of health threats to be contained. If improving global health benefits all humanity, the benefit is more apparent in wealthier areas and the burden more apparent in developing nations.

During the first decade of the twenty-first century, Asia was repeatedly plagued by outbreaks of avian influenza (especially H5N1), which required the culling of vast bird populations. Indonesia has been the epicentre of the global avian flu problem, making the country of special interest to medical

[17] See Sarah Hodges, 'The Global Menace', *Social History of Medicine* 25, no. 3 (2012), 719–28; and Warwick Anderson, 'Making Global Health History: The Postcolonial Worldliness of Biomedicine', *Social History of Medicine* 27, no. 2 (2014), 273–84.

[18] See, for example, Anne-Emmauelle Birn, 'Gates's Grandest Challenge: Transcending Technology as Public Health Ideology', *Lancet* 366, no. 9484 (6 August 2005), 514–19. For a trenchant critique on global health in Africa, see Johanna Tayloe Crane, *Scrambling for Africa: AIDS, Expertise, and the Rise of American Global Health Science* (Ithaca, NY: Cornell University Press, 2013).

[19] See also Anne-Emanuelle Birn, 'The Stages of International (Global) Health: Histories of Success or Successes of History?', *Global Public Health* 4, no. 1 (2009), 50–68; and João Biehl and Adriana Petryna, *When People Come First: Critical Studies in Global Health* (Princeton, NJ: Princeton University Press, 2013); Peter Redfield, *Life in Crisis: The Ethical Journey of Doctors without Borders* (Berkeley: University of California Press, 2013); Andrew Lakoff and Stephen J. Collier, *Biosecurity Interventions: Global Health and Security in Question* (New York: Columbia University Press, 2008).

[20] Jeremy Greene, Marguerite Thorp Basilico, Heidi Kim, and Paul Farmer, 'Colonial Medicine and Its Legacies', in *Reimagining Global Health: An Introduction*, ed. Paul Farmer, Jim Yong Kim, Arthur Kleinman, and Matthew Basilico (Berkeley: California University Press, 2013), 42.

researchers and international health organisations. In Indonesia, birds and humans live in close proximity, causing physicians to speculate that the virus could spread to the human population. This has indeed occurred, albeit rarely, and 'avian' flu in humans has a fatality rate of 88 per cent.[21] Containment strategies and research efforts by international health organisations therefore have intensified, with their centre in Indonesia. In 2007, however, the Indonesian minister of health Siti Fadilah Supari announced that her country would no longer participate in the Global Influenza Surveillance Network or share strains of the H5N1 virus internationally.[22] She argued that Indonesian samples had been provided to the pharmaceutical industry without the country's permission and that medications that had been developed from them were patented and unaffordable to most Indonesians. She was not prepared to support international research initiatives that would not benefit Indonesians. Although this announcement was widely condemned within Indonesia and internationally, it demonstrates that the demands of global health do not necessarily coincide with the interests of individual nations. Such national assertion is rare in the history of global health, but in this case it proved effective: the WHO has created a framework for the sharing of avian influenza samples that attempts to overcome inequities. The framework stipulates that medications or vaccines must be made affordable to the populations of countries that have provided samples or other forms of assistance to researchers.[23]

The emphases in global health on private, at times for-profit, initiatives resonate well in contemporary Indonesia, where private practices, private hospitals, and private health insurance schemes, all barely regulated, have proliferated in the past decade.[24] These private initiatives tend to cluster in urban areas, targeting wealthier patients who can afford the fees.[25] Midwives, who practised in rural areas during the Suharto era, have moved en masse to the cities to set up private

---

[21] On the avian flu in Indonesia, see Celia Lowe, 'Viral Clouds: Becoming H5N1 in Indonesia', *Cultural Anthropology* 25, no. 4 (2010), 625–49; Celia Lowe, 'Preparing Indonesia: H5N1 Influenza through the Lens of Global Health', *Indonesia*, no. 90 (2010), 147–70. See also Natalie Porter, 'Risky Zoographies: The Limits of Place in Avian Flu Management', *Environmental Humanities* 1 (2012), 103–21.

[22] Kennas Mullis, 'Playing Chicken with Bird Flu: "Viral Sovereignty", the Right to Exploit Natural Genetic Resources, and the Potential Human Rights Ramifications', *American University International Law Review* 24, no. 5 (2009), 943–67; and Rachel Irwin, 'Indonesia, H5N1, and Global Health Diplomacy', *Global Health Governance* 3, no. 2 (2010), http://blogs .shu.edu/ghg/files/2011/11/Irwin_Indonesia-H5N1-and-Global-Health-Diplomacy_Spring-2010.pdf; accessed on 12 July 2015.

[23] World Health Organization, *Pandemic Influenza Preparedness Framework for the Sharing of Influenza Viruses and Access to Vaccines and Other Benefits* (Geneva: World Health Organization, 2011).

[24] Stein Kristiansen and Purwo Santoso, 'Surviving Decentralisation?: Impacts of Regional Autonomy on Health Service Provision in Indonesia', *Health Policy* 77 (2006), 247–59.

[25] Paul C. Webster, 'Indonesia: Stratified Health the Norm', *Canadian Medical Association Journal* 185, no. 2 (5 February 2013), E99–E100.

practices.[26] Physicians, nurses, and midwives working in the public system continue to maintain private practices to supplement their income, and many primarily focus on their private patients. In 2014, the Indonesian government commenced a roll-out of a national health insurance scheme, which is expected to cover all citizens by 2018. The combination of a national insurance scheme and a crucial shortage of health care facilities, especially outside urban areas, prompted a report from the financial consultancy firm Ernst & Young encouraging international investment in Indonesia's health sector.[27] The authors cite earlier findings of the World Bank that the 'lack of qualified physicians and nurses is the major challenge' in Indonesian health care today, and that 'rural areas are severely underserved.'[28] The report suggests that private hospitals and physicians in private practice are ideally situated to address these shortcomings. With the recent economic integration of the member nations of the Association of Southeast Asian Nations (ASEAN), it will become possible to hire physicians from other member states to work in Indonesia. The Indonesian Medical Association and the Ministry of Health have warned of the consequences of this aspect of the global flow of medical provision.[29]

The recent shift to global health together with Indonesian decentralisation policies has eroded the position of Indonesia's national physicians. Global health organisations generally do not linger to assist state governments in strengthening health care services, preferring to bypass them. The emphasis on private initiative in health care acts as a disincentive for Indonesia's physicians to participate in community health clinics and social medicine programs. The recent introduction of private health care institutions, which chiefly benefits wealthier Indonesians who can afford the fees, is increasing health disparity between rich and poor. With the fragmentation of the state and decreased interest, within and outside Indonesia, in public health care institutions, the prominence of Indonesia's physicians on the national scene is eroding. Whether the recent introduction of universal health insurance will alter or reverse this trend is hard to predict.

After independence, Indonesia's physicians no longer had to work within the confines of the colonial state. As national physicians, they built Indonesia's health care infrastructure in close cooperation with the state and with the

---

[26] Webster, 'Midwife and Maternal Mortality'.
[27] Ernst & Young, *Ripe for Investment: The Indonesian Health Care Industry Post Introduction of Universal Health Coverage* (London: Ernst & Young Global Limited, 2015).
[28] Ernst & Young, *Ripe for Investment*, 6, 9.
[29] See, for example, Wahyudi Soeriaatmadja, 'Singapore Doctors Upset Peers in Indonesia', *Jakarta Globe*, 21 October 2013; Wahyudi Soeriaatmadja, 'Indonesia Row over Hiring of Foreign Doctors', *The Strait Times*, 21 October 2013; Amanda Siddharta, 'Healthcare within Borders', *Tempo* (English) (3 May 2015), 64–66.

assistance of various international health organisations. From the turn of the twentieth century, when global health overtook international health, foreign health organisations increasingly bypassed or displaced Indonesian physicians, thereby weakening their position both nationally and internationally. Critics have argued that global health initiatives view the developing world as a reservoir of disease threats to the West that should be contained. Global health again discredits national physicians as experts, preferring to rely on outside 'experts'. In many ways, the practice of global health appears to replicate colonial medicine, which – as we have seen – focused on containing specific diseases threatening European populations and accorded Indonesian physicians a limited role. Thus, colonial modes and manners – expressed now in the language of biosecurity and humanitarianism, and shaped by assumptions about competence, expertise, and dedication – continue to insinuate themselves into our contemporary world.

Bibliography

ARCHIVES CONSULTED

Archives of the KITLV/Royal Institute of Southeast Asian and Caribbean Studies, Leiden
Special Collections, University of Leiden Library
Special Collections, University of Amsterdam Library
Archives of the KIT/Royal Tropical Institute, Amsterdam
Archives of the International Institute of Social History, Amsterdam
National Archives of the Netherlands, The Hague
Indonesian National Archives, Jakarta
Archives at the University of California at San Francisco
Rockefeller Archive Centre
Archives, US National Library of Medicine
Special Collections, Library of the Faculty of Medicine, University of Indonesia
Special Collections, Library of the Faculty of Medicine, Airlangga University

NEWSPAPERS AND PERIODICALS CONSULTED

Bataviaasch Nieuwsblad
De Indische Courant
Het Nieuws van den Dag voor Nederlandsch Indië
Soerabaiasch Handelsblad
Sumatra Post
Handelingen van de Volksraad, 1918–42

PRIMARY SOURCES

A. 'STOVIA Schetsen, 1913–1923'. In *STOVIA Almanak 1924*, edited by Bahder Djohan, A. Ramali, A. Gafar, R. Mochtar, Soekandar, M. A. Hanafiah, Zainoedin, Loekmono, and Darwis, 168–80. Weltevreden: Kolff, 1924.

A. [Mohamad Amir]. 'Op den Uitkijk'. *Jong Sumatra* 4 (1921): 150–53.

A. H. 'Zorgen'. In *STOVIA Almanak 1925*, edited by Bahder Djohan, 159–61. Weltevreden: Kolff, 1925.

A. H. M. 'Quo Vadis'. *Orgaan der Vereeniging van Indische Geneeskundigen* 1, no. 2 (1918): 22–23.

A. R. 'Wanneer Pluizer zijn Slag Slaat'. In *STOVIA Almanak 1923*, edited by Bahder Djohan, Oesman Saleh, P. Pinontoan, Raden Ito, Djamaloedin, Soewandhi, and Soekendar, 197–200. Weltevreden: Kolff, 1923.

Adviseur voor Inlandsche Zaken [G. A. J. Hazeu]. *Sarekat Islam Congres (4e Nationale Congres), 26 Oct–2 Nov. 1919, Soerabaja*. Batavia: Landsdrukkerij, 1919.

'Aether-Trillingen'. In *NIAS Lustrum Almanak 1933–1934*, edited by Dj. Siregar, Soeharso, and C. Schreuder, 218–20. Surabaya: NIAS, 1934.

Alken, J. 'De School Voor Docter Djawa'. *Indisch Genootschap* (28 February 1882): 1–4.

Amir, Mohamad. 'Familieplichten'. *Jong Sumatra* 1 (1918): 136–40.

'Godsdienst en Spes-Patria'. *Jong Sumatra* 1 (1918): 161–65.

'De Hindoe's op Sumatra'. *Jong Sumatra* 1 (1918): 57–60.

'De Vrouwenbeweging ter Sumatra's Westkust'. *Jong Sumatra* 2 (1919): 2–8, 49–52.

'Letterkundige Verpoozingen'. *Jong Sumatra* 2 (1919): 133–34.

'Iets over de Sumatranen als Zeevarend Volk'. In *Gedenk-Nummer van Jong Sumatra*, 36–43. Weltevreden: Jong Sumatranen Bond, 1923.

'Sumatra's Eenheid: Bijdrage tot een Dynamisch-Psychologische Her-Stelling van het Probleem'. In *Gedenk-Nummer van Jong Sumatra*, 17–20. Weltevreden: Jong Sumatranen Bond, 1923.

'Prae-Advies Dr. Amir: Een Eigen Vaktijdschrift Voor den Indonesischen Arts'. *Bulletin van den Bond van Indische Geneeskundigen* 14, no. 3 (1925): 9–10.

'De Medische Hoogeschool te Batavia'. *Opbouw* 8 (1926): 932–45.

'Rondom een Indisch Jeugd-Congres'. *Opbouw* 10 (1927): 73–82.

Bijdrage tot de Kliniek en Therapie der Deflexieliggingen. Utrecht: Smits, 1928.

Boenga Rampai, edited by Mohamad Amir and M. Sarqawi. Medan: Centrale Courant en Boekhandel, 1940.

'Dr Abdul Rivai'. In *Boenga Rampai*, edited by Mohamad Amir and M. Sarqawi, 179–85. Medan: Centrale Courant en Boekhandel, 1940.

'Kemadjuan'. In *Boenga Rampai*, edited by Mohamad Amir and M. Sarqawi, 107–08. Medan: Centrale Courant en Boekhandel, 1940.

'Announcement [of the Founding of Ikatan Dokter Indonesia]'. *OSR News* 2, no. 11 (1950): 141–42.

Apituley, H. J. D., R. Tumbelaka, H. F. Lumentut, Radjiman, M. Brenthel, Moh. Salih, Ph. Laoh, and Abdul Rivai. *Eenige Opmerkingen naar aanleiding van de Voorstellen tot Reorganisatie van den Civiel Geneeskundigen Dienst in Nederl. Oost-Indië*. Amsterdam: Eisendrath, 1910.

Asharie. 'Stimulantia'. *Orgaan der Vereeniging van Inlandsche Geneeskundigen* 4, no. 1–2 (1914): 1–5.

Asharie and D. J. Siahaija. 'Gewone Vergadering op Zondag den 7en Juni 1914 in het Polikliniek Lokaal van de STOVIA'. *Orgaan der Vereeniging van Inlandsche Geneeskundigen* 4, no. 4–5 (1914): 4–5.

'Assistentenavond'. *NIAS Orgaan* 3, no. 2 (1930): 16.

Astrohadikoesoemo, Goelarso. 'Onze Eigen Geneesmiddelen'. *Medisch Tribune* 28, no. 2 (1940): 35–36.

'Sedikit Pemandangan tentang Obat-Obat Kita oentoek Diselidiki'. In *Het Tweede Congres van de Vereeniging van Indonesische Geneeskundigen*, 200–21. Batavia: Kenanga, 1940.

Atmosoeprodjo, Mochtar. 'Jong-Java en de Politiek'. In *Gedenkboek Jong Java 1915 – 7 Maart – 1930: Kitab Peringatan Jong-Java*, edited by Koentjoro Poerbopranoto, Soegandi Pringgoatmodjo, Soedarso, Joesoepadi Danoehadiningrat, and Moewardi, 67–73. Jakatera: Pedoman Besar Jong-Java, 1930.

Augustin, P. L. *Iets over Rechten en Plichten van den Inlandschen Arts*. Batavia: Kolff, 1914.

'De Oud-Leerlingen van de STOVIA en de Volksraad'. *Orgaan der Vereeniging van Indische Geneeskundigen* 8, no. 1–2 (1918): 9–12.

Aulia. 'Beberapa Pikiran tentang Terapi atau Pengobatan dengan Makanan Mentah'. *Berita Ketabiban* 1, no. 1-2-3 (2604 [1944]): 68–77.

Bakar, Aboe. 'Herinneringen en Overpeinzingen'. In *Ontwikkeling van het Geneeskundig Onderwijs te Weltevreden, 1851–1926*, edited by A. de Waart, 329–33. Weltevreden: Kolff, 1926.

'Bantoean Djawa Izi Hookoo Kai Kepada "Komisi Makanan Dimasa Perang" dan Kepada "Komisi Jamoe-Jamoe".' *Berita Ketabiban* 1, no. 4-5-6 (2604 [1944]): 10–12.

Beberapa Toemboeh-Toemboehan Obat jang Berfaedah jang Terdapat di Djawa. Djakarta: Djawa Gunseikanbu Naimubu Eiseikyoku, 1945.

'Berichten uit Nederland'. *Bulletin van den Bond van Indische Geneeskundigen* 14, no. 3 (1925): 13.

Bestuur [of the NIAS Association]. 'Bij het Vertrek van Dr. Soewarno'. *NIAS Orgaan* 4, no. 3 (1930): 6.

'Dokter Soerjatin Hoofd-Indisch-Arts'. *NIAS Orgaan* 4, no. 3 (1930): 7.

'De NIAS Vereeniging'. In *NIAS Jaarboek 1932*, edited by Moersito, Soehardo, S. Rachmat, Sosodoro, K. A. Tan, Mohamad, and Djafar Siregar 93–111. Surabaya: Kolff, 1932.

Bijker, J. *Rapport der Commissie tot Voorbereiding eener Reorganisatie van den Burgerlijken Geneeskundigen Dienst*. Batavia: Landsdrukkerij, 1908.

Boeka [P. C. C. Hansen]. 'Naar aanleiding van het Belangrijke Boek van Dr. Kohlbrugge'. *Indische Gids* 30 (1908): 480–87.

Boeke, J. 'Prae-Advies'. In *Prae-Adviezen van het Eerste Koloniaal Onderwijscongres*, 76–87. The Hague: Korthals, 1916.

Boeke, J. H. *Dualistische Economie*. Leiden: Van Doesburgh, 1930.

[Boenjamin, Raden]. 'Aan Onze Stamgenoten!' *Oedyånå pårå Prajitnå* 1, no. 1 (1909): 1.

Bond van Indonesische Artsen, Afdeeling Nederland. *Verweerschrift tegen de Rede van Dr. F. H. van Loon over 'De Psychische Eigenschappen der Maleische Rassen'*. Amsterdam: Hesse, 1924.

'Bondsbelangen: Het Aanstaande Congres van Onze Vereeniging'. *Orgaan der Vereeniging van Indische Geneeskundigen* 18, no. 5–6 (1930): 77.

Bonne, C. 'Uitzending van Artsen uit Nederland'. *Medisch Maandblad* 2, no. 17 (1947): 336.

Carp, E. A. D. E., Anthonius Henri Fortanier, and T. A. Kandou. *Psychosen op Exogenen Grondslag en Geestelijke Defecttoestanden*. Amsterdam: Scheltema & Holkema, 1937.

Colijn, Hendrikus. *Koloniale Vraagstukken van Heden en Morgen*. Amsterdam: Standaard, 1928.

'Continuing Student Agitation in Indonesia'. *Minerva* 5, no. 1 (1966): 116–23.

Corner, Lorraine and Y. Rahardjo. 'New Direction in Health Policy in Indonesia: The Need for a Demand-Oriented Perspective'. In *Health and Development in Southeast Asia*, edited by Paul Cohen and John Purcal, 77–103. Canberra: Australian National University, 1995.

Datoe Hitam. 'Iets over Adat en Traditie in Verband met de Jongeren'. *NIAS Orgaan* 1, no. 2 (1926): 31–33.

'De Bond en de Wetenschap'. *Bulletin van den Bond van Indische Geneeskundigen* 14, no. 3 (1925): 12.

'De Kwestie van het Doctoraal-Examen'. *Orgaan der Vereeniging van Indische Geneeskundigen* 21, no. 3–4 (1932): 28–29.

De Langen, C. D. 'Aan de Lezers!' *Tijdschrift voor Inlandsche Geneeskundigen* 23, no. 1 (1915): 1–4.

    'Beroepsbelangen'. *Orgaan der Vereeniging van Indische Geneeskundigen* 16, no. 1 (1927): 11–15.

'De Nederlandsch-Indische Artsenschool (NIAS) te Soerabaja'. In *NIAS Jaarboek 1932*, edited by Moersito, Soehardo, S. Rachmat, Sosodoro, K. A. Tan, Mohamad and Djafar Siregar, 53–58. Surabaya: Kolff, 1932.

'De NIAS Vereeniging'. In *NIAS Jaarboek 1932,* edited by Moersito, Soehardo, S. Rachmat, Sosodoro, K.A. Tan, Mohamad, and Djafar Siregar, 93–111. Surabaya: Kolff, 1932.

'De Psychische Eigenschappen der Maleische Rassen'. *Orgaan der Vereeniging van Indische Geneeskundigen* 13, no. 1 (December 1924): 36–40.

'De Verbreking van het Dienstverband'. *Orgaan der Vereeniging van Indische Geneeskundigen* 21, no. 1–2 (1933): 5–7.

Derde-jaars student. 'Roemloos Einde'. In *STOVIA Almanak 1924*, edited by Bahder Djohan, A. Ramali, A. Gafar, R. Mochtar, Soekandar, M.A. Hanafiah, Zainoedin, Loekmono, and Darwis, 188–94. Weltevreden: Kolff, 1924.

Dewantara, Ki Hadjar. 'Some Aspects of National Education and the Taman Siswa Institute of Jogjakarta'. *Indonesia*, no. 5 (1967): 150–68.

Dewantara, Ki Hadjar and Wurjaningrat. *20 Mei Pelopor 17 Augustus*. Bandung: Djapenpro Djabar, 1950.

'Dilettantisme of Wetenschap?' *Indonesia Merdeka* 2 (1924): 48.

Dinger, J. E., Raden Soekonto, and J. W. Tesch. 'Investigation into the Epidemiology of Diphtheria in the Hygiene Study Ward at Batavia'. *Documenta Neerlandica et Indonesica de Morbis Tropicis* 1, no. 1 (1949): 3–33.

Djajadiningrat, P. A. Achmad. *Herinneringen van Pangeran Aria Achmad Djajadiningrat*. Batavia: Kolff, 1936.

Djawa Izi Hookoo Kai, Osamu Serei No 28: Peratoeran Dasar, Peratoeran Khusus. Jakarta: Gunseibanku, 2604 [1944].

Djoehari and Asharie. 'Gewone Vergadering Gehouden op de 1ste Augutus 1915 in the Polikliniek Zaal der STOVIA'. *Orgaan der Vereeniging van Inlandsche Geneeskundigen* 5–6, no. 6–1 (1916): 11.

    'Gewone Vergadering Gehouden op de 18e Juli 1915 in the Polikliniek Zaal der STOVIA'. *Orgaan der Vereeniging van Inlandsche Geneeskundigen* 5–6, no. 6–1 (1916): 8–10.

Djohan, Bahder. 'De Maleische Taal en Hare Toekomst'. *Jong Sumatra* 1 (1918): 164–71.

    'De Strijd der Padries'. In *Gedenk-Nummer van Jong Sumatra*, 58–63. Weltevreden: Jong Sumatranen Bond, 1923.

    'School tot Opleiding van Indische Artsen: Verslag over 1923'. In *STOVIA-Almanak 1924*, 69–84. Weltevreden: Kolff, 1924.

'Algemeen Verslag over het Jaar 1924'. In *STOVIA Almanak 1925*, edited by Bahder Djohan, A. Ramali, A. Gafar, R. Mochtar, Soekandar, M. A. Hanafiah, Zainoedin, Loekmono, and Darwis, 56–85. Weltevreden: Kolff, 1925.

'Algemeen Verslag over het Jaar 1925'. In *STOVIA Almanak 1926*, edited by Bahder Djohan, Ahmad Ramali, Abdoel Gafar, Soekendar, Darwis, Loekmono, and Zainoedin, 85–98. Weltevreden: Kolff, 1926.

'Verslag over 1930'. *Orgaan der Vereeniging van Indische Geneeskundigen* 18, no. 11–12 (1930): 145–51.

'Verslag over 1938'. *Medisch Tribune* 27, no. 3 (1939): 17–22.

'Indonesich-Medische Taal'. *Medisch Tribune* 27, no. 12 (1939): 17.

'Verslag over het 1e Congres van de Vereeniging van Indonesische Geneeskundigen, December 1938 te Semarang'. *Medisch Tribune* 27, no. 3 (1939): 7–16.

'Beknopt Verslag van het 2e Congres'. *Medisch Tribune* 28, no. 4 (1940): 97–103.

Djohan, Bahder, ed. *STOVIA-Almanak 1925*. Weltevreden: Kolff, 1925.

Djohan, Bahder, A. Ramali, A. Gafar, R. Mochtar, Soekandar, M. A. Hanafiah, Zainoedin, Loekmono, and Darwis, eds. *STOVIA-Almanak voor het Jaar Negentien-Honderd Vier-en-Twintig*. Weltevreden: Kolff, 1924.

Djohan, Bahder, Ahmad Ramali, Abdoel Gafar, Soekendar, Darwis, Loekmono, and Zainoedin, eds. *STOVIA-Almanak voor het Jaar Negentien-Honderd Zes-en-Twintig*. Weltevreden: Kolff, 1926.

Djohan, Bahder, Oesman Saleh, P. Pinontoan, Raden Ito, Djamaloedin, Soewandhi, and Soekendar, eds. *STOVIA-Almanak voor het Jaar Negentien-Honderd Drie-en-Twintig*. Weltevreden: Kolff, 1923.

Djojohadikusumo, Margono. *Herinneringen uit 3 Tijdperken: Een Geschreven Familie-Overlevering*. Jakarta: Indira, 1970.

Djukanovic, Voyo and Edward P. Mach, eds. *Alternative Approaches to Meeting Basic Health Needs of Populations in Developing Countries*. Geneva: World Health Organization, 1975.

Douwes Dekker, E. F. E. 'De Indische Partij: Verslag der Progaganda-Deputatie'. *Het Tijdschrift* 2, no. 4 (15 October 1912): 97–146.

'Mijn Ontmoeting met Soetomo'. *Kritiek en Opbouw* (1, 16 October 1938): 246–48, 64–65.

Douwes Dekker, E. F. E., Tjipto Mangoenkoesoemo, and Raden Mas Soewardi Soerjaningrat. *Onze Verbanning*. Schiedam: De Indiër, 1913.

Douwes Dekker, E. F. E. and Harumi Wanasita. *70 Jaar Konsekwent*. Bandoeng: A. C. Nix, 1949.

Een Geneesheer in Indië [Cornelis Swaving]. *Twee Voorstellen in het Belang van de Nederlandsche Bezittingen in Oost-Indië*. Groningen: Wolters, 1850.

Een Indisch Geneesheer. *Indische Ziekten: Practische Handleiding ter Voorkoming van de Voornaamste in Nederlandsch-Indië Heerschende Ziekten*. Amsterdam: De Bussy, 1906.

Een oude. 'Ontgroenen!' In *NIAS Lustrum Almanak 1933–1934*, edited by D. J. Siregar, Soeharso, and C. Schreuder, 266–68. Surabaya: NIAS, 1934.

Engelen, O. E., Aboe Bakar Loebis, Abdullah Ciptoprawiro, Soejono Joedodibroto, Oetarjo, and Idris Siregar. *Lahirnya Satu Bangsa dan Negara*. Jakarta: Penerbit Universitas Indonesia, 1997.

'Enkele Opmerkingen naar aanleiding van de Rede van Dr. F. H. van Loon'. *Indonesia Merdeka* 2 (1924): 51–66.

Fanon, Frantz. *Black Skin, White Masks*. Translated by Charles Lam Markmann. New York: Grove Press, 1967.

   The Wretched of the Earth. Translated by Constance Farrington. New York: Grove Press, 1965.

'Fantasy'. In *STOVIA Almanak 1925*, edited by Bahder Djohan, A. Ramali, A. Gafar, R. Mochtar, Soekandar, M. Hanafiah, Zainoedin, Loekmono, and Darwis 150–52. Weltevreden: Kolff, 1925.

Fauna. 'Kemadjuan'. *Jong Sumatra* 1 (1918): 221–24.

Fruin-Mees, Willemine. *Geschiedenis van Java: Het Hindoetijdperk*. Weltevreden: Commissie voor de Volkslectuur, 1919.

Gandiwan, D. I. 'Bij een Mijlpaal'. In *STOVIA Almanak 1923*, edited by Bahder Djohan, Oesman Saleh, P. Pinontoan, Raden Ito, Djamaloedin, Soewandhi, and Soekendar, 210. Weltevreden: Kolff, 1923.

'Geestelijk Leven op de NIAS'. *NIAS Orgaan* 11, no. 1-2-3 (1938): 19–20.

'Gids voor Inlandsche Geneeskundigen'. *Orgaan der Vereeniging van Inlandsche Geneeskundigen* 2, no. 1 (1911): 1–2.

Gonggopoetro, Pirngadi. 'Ontslagen'. In *STOVIA Almanak 1923*, edited by Bahder Djohan, Oesman Saleh, P. Pinontoan, Raden Ito, Djamaloedin, Soewandhi, and Soekendar 189–96. Weltevreden: Kolff, 1923.

Gunseikan, J. M. 'Nasehat dan Petoendjoek'. *Berita Ketabiban* 1, no. 1-2-3 (2604 [1944]): 5.

Haasse, Hella S. *The Black Lake*. Translated by Ina Rilke. London: Portobello, 2012 [1948].

Hadibroto, Soemitro. *Het Trachoom op de Volksscholen te Batavia*. Batavia: Kolff, 1937.

Haga, J. 'Geneeskundige Dienst in Ned.-Indië'. *Indische Gids* 30 (1908): 25–32.

   'Reorganisatie van den Geneeskundigen Dienst in Ned.-Indië'. *Indische Gids* 31 (1909): 457–64.

Hakim, Abdul. 'Meditaties over Solidariteit en Broederzin onder de Inlandsche Geneesheeren'. *Orgaan der Vereeniging van Inlandsche Geneeskundigen* 5, no. 1-2-3-4 (1915): 33–35.

Hanafiah, Mohammad Ali. *Drama Kedokteran Terbesar*. Jakarta: Yayasan Gedung-gedung Bersejarah Jakarta, 1976.

Hanifah, Abu. 'Gedachten over den Indonesischen Arts en de Maatschappij'. *Medisch Tribune* 28, no. 11 (1940): 277–88.

Harahap, Parada. *Riwajat Dr. A. Rivai*. Medan: Indische Drukkerij, 1939.

[Hatta, Mohammad]. 'Het Psychologische Conflict'. *Hindia Poetra* 1 (1923): 65–69.

Hatta, Mohammad. 'Indonesia Free'. In *Portrait of a Patriot: Selected Writings*, 205–97. The Hague: Mouton, 1972 [1928].

Hatta, Mohammad and C. P. J. van der Peet. *Verspreide Geschriften*. 2 vols. Jakarta: Penerbitan dan Balai Buku Indonesia, 1952.

Hendarmin. 'Mempertegoeh Djasmani'. *Berita Ketabiban* 1, no. 1-2-3 (2604 [1944]): 58–59.

Hendrate, L. 'A Model for Community Health Care in Rural Java'. *Development Digest* 19, no. 1 (1981): 107–14.

'Herderszangen'. In *STOVIA Almanak 1923*, edited by Bahder Djohan, Oesman Saleh, P. Pinontoan, Raden Ito, Djamaloedin, Soewandhi, and Soekendar 165–66. Weltevreden: Kolff, 1923.

Het Eerste Congres van de Vereeniging van Indonesische Geneeskundigen Gehouden op 24, 25, en 26 December 1938 te Semarang. Batavia: Kenanga, 1938.

'Het Eerste Javaansche Congres'. *Jong Indië* 1, no. 15 (10 October 1908): 129–31, 141–42.

'Het Nieuwe Kleed'. *Bulletin van den Bond van Indische Geneeskundigen* 14, no. 2 (1925): 1.

'Het Steunfonds'. *Orgaan der Vereeniging van Indische Geneeskundigen* 21, no. 1–2 (1933): 3–4; no. 5–6 (1933): 33–34.

'Het Vertrek van C. D. de Langen'. *Orgaan der Vereeniging van Indische Geneeskundigen* 15, no. 1 (1926): 64–66.

'Historisch Overzicht van de Voorstellen tot Reorganisatie van den Burgerlijken Geneeskundigen Dienst'. In *Rapport der Commissie tot Voorbereiding eener Reorganisatie van den Burgerlijken Geneeskundigen Dienst*, edited by J. Bijker, 169–98. Batavia: Landsdrukkerij, 1908.

Hoofdbestuur. 'Geachte Collega's!' *Orgaan der Vereeniging van Inlandsche Geneeskundigen* 3, no. 3 (1912): 39–41.

'Het Indisch Ontwerp 1913'. *Bond van Geneesheeren in N.-I.*, no. 52–53 (1912): 1–29.

'De Salaris-Vermindering'. *Orgaan der Vereeniging van Indische Geneeskundigen* 19, no. 3–4 (1931): 47.

'Verslag over 1932'. *Orgaan der Vereeniging van Indische Geneeskundigen* 21, no. 3–4 (1932): 11–16.

'Verslag over de Viering van het 25-Jaar Bestaan Onzer Vereeniging te Batavia-Centrum'. *Orgaan der Vereeniging van Indische Geneeskundigen* 26, no. 1–2 (1938): 1–9.

'Hoofdbestuursmededeelingen'. *Orgaan der Vereeniging van Indische Geneeskundigen* 21, no. 1–2 (1933): 1–2.

Huizinga, J. *Herfsttij der Middeleeuwen*. Haarlem: Tjeenk Willink, 1919.

Hydrick, John Lee. 'Health Education by the Public Health Service of the Netherlands East Indies'. *Mededeelingen van den Burgelijken Geneeskundigen Dienst* 16 (1927): 476–89.

Intensive Rural Hygiene Work and Public Health Education of the Public Health Service of Netherlands India. Batavia: Author, 1937.

'Indonesian Universities in Transition: Catching up and Opening Up'. *Bulletin of Indonesian Economic Studies* 48, no. 2 (2012): 229–51.

'The Indonesian University Situation'. *Minerva* 4, no. 3 (1966): 433–46.

Indonesiche Vereeniging. *Gedenkboek 1908–1923*. The Hague: Indonesiche Vereeniging, 1924.

'Infaam!' *Orgaan der Vereeniging van Inlandsche Geneeskundigen* 3, no. 4–5 (1912): 63–68.

'Ingezonden: De Artsenpositie in Indonesië, II'. *Nederlands Tijdschrift voor Geneeskunde* 91, no. 52 (27 December 1947): 3756.

J. L. 'Fragment uit 't Schoolleven'. In *STOVIA Almanak 1926*, edited by Bahder Djohan, Ahmad Ramali, Abdoel Gafar, Soekendar, Darwis, Loekmono, and Zainoedin, 253–58. Weltevreden: Kolff, 1926.

'Samenleving'. In *STOVIA Almanak 1926*, edited by Bahder Djohan, Ahmad Ramali, Abdoel Gafar, Soekendar, Darwis, Loekmono, and Zainoedin, 273–79. Weltevreden: Kolff, 1926.

Ja-Ben [Tjiang Kok Mas]. 'Van Groen naar Rood'. In *NIAS Lustrum Almanak 1933– 1934*, edited by Dj. Siregar, Soeharso, and C. Schreuder, 243–47. Surabaya: NIAS, 1934.

'Jaarverslag betreffende den Bond van Inlandsche Geneeskundigen over 1913'. *Orgaan der Vereeniging van Inlandsche Geneeskundigen* 4, no. 1–2 (1913): 19.

'Jaarverslag over 1937'. *Orgaan der Vereeniging van Indische Geneeskundigen* 25 (1937): 1–4.

Jenney, E. Ross. 'Public Health in Indonesia'. *Public Health Reports* 68, no. 4 (1953): 409–15.

'Technical Assistance for Public Health in the Republic of Indonesia'. *Public Health Reports* 68, no. 7 (1953): 707–13.

Job. 'Bij de Uitdragers'. In *STOVIA Almanak 1925*, edited by Bahder Djohan, A. Ramali, A. Gafar, R. Mochtar, Soekandar, M. A. Hanafiah, Zainoedin, Loekmono, and Darwis, 164–69. Weltevreden: Kolff, 1925.

Joesoef, Mohamad. 'Notulen van de Algemeene Ledenvergadering, Gehouden in 't Nieuwe Stovia-Gebouw te Salemba op den 25en Juni 1922'. *Orgaan der Vereeniging van Indische Geneeskundigen* 12, no. 1 (1923): 2–4.

'John Lee Hydrick, MD'. *Medisch Tribune* 27, no. 8 (1939): 3–7.

Johnny. 'Bekentenissen'. In *STOVIA Almanak 1925*, edited by Bahder Djohan, A. Ramali, A. Gafar, R. Mochtar, Soekandar, M. A. Hanafiah, Zainoedin, Loekmono, and Darwis, 155–58. Weltevreden: Kolff, 1925.

Jong-Java: Congresnummer 7e Jong-Java Congres. Weltevreden: Indonesische Drukkerij, 1925.

Jubileumnummer 1911–1936: Orgaan Vereeniging van Indische Geneeskundigen. Batavia: Kolff, 1937.

K. [Kayadoe]. 'Ons Tijdschrift'. *Bulletin van den Bond van Indische Geneeskundigen* 14, no. 3 (1925): 21–23.

Kaiser, L. 'In Memoriam Mevr. Dr. J. C. Soewarno-van der Kaaden'. *Nederlands Tijdschrift voor Geneeskunde* 109, no. 5 (1965): 243–44.

Kandou, T. A. 'De Civilisatie van Celebes door Minahassers'. *Orgaan van de Studeerenden Vereeniging Minahassa* 1, no. 3 (1918): 40–43.

'De Evolutie bij de Minahassers'. *Orgaan van de Studeerenden Vereeniging Minahassa* 1, no. 1 (1918): 9–16.

'De Minahassers en 't Nederlands'. *Orgaan van de Studeerenden Vereeniging Minahassa* 1, no. 2 (15 March 1918): 24–29.

'Minahassa's Studeerende Jongelingschap en haar Toekomstige Taak'. *Orgaan van de Studeerenden Vereeniging Minahassa* 1, no. 8 (February 1919): 113–17.

'Rede ter Opening van de Eerste Jaarvergadering der Studeerenden-Vereeniging Minahassa'. *Orgaan van de Studeerenden Vereeniging Minahassa* 1, no. 9 (March 1919): 129–34.

Karels, René. *Mijn Aardse Leven Vol Moeite en Strijd: Raden Mas Noto Soeroto, Javaan, Dichter, Politicus, 1888–1951* (Leiden: KITLV Press, 2010).

Karsten, Thomas. 'Rassenwaan en Rassenbewustzijn'. *De Taak* 1, no. 18 (1 December 1917): 205–06.

Kartono, Sosro, Noto Soeroto, and Soewardi Soerjaningrat, eds. *Soembangsih: Gedenkboek Boedi Oetomo, 1908–1918*. Amsterdam: Tijdschrift Nederlandsch Indië Oud & Nieuw, 1918.

Kayadoe, Jeremias. 'Waarschuwing'. *Orgaan der Vereeniging van Inlandsche Geneeskundigen* 5–6, no. 6–1 (1916): 27–28.

'Uit Roerige Jaren'. In *Jubileumnummer 1911–1936*, 6–13. Batavia: Kolff, 1937.

'Enkele Medische Problemen Hier te Lande'. In *Het Eerste Congres van de Vereeniging van Indonesische Geneeskundigen*, 16–25. Batavia: Kenanga, 1938.

Ketterer, Warren A. 'Economic Benefits of Malaria Control in the Republic of Indonesia'. *Public Health Reports* 68, no. 11 (1953): 1056–58.

'Village Polyclinics in Middle Java'. *Public Health Reports* 68, no. 6 (1953): 558–62.

Kits van Waveren, E. 'De Artsenpositie in Indonesië'. *Nederlands Tijdschrift voor Geneeskunde* 91, no. 48 (29 November 1947): 3430–69.

Kodijat, Raden. 'Specialistische Kliniek'. In *Het Tweede Congres van de Vereeniging van Indonesische Geneeskundigen*, 5–18. Batavia: Kenanga, 1940.

Kohlbrugge, J. H. F. *Blikken in het Zieleleven van den Javaan en zijner Overheerschers*. Leiden: Brill, 1907.

'Hygiënische Toestanden in de Desa'. *Indisch Genootschap* (12 February 1907): 189–205.

'Psychologische Koloniale Politiek'. *Vereeniging Moederland en Koloniën* 8, no. 2 (1907): 1–44.

'Welken Weg Moeten Wij Volgen Om den Javaan te Ontwikkelen?' *Vereeniging Moederland en Koloniën* 8, no. 7 (1908): 3–71.

'Zielkunde als Grondslag van Koloniaal Beleid'. *De Militaire Gids* 27 (1908): 229–51.

'Het Rapport der Commissie, tot Voorbereiding eener Reorganisatie van den Burgelijken Geneeskundigen Dienst in N. I., Critisch Beschouwd'. *Indische Gids* 31 (1909): 312–25.

De Inlandsche Beweging en de Onrust in Indië. Utrecht: Oosthoek, 1927.

Koloniaal Onderwijscongres. *Stenografisch Verslag van het Verhandelde op het Derde Koloniaal Onderwijscongres*. Groningen: Wolters, 1924.

Laoh, Ph. *Iets over de Aetiologie, Prophylaxis en Therapie der Beri-Beri: Bijdragen tot de Kennis der Infectie-Ziekten*. Batavia: Kolff, 1903.

Latif, S. M. 'Dr. A. Rivai'. In *Dr. A. Rivai Sepintas Lalu*, edited by Hilda Rivai and S. M. Latif, 9–40. N.p.: n.p., 1938.

Latumeten, Jonas Andreas. *Over de Kernen van den Nervus Oculomotorius*. Utrecht: Den Boer, 1924.

League of Nations Health Organisation. *Intergovernmental Conference of Far-Eastern Countries on Rural Hygiene: Report of the Preparatory Committee*. Geneva: League of Nations Health Organisation, 1937.

Lectures of the World Health Organization Visiting Team of Medical Scientists to Indonesia. Djakarta: Ikatan Dokter Indonesia, 1953.

Leimena, J. *Membangun Kesehatan Rakjat*. Djakarta: Noordhoff-Kolff, 1952.

The Upbuilding of Public Health in Indonesia. Djakarta: Pertjetakan Negara, 1952.

Some Aspects of Health Protection to Local Areas in Indonesia. Djakarta: Ministry of Health, 1953.

'World Health and World Community'. *Ecumenical Review* 8, no. 4 (1956): 407–09.

Lévy-Bruhl, Lucien. *Primitive Mentality*. London: George Allen & Unwin, 1923.

    How Natives Think. London: George Allen & Unwin, 1926.

    The Soul of the Primitive. London: George Allen & Unwin, 1928.

M. 'Bij de Olifanten van Soerakarta'. In *STOVIA Almanak 1923*, edited by Bahder Djohan, Oesman Saleh, P. Pinontoan, Raden Ito, Djamaloedin, Soewandhi, and Soekendar, 183–84. Batavia: Kolff, 1923.

    'De Medische Wetenschap'. In *STOVIA Almanak 1923*, edited by Bahder Djohan, Oesman Saleh, P. Pinontoan, Raden Ito, Djamaloedin, Soewandhi, and Soekendar, 180. Weltevreden: Kolff, 1923.

Mams. 'De Eerste Ontgroeningsavond'. In *NIAS Lustrum Almanak 1933–1934*, edited by Dj. Siregar, Soeharso, and C. Schreuder, 249–52. Surabaya: NIAS, 1934.

Manap, A. 'In Memoriam R. Soetedjo'. *NIAS Orgaan* 11–12, no. 4-1-2 (1938): 48–49.

Mangoendiningrat, K. R. T. Saleh. 'Ketabiban didalam Bangsa Indonesia ditanah Djawa'. In *Het Tweede Congres van de Vereeniging van Indonesische Geneeskundigen*, 222–47. Batavia: Kenanga, 1940.

Mangoenkoesoemo, Goenawan. 'De Geboorte van Boedi-Oetomo'. In *Soembangsih: Gedenkboek Boedi-Oetomo 1908 – 20 Mei – 1918*, edited by Sosro Kartono, Noto Soeroto, and Suwardi Surjaningrant, 9–14. Amsterdam: Nederlandsch-Indië Oud en Nieuw, 1918.

    'What Heeft Indonesië Noodig?'. *Hindia Poetra* 1, no. 9 (1919): 193–97; no. 10 (1919): 209–12.

Mangoenkoesoemo, Tjipto. 'Eenheid'. *Het Tijdschrift*, 15 February 1912, 400–04.

    'Ervaringen uit het Leven: Kracht Boven Recht'. *De Expres*, 30 September 1912, 1.

    'Geestelijke Immobiliteit Ge-eischt.' *Het Tijdschrift*, 1 September 1912, 15–19.

    Open Brief aan Mijne Landgenoten. Kepandjen: Author, 1912.

    'Het Indisch Nationalisme en zijn Rechtvaardiging'. In *Javaansch of Indisch Nationalisme: Pro en Contra*, edited by R. M. S. Soeriokoesoemo, A. Muhlenfeld, Tjipto Mangoenkoesoemo, and J. B. Wens, 15–35. Semarang: H. A. Benjamins, 1918.

    'Iets over Javaansche Cultuurontwikkeling: Prae-Advies'. In *Congres Voor Javaansche Cultuur-Ontwikkeling*, 1–29. Semarang: Misset, 1918.

Mansoer, Tengkoe. *De Lachgasnarcose in de Heelkunde*. Leiden: Patria, 1928.

Martoatmodjo, Raden Boentaran. *Bijdrage tot de Studie van het 'Ultravirus Tuberculeux'*. Leiden: Boekhandel S. Garnade, 1931.

    'Openingsrede'. *Medisch Tribune* 29, no. 5 (1941): 119–22.

    'Pemadangan Singkat Perihal Kesehatan dan Makanan Rakjat dll'. *Berita Ketabiban* 1, no. 4-5-6 (2604 [1944]): 43–52.

Marzoeki. 'Notulen van de Ledenvergadering, Gehouden in de Conferentiekamer van het Nieuwe Stoviagebouw, Salemba, op 19 Nov. 1922'. *Orgaan der Vereeniging van Indische Geneeskundigen* 12, no. 1 (1923): 7–11.

    'Mededeelingen van de Redactie'. *Orgaan der Vereeniging van Indische Geneeskundigen* 12, no. 1 (1923): 1.

The Medical Faculty, Its Allied Departments and Its Relation to the National University of Indonesia: A Brief Report Prepared by the Ministry of Health, Republic of Indonesia. Yogyakarta: Ministry of Health, RI, 1950.

'Mijlpalen'. *NIAS Orgaan* 11, no. 1-2-3 (1938): 23–25.

Mochtar, Achmad. *Onderzoekingen omtrent Eenige Leptospiren-Stammen.* Amsterdam: Universiteitsboekhandel, 1927.

'Dysenterie di Djawa'. *Berita Ketabiban* 1, no. 1-2-3 (2606 [1944]): 38–43.

Mochtar, Raden. 'De Decentralisatie van den Dienst der Volksgezondheid'. In *Het Eerste Congres van de Vereeniging van Indonesische Geneeskundigen*, 44–55. Batavia: Kenanga, 1938.

'Intensief Hygienewerk en Medisch-Hygienische Propaganda'. *Medisch Tribune* 27, no. 10 (1939): 16–21; no. 12 (1939): 4–12.

Obat-Obat dari Bahan-Bahan Negeri Sendiri. Djakarta: Balai Poestaka, 1945.

'Modern Evangelie: Penneprikjes naar aanleiding van v. Loon's Rede in den Haag op 14 Juni 1924'. *Indonesia Merdeka* 2 (1924): 66–68.

Moersito, Soehardo, S. Rachmat, Sosodoro, K. A. Tan, Mohamad, and Djafar Siregar, eds. *Jaarboek 1932 Uitgegeven door de NIAS Vereeniging te Soerabaja.* Surabaya: Kolff, 1932.

Moewardi. 'Kepandoean dalam Jong-Java'. In *Gedenkboek Jong Java 1915 – 7 Maart – 1930: Kitab Peringatan Jong-Java*, edited by Koentjoro Poerbopranoto, Soegandi Pringgoatmodjo, Soedarso, Joesoepadi Danoehadiningrat, and Moewardi, 141–80. Jakatera: Pedoman Besar Jong-Java, 1930.

'Verslag van het Secretariaat, Uitgebracht aan het Congres te Solo'. *Medisch Tribune* 28, no. 5 (1940): 125–48.

Mr. 'Jong-Java 1915–1922'. In *Jong-Java's Jaarboekje, 1923*, edited by Hoofdbestuur Studeerenden Vereeniging Jong-Java, 115–29. Weltevreden: Kolff, 1923.

Ms [A. Maramis]. 'De Exodus van Minahassers'. *Orgaan van de Studeerenden Vereeniging Minahassa* 1, no. 3 (1918): 33–38.

'De Geestelijke Opleving in de Minahassa'. *Orgaan van de Studeerenden Vereeniging Minahassa* 1, no. 1 (1918): 19–21.

MSh. 'Menjehatkan Bangsa'. *Berita Ketabiban: Madjallah dari Djawa Izi Hookoo Kai* 1, no. 1-2-3 (2604 [1944]): 59–60.

Mullis, Kennas. 'Playing Chicken with Bird Flu: "Viral Sovereignty", the Right to Exploit Natural Genetic Resources, and the Potential Human Rights Ramifications'. *American University International Law Review* 24, no. 5 (2009): 943–67.

'Nogmaals Dr. van Loon!' *Orgaan der Vereeniging van Indische Geneeskundigen* 13, no. 1 (December 1924): 41–46.

Nugroho, Gunawan. 'A Community Development Approach to Raising Health Standards in Central Java, Indonesia'. In *Health by the People*, edited by Kenneth W. Newell, 91–111. Geneva: World Health Organization, 1975.

'Ons Clubhuis'. In *NIAS Jaarboek 1932*, edited by Moersito, Soehardo, S. Rachmat, Sosodoro, K. A. Tan, Mohamad, and Djafar Siregar, 112–24. Surabaya: Kolff, 1932.

'Ons Eerste Congres'. *Medisch Tribune* 27, no. 3 (1939): 5–6.

Orion. 'Het Standaardwerk'. In *STOVIA-Almanak 1923*, edited by Bahder Djohan, Oesman Saleh, P. Pinontoan, Raden Ito, Djamaloedin, Soewandhi, and Soekendar, 172–75. Weltevreden: Kolff, 1923.

Otede. 'Geneeskunde en de Inlandsche Bevolking'. *NIAS Orgaan* 1, no. 2 (1926): 34–36.

Partaningrat, Raden Mas Wirasmo. 'Positie en Instructie van den Regentschapsgeneeskundige'. In *Het Tweede Congres van de Vereeniging van Indonesische Geneeskundigen*, 64–95. Batavia: Kenanga, 1940.

'Pelantikan dan Pendirian Badan Persiapan Djawa Izi Hookoo Kai'. *Berita Ketabiban* 1, no. 1-2-3 (2606 [1944]): 6–9.

'Pemboekaan'. *Berita Ketabiban* 1, no. 1-2-3 (2604 [1944]): 26–28.

'Pemboekaan Pendirian "Izi Hookoo Kai" dengan Resmi pada tanggal 30 VIII 2603'. *Berita Ketabiban* 1, no. 1-2-3 (2604 [1944]): 17–18.

'Persidangan Oemoem Izi Hookoo Kai'. *Berita Ketabiban* 1, no. 1-2-3 (2604 [1944]): 44–53.

Pirngadi. 'Afscheid'. *Jong Java* 11, no. 19–20 (1–15 October 1926): 3–4.

    'Medisch Dispuut Gezelschap'. In *STOVIA Almanak 1924*, edited by Bahder Djohan, A. Ramali, A. Gafar, R. Mochtar, Soekandar, M. A. Hanafiah, Zainoedin, Loekmono, and Darwis, 143–48. Weltevreden: Kolff, 1924.

Poerbapranato, Koentjoro. 'Het Offer van Jong-Java aan het Altaar van het Vaderland'. In *Gedenkboek Jong Java 1915 – 7 Maart – 1930: Kitab Peringatan Jong-Java*, edited by Koentjoro Poerbopranoto, Soegandi Pringgoatmodjo, Soedarso, Joesoepadi Danoehadiningrat, and Moewardi, 41–56. Jakatera: Pedoman Besar Jong-Java, 1930.

Poerwosoewardjo, Raden. 'De Organisatie van den Regentschapsgezondheidsdienst'. In *Het Eerste Congres van de Vereeniging van Indonesische Geneeskundigen*, 74–90. Batavia: Kenanga, 1938.

Poesponegoro, Soedjono Djoened. *Laporan Perkembangan Pendidikan Dokter pada Fakultas Kedokteran Universitas Indonesia Djakarta/Report on the Development of Medical Education at the Faculty of Medicine, University of Indonesia, Djakarta*. Jakarta: Fakultas Kedoktoran Universitas Indonesia, 1960.

Pohan, Aminoeddin. 'Een Reorganisatie van den Jong Sumatranenbond'. *Jong Batak* 1, no. 2 (1926): 30–33.

    'Rede op de Oprichtingsvergadering'. *Jong Batak* 1, no. 1 (1926): 7–10.

'Politics in the World of Science and Learning: Indonesia'. *Minerva* 4, no. 2 (1965): 302.

'Politiek en Psychologie, Vervolg'. *PEB* 5, no. 8 (28 February 1924): 99–100.

Prawiranegara, Isis. *Oebar Kampoeng*. Djakarta: Djawa Goenseibankoe, 2603 [1943].

Prawirohardjo, Sarwono. 'Nasib Studiefonds Kita dikemoedian Hari'. In *Gedenkboek Jong Java 1915 – 7 Maart – 1930: Kitab Peringatan Jong-Java*, edited by Koentjoro Poerbopranoto, Soegandi Pringgoatmodjo, Soedarso, Joesoepadi Danoehadiningrat, and Moewardi, 183–205. Jakatera: Pedoman Besar Jong-Java, 1930.

Primary Health Care (Village Community Health Development) in Indonesia. Jakarta: Ministry of Health, RI, 1978.

'Psychiatrisch Fascisme'. *De Taak* 7, no. 311 (15 January 1924): 1809–11.

R. G. H. 'S. C. S. (Sumatraansch Commensalenhuis STOVIA)'. In *STOVIA Almanak 1923*, edited by Bahder Djohan, Oesman Saleh, P. Pinontoan, Raden Ito, Djamaloedin, Soewandhi, and Soekendar, 147–55. Weltevreden: Kolff, 1923.

Rachman, Abdoel. 'Jong Sumatra, Heil U!' *Wederopbouw* 1, no. 1 (1918): 11–14.

Raden Djenal Asikin Widjaja Koesoemah. *Bijdrage tot de Kennis van de Bloedbilirubineverhoudingen bij Gezonden en Zieken in de Tropen*. Batavia: Kolff, 1932.

Ramali, A. 'Pengobatan Penjakit Diabetes Mellitus dengan Obat Rempah-Rempah'. *Berita Ketabiban: Madjallah dari Djawa Izi Hookoo Kai* 1, no. 1-2-3 (2604 [1944]): 90–98.

Ramali, Ahmad and K. St. Pamoentjak. *Kamus Kedoktoran: Arti dan Keterangan Istilah*. Djakarta: Djambatan, 1953.

'Rampant Disorder: Indonesia'. *Minerva* 5, no. 2 (1966): 300–01.

Rasjid, Abdul. 'Beschouwingen over de Positie van den Ind.-Arts'. In *Het Eerste Congres van de Vereeniging van Indonesische Geneeskundigen*, 26–37. Batavia: Kenanga, 1938.

'Beginselverklaring'. *Medische Tribune* 27, no. 4 (1939): 2–4.

'Oproep'. *Medisch Tribune* 28, no. 5 (1940): 123–25.

'Rede, Uitgesproken op de in Sept j.l. Gehouden Vergadering van de Afdeeling Batavia'. *Medische Tribune* 28, no. 10 (1940): 248–75.

'Kata Pengantar'. *Berita Ketabiban* 1, no. 1-2-3 (2604 [1944]): 2–4.

'Pedato dari Dr. Abdul Rasjid'. *Berita Ketabiban* 1, no. 1-2-3 (2604 [1944]): 9–11.

'Tabib Indonesia dan Pendirian *Izi Hookoo Kai*'. *Berita Ketabiban* 1, no. 1-2-3 (2604 [1944]): 61–62.

Remboelan. 'Treurig'. *NIAS Orgaan* 1, no. 3 (1926): 48.

Ripe for Investment: The Indonesian Health Care Industry Post Introduction of Universal Health Coverage. London: EY, 2015.

Rivai, Abdul. 'Demoralisatie van den Javaan'. *Oost en West* 1, no. 6 (30 May 1901): 2–3.

'Holland, de Inlanders en nog Iets'. *Koloniaal Weekblad* 6, no. 18 (1906): 2–5.

'Over den Invloed van de Flagellaten op de Zelfreiniging van het Bassinwater'. *Geneeskundige Bladen uit Kliniek en Laboratorium voor de Praktijk* 14, no. 9 (1909): 305–441.

'Rede over het "Kostbaar Geschenk".' *Orgaan der Vereeniging van Indische Geneeskundigen* 12, no. 2 (1923): 19–26.

Student Indonesia di Eropa. Jakarta: Gramedia, 2000 [1928].

Rivai, Abdul, J. T. Terburgh, A. E. Sitsen, and A. de Waart. *Het Hooger Onderwijs Vraagstuk, Speciaal in Veband met het Geneeskundig Onderwijs in Nederlandsch-Indië*. Orgaan van Indische Artsen (Special Issue). Batavia: VIG, 1919.

Rivai, Hilda and S. M. Latif. *Dr. A. Rivai Sepintas Laloe*. N.p.: n.p., 1938.

Roem. 'Nogmaals: Collega's Vereenigt U!'. *Orgaan der Vereeniging van Inlandsche Geneeskundigen* 2, no. 3 (1911): 21–25.

Rokx, Claudia, John Giles, Elan Satriawan, Puti Marzoeki, Pandu Harimurti, and Elif Yavuz. *New Insights into the Provision of Health Services in Indonesia: A Health Workforce Study*. Washington, DC: World Bank, 2010.

Roll, H. F. *Jaarlijksch Verslag der School tot Opleiding van Inl. Artsen te Weltevreden over den Cursus 1902/1903*. Batavia: Landsdrukkerij, 1903.

Is Reorganisatie van de School tot Opleiding van Inlandsche Artsen te Weltevreden Nogmaals Nodig? Dordrecht: Morks & Geuze, 1909.

S. 'Toen Hij Nog NIASser Was'. In *NIAS Jaarboek 1932*, edited by Moersito, Soehardo, S. Rachmat, Sosodoro, K. A. Tan, Mohamad, and Djafar Siregar, 207–15. Surabaya: Kolff, 1932.

'De Positie van de Medische Scholen in Indonesië'. In *NIAS Lustrum Almanak 1933–1934*, edited by Dj. Siregar, Soeharso, and C. Schreuder, 20–26. Batavia: Kolff, 1934.

Samallo, Jacob. 'Herinneringen uit het Leven van de Élèves der STOVIA 25 Jaar Geleden'. In *Ontwikkeling van het Geneeskundig Onderwijs te Weltevreden, 1851–1926*, edited by A. de Waart, 289–94. Weltevreden: Kolff, 1926.

Sambijono, Satrijo, Hasan Basri Saanin, and Go Sie Lok. *NIAS-STOVIT Lustrum Almanak 1938*. Soerabaja: Kolff, 1938.

Sardjito, M. 'De Toelating van Indische Geneeskundigen, Abituriënten van de STOVIA en de NIAS tot de Universiteit en Hoogeschool'. *NIAS Orgaan* 11, no. 1-2-3 (1938): 6–18.

　　The Development of the Universitas Gadjah Mada. Yogyakarta: Universitas Gadjah Mada, 1955.

[Sastroamidjojo], Raden Seno. 'Ons Tijdschrift'. *Tijdschrift voor Indische Geneeskundigen* 27, no. 2 (1919): 1–6.

　　'Algemeen Ziekenhuis'. In *Het Tweede Congres van de Vereeniging van Indonesische Geneeskundigen*, 19–34. Batavia: Kenanga, 1940.

　　Obat Asli Indonesia. Djakarta: Kebangsaan Pustaka Rakjat, 1948.

Satiman. 'Onze Vereeniging Tri Koro Dharmo'. In *Maju Setapak*, edited by Pitut Soeharto and A. Zainoel Ihsan. Jakarta: Aksara Jayasakti, 1981 [1916].

　　'Bij de Oprichting van Jong-Java'. In *Gedenkboek Jong Java 1915 – 7 Maart – 1930: Kitab Peringatan Jong-Java*, edited by Koentjoro Poerbopranoto, Soegandi Pringgoatmodjo, Soedarso, Joesoepadi Danoehadiningrat, and Moewardi, 59–64. Jakatera: Pedoman Besar Jong-Java, 1930.

Satō, T. 'Menjehatkan Rochani dan Djasmani Pendoedoek'. *Berita Ketabiban* 1, no. 1-2-3 (2604 [1944]): 56–57.

Scherp, A. J. H. 'De Inrichting der Gouvernements-Internaten Voor Inlandsche Jonglieden in Nederlands-Indië in Verband met de Zedelijke Vorming der Leerlingen'. *Indisch Genootschap* (26 March 1907): 219–41.

Sejarah Kesehatan Nasional Indonesia. 3 vols. Jakarta: Departement Kesehatan RI, 2009.

Senduk, R. C. L. '1918–1928'. *Jong Celebes* 4, no. 3–4 (1928): 2.

Sh. 'Bij 't Portret van Dr. Th. G. van Vogelpoel'. In *STOVIA Almanak 1926*, edited by Bahder Djohan, Ahmad Ramali, Abdoel Gafar, Soekendar, Darwis, Loekmono, and Zainoedin, 151–56. Weltevreden: Kolff, 1926.

Siregar, Dj., Soeharso, and C. Schreuder, eds. *NIAS Almanak, Lustrumnummer 1933–1934*. Batavia: Kolff, 1934.

Siregar, Gindo. 'Het Bestaansrecht van een Jong Bataks Bond'. *Jong Batak* 1, no. 1 (1926): 3–6.

Sitanala, J. B. 'Beschouwt de Oosterling "Arbeid" als een "Vloek" des Heeren?' In *Het Eerste Congress van de Vereeniging van Indonesische Geneeskundigen*, 143–84. Batavia: Kenanga, 1938.

Sjaaf, Mohamad. *Vezelverloop in Netvlies en Oogzenuw*. Amsterdam: Buijten & Schipperheijn, 1923.

Smyth, Francis Scott. 'University of California Medical Science Teaching in Indonesia'. *Journal of Medical Education* 32, no. 5 (1957): 344–49.

　　'Health and Medicine in Indonesia'. *Journal of Medical Education* 38, no. 8 (1963): 693–96.

Sn. [Seno Sastroamidjojo]. 'De Indonesische Geneeskundige en zijn Gemeenschap'. *Medisch Tribune* 29, no. 7 (1941): 187–97.

Snouck Hurgronje, Christiaan. 'Blikken in het Zieleleven van den Javaan?' *De Gids* 71, no. 3 (1908): 423–47.

　　Ambtelijke Adviezen van C. Snouck Hurgronje 1889–1936, edited by Emile Gobée and Cornelis Adriaanse, Vol. 2. The Hague: Nijhoff, 1959.

Soangkoepon and Abdul Rasjid. *Redevoeringen van de Leden van den Volksraad de Heeren Abdul Firman Gelar Maharadja Soangkoepon en Abdul Rasjid Gelar Maharadja Mahkota Soangkoepon over het Zittingsjaar 1936–1937.* Buitenzorg: Buitenzorgsche Drukkerij, 1937.

Soewarno, Mas. 'Iets over Kampogen'. *Nederlands Tijdschrift voor Geneeskunde* 90 (1946): 213–16.

Soebandrio. *Pangaruh Revolusi Indonesia Didunia.* Jakarta: Departemen Luar Negeri RI, 1962.

Soedjatmoko. *An Introduction to Indonesian Historiography.* Ithaca, NY: Cornell University Press, 1965.

Southeast Asia Today and Tomorrow. Honolulu, HI: East-West Center Press, 1969.

Development and Freedom. New Delhi: Centre for Policy Research, 1980.

The Primacy of Freedom in Development. Lanham, MD: University Press of America, 1985.

Menjadi Bangsa Terdidik Menurut Soedjatmoko. Jakarta: Kompas, 2010.

Soedjatmoko, Selo Soemardjan and Kenneth W. Thompson. *Culture, Development, and Democracy: The Role of the Intellectual.* Tokyo: United Nations University Press, 1994.

Soeharto, Raden. 'Kewadjiban Tabib Dizaman Pembangoenan'. *Berita Ketabiban* 1, no. 1-2-3 (2604 [1944]): 64–66.

Soekardie, Raden. 'Uit het Leven van een Indisch Geneeskundige Nu 25 Jaar Geleden: Door Ziekte Gered'. In *Ontwikkeling van het Geneeskundig Onderwijs te Weltevreden, 1851–1926,* edited by A. de Waart, 296–97. Weltevreden: Kolff, 1926.

Soekarno. 'Pidato'. *Berita Ketabiban* 1, no. 1-2-3 (2604 [1944]): 28.

Lahirnja Pantjasila: Filsafah Indonesia Tertjakup dalam Pantjasila. Bandung: Duar-r, 1961.

Sukarno: An Autobiography as Told to Cindy Adams. Indianapolis, IN: Bobbs-Merrill, 1965.

Soekiman. 'De Beteekenis van het Javaansche Cultuur Congres'. *Jong Java* 3, no. 11 (1918): 159–64.

'Rede Uitgesproken ten Tweeden Jong-Java Congresse'. *Jong-Java* 3, no 12 (1918): 223–27.

Soem, Noeroe'l. 'Moeder!: Lief en Leed van een NIASser'. In *NIAS-STOVIT Lustrum Almanak 1938,* edited by Sambijono, Satrijo, Hasan Basri Saanin, and Go Sie Lok, 105–09. Soerabaja: Kolff, 1938.

Soemedi. 'De Noodzakelijkheid van een Goede Opleiding'. In *Het Tweede Congres van de Vereeniging van Indonesische Geneeskundigen,* 125–43. Batavia: Kenanga, 1940.

'Soerat Soempah'. *Berita Ketabiban* 1, no. 1-2-3 (2604 [1944]): 25.

[Soerjaningrat, Raden Mas Soewardi]. *Als Ik Eens Nederlander Was.* Bandoeng: Inlandsch Comité tot Herdenking van Neêrlands Honderdjarige Vrijheid, 1913.

'Welke Plaats Behooren bij het Onderwijs in te Nemen, Eensdeels de Inheemsche Talen (ook het Chineesch en Arabisch), Anderdeels het Nederlandsch?: Prae-Advies'. In *Prae-Adviezen van het Eerste Koloniaal Onderwijscongres,* 33–72. The Hague: Korthals, 1916.

Levensschets van Wahidin Soedirohoesodo. The Hague: Hadi Poestaka, 1922.

Soetomo, Raden. 'Een Gemotiveerde Grief'. *Orgaan der Vereeniging van Inlandsche Geneeskundigen* 3, no. 3 (1912): 43.

'Mijn Standpunt'. *Orgaan der Vereeniging van Indische Geneeskundigen* 8, no. 1–2 (1918): 2–3, 6–8.

'Ter Overweging'. *Orgaan der Vereeniging van Indische Geneeskundigen* 12, no. 1 (1923): 11–12.

Towards a Glorious Indonesia: Reminiscences and Observations of Dr. Soetomo. Translated by Suharni Soemarmo and Paul W. van der Veur. Athens: Ohio University Center for International Studies, 1987.

Soetopo. 'Bij de Viering van het Derde Lustrum van de NIAS te Soerabaia'. *NIAS Orgaan* 3, no. 1 (1928): 53.

Soewandi. 'Jong-Java en Sport'. In *Gedenkboek Jong Java 1915 – 7 Maart – 1930: Kitab Peringatan Jong-Java*, edited by Koentjoro Poerbopranoto, Soegandi Pringgoatmodjo, Soedarso, Joesoepadi Danoehadiningrat, and Moewardi, 118–21. Jakatera: Pedoman Besar Jong-Java, 1930.

Soewarno, Mas. *Over Eenige Vormen van Irisdepigmentatie.* Amsterdam: De Bussy, 1919.

'Dr. R. Soetomo + (1888–1938)'. *NIAS Orgaan* 11/12, no. 4-1-2 (1938): 41–44.

Soewarno-van der Kaaden, Johanna Cornelia. *Nonna Dokter.* Bussum: Van Dishoek, 1936.

De Weg naar Pelantoegan. Leiden: Stafleu, 1936.

De Bonte Slendang. Bussum: Van Dishoek, 1942.

'Sport- en Kunstvereeniging'. In *STOVIA Almanak 1925*, edited by Bahder Djohan, A. Ramali, A. Gafar, R. Mochtar, Soekandar, M. A. Hanafiah, Zainoedin, Loekmono, and Darwis, 109–11. Weltevreden: Kolff, 1925.

'"STOVIA"-Herinneringen uit den "Goeden" Ouden Tijd'. In *STOVIA Almanak 1926*, edited by Bahder Djohan, Ahmad Ramali, Abdoel Gafar, Soekendar, Darwis, Loekmono, and Zainoedin, 235–39. Weltevreden: Kolff, 1926.

'Students' Role in Indonesian Political Changes'. *Minerva* 4, no. 4 (1966): 584–85.

Sursum Corda. 'De Vreemdeling'. In *STOVIA Almanak 1924*, edited by Bahder Djohan, A. Ramali, A. Gafar, R. Mochtar, Soekandar, M. A. Hanafiah, Zainoedin, Loekmono, and Darwis, 201–04. Weltevreden: Kolff, 1924.

Swaving, C. 'Voorstel tot Verbetering van den Burgerlijken Geneeskundigen Dienst in Nederlandsch-Indië'. *Nederlands Tijdschrift voor Geneeskunde* 17 (1873): 549–53.

Tabib. 'Vacantie-Indrukken: De Stads-Hygiëne van Semarang'. *NIAS Orgaan* 4, no. 2 (1929): 11–14.

Tangkau, W. J. T. 'Woord van Opwekking'. *Orgaan der Vereeniging van Inlandsche Geneeskundigen* 5, no. 1-2-3-4 (1915): 22–25.

Tehupeiory, J. E. 'Enkele Mededeelingen uit Mijne Verloskundige Praktijk'. *Tijdschrift van Inlandsche Geneeskundigen* 11, no. 7, 8, 9, 10 (1903): 97–113.

Onder de Dajaks in Centraal-Borneo: Een Reisverhaal. Batavia: Kolff, 1906.

De Inlander Voor en Na de Stichting van het Algemeen Nederlandsch Verbond. Amsterdam: Boon, 1908.

'Raden Adjeng Badaroesmi: Een Nimf uit de Preanger'. In *De Njai Moeder van Alle Volken*, edited by Maya Sutedja-Liem, 73–174. Leiden: KITLV Press, 2007.

Tehupeiory, W. K. 'Iets over de Inlandsche Geneeskundigen'. *Indisch Genootschap* (28 January 1908): 101–34.

'The Native Physicians [1908]'. In *Regents, Reformers, and Revolutionaries: Indonesian Voices of Colonial Days*, edited by Greta O. Wilson, 48–59. Honolulu: University of Hawaii Press, 1978.

'Reorganisatie van het Onderwijs aan de School tot Opleiding van Inlandsche Artsen te Weltevreden'. *Indische Gids* 31 (1909): 922–28.

'Onze Vereening: De Voorgeschiedenis van Hare Oprichting en Hare Kleuterjaren'. In *Jubileumnummer 1911–1936*, 1–5. Batavia: Kolff, 1937.

'Openingsrede'. In *Het Eerste Congres van de Vereeniging van Indonesische Geneeskundigen*, 12–15. Batavia: Kenanga, 1938.

Tesch, Johan W. *The Hygiene Study Ward Centre at Batavia: Planning and Preliminary Results, 1937–1941*. Leiden: Universitaire Pers, 1947.

Tjoh. 'Mensenkennis bij "de Baas".' *NIAS Orgaan* 1, no. 2 (1926): 27–29.

'NIAS Zoologie'. *NIAS Orgaan* 1, no. 2 (1926): 30–31.

'NIAS Zoologie, II'. *NIAS Orgaan* 1, no. 3 (1926): 58–59.

Tobing, F. L. 'Medisch Dispuut Gezelschap'. In *STOVIA Almanak 1925*, edited by Sambijono, Satrijo, Hasan Basri Saanin, and Go Sie Lok, 134–37, Weltevreden: Kolff, 1925.

'Toespraak van de Vertegenwoordiger der NIASsers tot den Directeur van de Jubileerende Scholen'. In *NIAS-STOVIT Lustrum Almanak 1938.* edited by Sambijono, Satrijo, Hasan Basri Saanin, and Go Sie Lok, 9–20, Soerabaja: Kolff, 1938.

'Tonari-Gumi dan Kesehatan'. *Berita Ketabiban* 1, no. 4-5-6 (2604 [1944]): 13–18.

Tönnies, Ferdinand. *Gemeinschaft und Gesellschaft: Grundbegriffe der Reinen Soziologie*. 2nd edn. Berlin: Karl Curtius, 1912.

Topee, G. L. 'Rede'. *Het Tijdschrift*, 15 October 1912, 114–21.

Travaglino, P. H. M. 'De Psychose van den Inlander in Verband met zijn Karakter'. *Geneeskundig Tijdschrift voor Nederlandsch-Indië* 60 (1920): 99–111.

'Het Karakter van den Inlander'. *PEB* 5, no. 27, 28 (1920): 343–47, 357–60.

'Politiek en Psychologie'. *PEB* 5, no. 8 (21 February 1924): 86–93.

'De Sociale Beteekenis der Schizophrenie Voor de Inlandsche Samenleving'. *Mededeelingen van den Dienst der Volksgezondheid in Nederlandsch-Indië* 14, no. 2 (1925): 125–31.

'De Schizophrenie en de Javaanse Psyche'. *Psychiatrische en Neurologische Bladen* 31 (1927): 416–25.

'Trilbeelden'. In *STOVIA Almanak 1926*, edited by Bahder Djohan, Ahmad Ramali, Abdoel Gafar, Soekendar, Darwis, Loekmono, and Zainoedin, 240–45. Weltevreden: Kolff, 1926.

'Twee Lezenswaardige Geschriften'. *Hindia Poetra* 1 (1923): 47–48.

'Uit de Verslagen van de Vergaderingen van de Afdeeling West-Java'. *Orgaan der Vereeniging van Inlandsche Geneeskundigen* 2, no. 1 (1910): 7–10.

'Uit den Volksraad'. *Medisch Tribune* 27, no. 8 (1939): 8–24.

'Uit den Volksraad'. *Medisch Tribune* 29, no. 3 (1941): 73–84.

'Uit den Volksraad'. *Medisch Tribune* 29, no. 10 (1941): 245–59.

Universiteit van Indonesië: Gids Voor het Academiejaar 1949–1950. Batavia: Landsdrukkerij, 1949.

Van Bloklan. *Ratjikan Obat Djawa I*. Soerakarta: Albert Rusche & Company, 1898.

Ratjikan Djampi Djawi, Karanganipoen Njonjah van Bloklan Ing Djakarta; Kawedalaken Denging Wirjapanitra, Solo. Solo: Sadoe-Boedi, 2602 [1942].

Serat Primbon Oesada, Van Bloklan; Kadjawekaken Mawi Askara Latyn Dening Wirjapanitra. Solo: Sadoe-Boedi, 2602 [1942].

Van Blokland, Njonja W. *Doekoen Djawa: Oetawa Kitab dari Roepa-Roepa Obat njang terpake di Tanah Djawa.* Batavia: Van Dorp, 1885.

Van den Berg, L. W. C. *De Inlandsche Rangen en Titels op Java en Madoera.* 2nd edn. The Hague: Martinus Nijhoff, 1902.

Van der Burg, Cornelis Leonard. *Persoonlijke Gezondheidsleer Voor Europeanen, die naar Nederlandsch-Indië Gaan of Daar Wonen.* Amsterdam: De Bussy, 1895.

'Schets eener Geschiedenis der School Voor Inlandsche Geneeskundigen (Dokter Djawa) te Batavia'. *Indische Gids* 18 (1896): 1962–76.

Van Deventer, Conrad Theodor. 'Een Ereschuld'. *De Gids* 63 (1899): 205–57.

'Insulinde's Toekomst'. *De Gids* 72, no. 3 (July 1908): 69–99.

Van Eyken, A. J. H. *Voordracht over de Jong Javaansche Beweging.* The Hague: Korthuis, 1909.

Van Gennep, Arnold. 'Verplichte Rechtsbijstand in Civiele Zaken bij de Landraden en Residentiegerechten op Java en Madoera in Verband met Deunificatie van Recht'. *Indisch Genootschap* (27 December 1910): 59–112.

Van Hinloopen Labberton, D. *Theosofie in Verband met Boedi-Oetomo/Theosophie oentoek Boedi-Oetomo.* Batavia: Boekhandel & Drukkerij Kho Tjeng Bie, 1909.

Geïllustreerd Handboek van Insulinde. Amsterdam: Vivat, 1910.

Van Loon, F. H. 'Acute Verwardheidstoestanden in Nederlands-Indië'. *Geneeskundig Tijdschrift voor Nederlandsch-Indië* 62 (1922): 658–90.

'De Psychische Eigenschappen der Maleische Rassen'. *Indisch Genootschap* (22 February 1924): 21–50.

'Het Onderwijs in de Zenuw- en Zielziekten'. In *Ontwikkeling van het Geneeskundig Onderwijs te Weltevreden, 1851–1926,* edited by A. de Waart, 209–14. Weltevreden: Kolff, 1926.

'Amok and Lattah'. *Journal of Abnormal & Social Psychology* 21, no. 4 (1927): 434–44.

'Protopathic-Instinctive Phenomena in Normal and Pathological Malay Life'. *British Journal of Medical Psychology* 8, no. 4 (1928): 264–76.

'Rassenpsychologische Onderzoekingen'. *Psychiatrische en Neurologische Bladen* 32 (1928): 190–26.

'Psychologische Beschouwing omtrent den Huidigen Toestand op Java'. *Nederlands Tijdschrift voor Geneeskunde* 90, no. 18 (4 May 1946): 425–30.

Van Wulfften Palthe, P. M. 'Het Ontstaan der No--duniversiteit van Nederlandsch-Indië'. *Nederlands Tijdschrift voor Geneeskunde* 90, no. 26 (29 June 1946): 748–50.

'Ingezonden: De Artsenpositie in Indonesië'. *Nederlands Tijdschrift voor Geneeskunde* 92, no. 2 (10 January 1947): 122.

'Ingezonden: Psychological Aspects of the Indonesian Problem'. *Nederlands Tijdschrift voor Geneeskunde* 93, no. 49 (3 December 1949): 4118–19.

Psychological Aspects of the Indonesian Problem. Leiden: Brill, 1949.

Van Wulfften Palthe, P. M. and P. A. Kerstens. *Opening Nood-Universiteit: Redevoeringen.* Batavia: J.B. Wolters, 1946.

'Verdere Opmerkingen naar aanleiding van de Rede van Dr. F. H. van Loon'. *Indonesia Merdeka* 2 (1924): 79–91.

'Vergadering van de Vereeniging van Ind. Geneeskundigen Gehouden den 27en Januari 1918'. *Orgaan der Vereeniging van Indische Geneeskundigen* 8, no. 1–2 (1918): 14–15.

'Verslag over 1934'. *Orgaan der Vereeniging van Indische Geneeskundigen* 24, no. 1–2 (1936): 2–4.

'Verslag over 1935'. *Orgaan der Vereeniging van Indische Geneeskundigen* 24, no. 1–2 (1936): 13–14.

'Verslag van de Oprichtingsvergardering'. *Jong Batak* 1, no. 1 (1926): 20–22.

'Verslag van de Voorvergardering van de JBB'. *Jong Batak* 1, no. 1 (1926): 22–23.

Vollenhoven, Cornelis van. *De Indonesiër en zijn Grond*. Leiden: Brill, 1919.

   De Ontdekking van het Adatrecht. Leiden: Brill, 1928.

von Römer, L. S. A. M. *Historical Sketches: An Introduction to the Fourth Congress of the Far Eastern Association of Tropical Medicine, to Be Held at Batavia from 6th to 13th August 1921*. Batavia: Javasche Boekhandel en Drukkerij, 1921.

'Voorwoord'. In *STOVIA Almanak 1925*. Edited by Bahder Djohan, A. Ramali, A. Gafar, R. Mochtar, Soekandar, MA. Hanafiah, Zainoedin, Loekmono, and Darwis, Weltevreden: Kolff, 1925.

Waart, A. de, ed. *Ontwikkeling van het Geneeskundig Onderwijs te Weltevreden, 1851–1926*. Weltevreden: Kolff, 1926.

Warouw, S. J. 'Nationalisme'. *Orgaan van de Studeerenden-Vereeniging Minahassa* 2, no. 2 (May 1922): 1–2.

   Resultaten van Trachoom-Onderzoek bij Enkele Bevolkingsgroepen in Nederlandsch Indië. Leiden: Dubbeldeman, 1935.

   Indonesië in Rijksverband. N.p.: n.p., 1946.

   Minahassa Strijdt voor Zelfbeschikkingsrecht en Vrijheid. The Hague: KKM, 1949.

Wellington, John S. 'Indonesian Physicians Studying Abroad'. *Journal of Medical Education* 43 (1968): 1183–91.

   'Medical Science and Technology'. In *Indonesia: Resources and Their Technological Development*, edited by Howard M. Beers, 165–73. Lexington: University Press of Kentucky, 1970.

Westplat, J. 'Urgente Rangverbetering Voor de Inlandsche Geneeskundigen'. *Orgaan der Vereeniging van Inlandsche Geneeskundigen* 3, no. 2 (1912): 5–7.

   'Een Compensatie in het Moeilijke Bestaan in den Ouden Dag'. *Orgaan der Vereeniging van Inlandsche Geneeskundigen* 4, no. 6 (1913): 77–79.

World Bank. 'The World Bank on the Social Impact of the Indonesian Crisis'. *Population and Development Review* 24, no. 3 (1998): 664–66.

World Health Organization. *Pandemic Influenza Preparedness Framework for the Sharing of Influenza Viruses and Access to Vaccines and Other Benefits*. Geneva: World Health Organization, 2011.

World Health Organization, Country Office for Indonesia. *WHO Country Cooperation Strategy 2007–2012: Indonesia*. New Delhi: WHO Regional Office for South-East Asia, 2008.

Wuller, F. H. 'Verslag van de Lotgevallen der Vereeniging van Inlandsche Geneeskundigen over het Jaar 1911'. *Orgaan der Vereeniging van Inlandsche Geneeskundigen* 3, no. 3 (1912): 35–38.

Z. 'Zoeken'. In *STOVIA Almanak 1924*, edited by Bahder Djohan, A. Ramali, A. Gafar, R. Mochtar, Soekandar, M. A. Hanafiah, Zainoedin, Loekmono, and Darwis, 199–200. Weltevreden: Kolff, 1924.

Zahar, S. B. 'Over den Positie van den Regentschapsarts'. In *Het Eerste Congres van de Vereeniging van Indonesische Geneeskundigen*, 56–68. Batavia: Kenanga, 1938.

'Pemeriksaan tentang Sakit Malaria dalam Bogor-Si dan Desa-Desa Sekitarnya'. *Berita Ketabiban* 1, no. 4-5-6 (2604 [1944]): 19–27.

'Zijn Eerste Nacht'. In *NIAS Jaarboek 1932*, edited by Moersito, Soehardo, S. Rachmat, Sosodoro, K. A. Tan, Mohamad, and Djafar Siregar, 197–201. Surabaya: Kolff, 1932.

SECONDARY SOURCES

Abdullah, Taufik. 'Modernization in the Minangkabau World: West Sumatra in the Early Decades of the Twentieth Century'. In *Culture and Politics in Indonesia*, edited by Claire Holt, Benedict R. O'G. Anderson, and James Siegel, 179–245. Ithaca, NY: Cornell University Press, 1972.

Indonesia: Towards Democracy. Singapore: Institute of Southeast Asian Studies, 2009.

Abeyasekere, Susan. 'Partai Indonesia Raja, 1936–42: A Study in Cooperative Nationalism'. *Journal of Southeast Asian Studies* 3, no. 2 (1972): 262–76.

One Hand Clapping: Indonesian Nationalists and the Dutch, 1939–1942. Melbourne: Centre of Southeast Asian Studies, Monash University, 1976.

'Health as a Nationalist Issue in Colonial Indonesia'. In *Nineteenth and Twentieth Century Indonesia: Essays in Honour of Professor J. D. Legge*, edited by David P. Chandler and M. C. Ricklefs, 1–14. Melbourne: Monash University Press, 1986.

Achmad, Januar. *Hollow Development: The Politics of Health in Soeharto's Indonesia*. Canberra: Australian National University, 1999.

Adam, Ahmat B. *The Vernacular Press and the Emergence of Modern Indonesian Consciousness*. Ithaca, NY: Southeast Asia Program, Cornell University, 1995.

Adam, Asvi Warman. *Sarwono Prawirohardjo: Pembangun Institusi Ilmu Pengetahuan di Indonesia*. Jakarta: Lembaga Ilmu Pengetahuan Indonesia, 2009.

Adams, Vincanne. *Doctors for Democracy: Health Professionals in the Nepal Revolution*. Cambridge: Cambridge University Press, 1998.

'Against Global Health: Arbitrating Science, Non-Science, and Nonsense through Health'. In *Against Health: How Health Became the New Morality*, edited by J. M. Metzl and A. Kirkland, 40–60. New York: New York University Press, 2010.

Agung, Ide Anak Agung Gde. *From the Formation of the State of East Indonesia towards the Establishment of the United States of Indonesia* Jakarta: Yayasan Obor Indonesia, 1996.

Alwi, Des. *Bersama Hatta, Syahrir, Dr. Tjipto & Iwa K. Soemantri di Banda Naira*. Jakarta: Dian Rakyat, 2002.

Friends and Exiles: A Memoir of the Nutmeg Isles and the Indonesian Nationalist Movement. Ithaca, NY: Southeast Asia Program, Cornell University, 2008.

Amrith, Sunil S. *Decolonizing International Health: India and Southeast Asia, 1930–1965*. Basingstoke: Palgrave Macmillan, 2006.

Andaya, Leonard Y. 'The Trans-Sumatra Trade and the Ethnicization of the "Batak".' *Bijdragen tot de Taal-, Land- en Volkenkunde* 158, no. 3 (2002): 367–409.

Anderson, Benedict R. O'G. *Some Aspects of Indonesian Politics under the Japanese Occupation, 1944–1945*. Ithaca, NY: Cornell University, Department of Far Eastern Studies, 1961.

'The Problem of Rice: Stenographic Notes on the Fourth Session of the Sanyo Kaigi, January 8, 2605, 10.00 A.M.'. *Indonesia*, no. 2 (1966): 77–123.

Java in a Time of Revolution: Occupation and Resistance, 1944–1946. Jakarta: Equinox, 2006 [1972].

Imagined Communities: Reflections on the Origin and Spread of Nationalism. Rev. and extended edn. London: Verso, 2006.

'Old State, New Society: Indonesia's New Order in Comparative Historical Perspective'. In *Language and Power: Exploring Political Cultures in Indonesia*, 94–120. Jakarta: Equinox, 2006.

Anderson, Warwick. *The Cultivation of Whiteness: Science, Health and Racial Destiny in Australia*. Melbourne: University of Melbourne Press, 2002.

Colonial Pathologies: American Tropical Medicine, Race, and Hygiene in the Philippines. Durham, NC: Duke University Press, 2006.

'Making Global Health History: The Postcolonial Worldliness of Biomedicine'. *Social History of Medicine* 27, no. 2 (2014): 372–84.

Anderson, Warwick and Hans Pols. 'Scientific Patriotism: Medical Science and National Self-Fashioning in Southeast Asia'. *Comparative Studies in Society and History* 54, no. 1 (2012): 93–113.

Anwar, Rosihan. *Against the Currents: A Biography of Soedarpo Sastrosatomo*. Jakarta: Pustaka Sinar Harapan, 2003.

'Dimensi Pendidikan Kedoktoran: Kepemimpinan, Humanisme, Kejuangan'. In *Sejarah Kecil: Petite Histoire Indonesia*, edited by Rosihan Anwar, Vol. 3, 3–14. Jakarta: Kompas, 2009.

Appiah, Kwame Anthony. *Cosmopolitanism: Ethics in a World of Strangers*. New York: Penguin, 2007.

Aritonang, Jan Sihar and Karel Adriaan Steenbrink, eds. *A History of Christianity in Indonesia*. Leiden: Brill, 2008.

Aspinall, Edward. 'Indonesia: Moral Force Politics and the Struggle against Authoritarianism'. In *Student Activism in Asia: Between Protest and Powerlessness*, edited by Meredith L. Weiss, Edward Aspinall, and Patricio M. Abinales, 153–79. Minneapolis: University of Minnesota Press, 2012.

Aspinall, Edward and Greg Fealy. *Local Power and Politics in Indonesia: Decentralisation & Democratisation*. Singapore: Institute of Southeast Asian Studies, 2003.

Aspinall, Edward and Eve Warburton. 'A Healthcare Revolution in the Regions'. *Inside Indonesia*, no. 111 (2013). www.insideindonesia.org/a-healthcare-revolution-in-the-regions-2.

Badgley, Robin F. and Samuel M. Wolfe. *Doctors Strike: Medical Care and Conflict in Saskatchewan*. New York: Atherton, 1967.

Baird, J. Kevin and Sangkot Marzuki. *War Crimes in Japan-Occupied Indonesia: A Case of Murder by Medicine*. Washington, DC: Potomac Books, 2015.

Balfas, M. *Dr. Tjipto Mangoenkoesoemo: Demokrat Sedjati*. Djakarta: Djambatan, 1952.

Bashford, Alison. *Imperial Hygiene: A Critical History of Colonialism, Nationalism, and Public Health*. Basingstoke: Palgrave MacMillan, 2004.

   'Global Biopolitics and the History of World Health'. *History of the Human Sciences* 19, no. 1 (2006): 67–88.

Becker, Howard S., Blanche Geer, Everett C. Hughes, and Anselm M. Strauss. *Boys in White: Student Culture in Medical School*. Chicago: University of Chicago Press, 1961.

Berman, Marshall. *All That Is Solid Melts into Air: The Experience of Modernity*. New York: Simon & Schuster, 1982.

Bhattacharya, Sanjoy. *Expunging Variola: The Control and Eradication of Smallpox in India, 1947–1977*. Hyderabad: Orient BlackSwan, 2006.

Bhattacharya, Sanjoy, Mark Harrison, and Michael Worboys. *Fractured States: Smallpox, Public Health and Vaccination Policy in British India, 1900–1947*. Hyderabad: Orient BlackSwan, 2005.

Bhattacharya, Sanjoy and Sharon Messenger, eds. *The Global Eradication of Smallpox*. Hyderabad: Orient BlackSwan, 2010.

Biehl, João and Adriana Petryna. *When People Come First: Critical Studies in Global Health*. Princeton, NJ: Princeton University Press, 2013.

Bijl, Paul. *Emerging Memory: Photographs of Colonial Atrocity in Dutch Cultural Remembrance*. Amsterdam: Amsterdam University Press, 2015.

Birn, Anne-Emmauelle. 'Gates's Grandest Challenge: Transcending Technology as Public Health Ideology'. *Lancet* 366, no. 9484 (6 August 2005): 514–19.

   Marriage of Convenience: Rockefeller International Health and Revolutionary Mexico. Rochester, NY: University of Rochester Press, 2006.

   'The Stages of International (Global) Health: Histories of Success or Successes of History?' *Global Public Health* 4, no. 1 (2009): 50–68.

Birn, Anne-Emanuelle and Theodore M. Brown. *Comrades in Health: U.S. Health Internationalists, Abroad and at Home*. New Brunswick, NJ: Rutgers University Press, 2013.

Birn, Anne-Emanuelle and Armando Solorzano. 'The Hook of Hookworm: Public Health and the Politics of Eradication in Mexico'. In *Western Medicine as Contested Knowledge*, edited by Andrew Cunningham and Bridie Andrews, 147–71. Manchester: Manchester University Press, 1997.

Boer, P. C. *The Loss of Java: The Final Battles for the Possession of Java Fought by Allied Air, Naval and Land Forces in the Period of 18 February–7 March 1942*. Singapore: National University of Singapore Press, 2011.

Boomgaard, Peter. 'Dutch Medicine in Asia, 1600–1900'. In *Warm Climates and Western Medicine: The Emergence of Tropical Medicine, 1500–1900*, edited by David Arnold, 42–64. Amsterdam: Rodopi, 1996.

   'The Development of Colonial Healthcare in Java: An Exploratory Introduction'. *Bijdragen tot de Taal-, Land- en Volkenkunde* 149, no. 1 (1997): 77–93.

   'Smallpox, Vaccination, and the *Pax Neerlandica*: Indonesia, 1550–1930'. *Bijdragen tot de Taal-, Land- en Volkenkunde* 159, no. 4 (2003): 590–617.

Borgers, A. H. *Doctor Willem Bosch (1798–1874) en zijn Invloed op de Geneeskunde in Nederlandsch Oost-Indië*. Utrecht: Kemink en Zoon, 1941.

Borowy, Iris and Anne Hardy. *Of Medicine and Men: Biographies and Ideas in European Social Medicine between the World Wars*. Frankfurt am Main: Peter Lang, 2008.

Bosma, Ulbe. *Karel Zaalberg: Journalist en Strijder Voor de Indo*. Leiden: KITLV Press, 1997.

'Citizens of Empire: Some Comparative Observations on the Evolution of Creole Nationalism in Colonial Indonesia'. *Comparative Studies in Society and History* 46, no. 4 (2004): 646–81.

Bouman, B. *Ieder Voor zich en de Republiek voor ons Allen: De Logistiek achter de Indonesische Revolutie, 1945–1950*. Amsterdam: Boom, 2006.

Bourchier, David. *Illiberal Democracy in Indonesia: The Ideology of the Family State*. New York: Routledge, 2014.

Brandt, Allan M. 'How AIDS Invented Global Health'. *New England Journal of Medicine* 368, no. 23 (6 June 2013): 2149–52.

Braude, Ann Deborah. *Radical Spirits: Spiritualism and Women's Rights in Nineteenth-Century America*. Boston, MA: Beacon Press, 1989.

Broto, Wasisto, Thomas Suroso, Rushdy Hoesein, and Abdul Syukur. *Sejarah Pembangunan Kesehatan Indonesia 1973–2009*. Jakarta: Kementrian Kesehatan Republik Indonesia, 2009.

Brown, Colin. *A Short History of Indonesia: The Unlikely Nation?* Sydney: Allen & Unwin, 2003.

Brown, E. Richard. 'Public Health in Imperialism: Early Rockefeller Programs at Home and Abroad'. *American Journal of Public Health* 66, no. 9 (1976): 897–903.

Rockefeller Medicine Men: Medicine and Capitalism in America. Berkeley: University of California Press, 1979.

Brown, Theodore M., Marcos Cueto, and Elizabeth Fee. 'The World Health Organization and the Transition from "International" to "Global" Public Health'. *American Journal of Public Health* 96, no. 1 (2004): 62–72.

Brown, Theodore M. and Elizabeth Fee. 'Rudolf Carl Virchow: Medical Scientist, Social Reformer, Role Model'. *American Journal of Public Health* 96, no. 12 (2006): 2102–05.

'The Bandoeng Conference of 1937: A Milestone in Health and Development'. *American Journal of Public Health* 98, no. 1 (2008): 40–43.

Brugmans, I. J. *Geschiedenis van het Onderwijs in Nederlandsch-Indië*. Groningen, Batavia: J. B. Wolters, 1938.

Burns, Peter. *The Leiden Legacy: Concepts of Law in Indonesia*. Leiden: KITLV Press, 2004.

'Custom, That Is before All Law'. In *The Revival of Tradition in Indonesian Politics: The Deployment of Adat from Colonialism to Indigenism*, edited by Jamie S. Davidson and David Henley, 68–86. London, New York: Routledge, 2007.

Carpenter, Kenneth J. *Beriberi, White Rice, and Vitamin B: A Disease, a Cause, and a Cure*. Berkeley: University of California Press, 2000.

Chakrabarty, Dipesh. *Provincializing Europe*. Princeton, NJ: Princeton University Press, 2000.

Chauvel, Richard. *Nationalists, Soldiers and Separatists: The Ambonese Islands from Colonialism to Revolt, 1880–1950*. Leiden: KITLV Press, 2008.

Cheah, Pheng. *Spectral Nationality: Passages of Freedom from Kant to Postcolonial Literatures of Liberation*. New York: Columbia University Press, 2003.

Connely, Matthew. *Fatal Misconception: The Struggle to Control World Population*. Cambridge, MA: Belknap Press of Harvard University Press, 2008.

Coté, Joost. 'Thomas Karsten's Indonesia: Modernity and the End of Europe, 1914–1945'. *Bijdragen tot de Taal-, Land- en Volkenkunde* 170 (2014): 66–98.

Coté, Joost and Hugh O'Neill. *The Life and Work of Thomas Karsten*. Amsterdam: Architectura & Natura, 2017.

Crane, Johanna Tayloe. *Scrambling for Africa: AIDS, Expertise, and the Rise of American Global Health Science*. Ithaca, NY: Cornell University Press, 2013.

Cribb, Robert. 'The Nationalist World of Occupied Jakarta, 1946–1949'. In *From Batavia to Jakarta: Indonesia's Capital 1930s to 1980s*, edited by Susan [Blackburn] Abeyasekere. Melbourne: Monash University, 1985.

Cribb, Robert, ed. *The Indonesian Killings of 1965–1966: Studies from Java and Bali*. Melbourne: Centre of Southeast Asian Studies, Monash University, 1990.

Gangsters and Revolutionaries: The Jakarta People's Militia and the Indonesian Revolution, 1945–1949. Sydney: Allen & Unwin, 1991.

'Development Policy in the Early 20th Century'. In *Development and Social Welfare: Indonesia's Experiences under the New Order*, edited by Jan-Paul Dirkse, Frans Hüsken, and Mario Rutten, 225–45. Leiden: KITLV Press, 1993.

'Legal Pluralism and Criminal Law in the Dutch Colonial Order'. *Indonesia*, no. 90 (2010): 47–66.

Cueto, Marcos. *Missionaries of Science: The Rockefeller Foundation and Latin America*. Bloomington: Indiana University Press, 1994.

'The Cycles of Eradication: The Rockefeller Foundation and Latin American Public Health, 1918–1940'. In *International Health Organizations and Movements, 1918–1939*, edited by Paul Weindling, 222–43. Cambridge: Cambridge University Press, 1995.

'The Origins of Primary Health Care and Selective Primary Health Care'. *American Journal of Public Health* 94, no. 11 (2004): 1864–74.

Cueto, Marcos and Steven Palmer. *Medicine and Public Health in Latin America: A History*. Cambridge: Cambridge University Press, 2014.

Cummings, William K. and Salman Kasenda. 'The Origin of Modern Indonesian Higher Education'. In *From Dependence to Autonomy: The Development of Asian Universities*, edited by Philip G. Altbach and Viswanathan Selvaratnam, 143–66. Dordrecht: Kluwer, 1989.

Curtin, Philip D. '"The White Man's Grave": Image and Reality, 1780–1850'. *Journal of British Studies* 1, no. 1 (1961): 94–110.

Davidson, Jamie S. and David Henley. *The Revival of Tradition in Indonesian Politics: The Deployment of Adat from Colonialism to Indigenism*. London, New York: Routledge, 2007.

De Graaff, Bob and Elsbeth Locher-Scholten. *J. P. Graaf van Limburg Stirum, 1873–1948: Tegendraads Landvoogd en Diplomaat*. Zwolle: Waanders, 2007.

De Jong, J. J. P. *Avondschot: Hoe Nederland zich Terugtrok uit zijn Aziatisch Imperium*. Amsterdam: Boom, 2011.

De Terugtocht: Nederland en de Dekolonisatie van Indonesië. Amsterdam: Boom, 2015.

Dibley, Michael J. and Meiwita Budiharsana. 'Keeping Women and Babies Healthy within an Unequal System'. *Inside Indonesia*, no. 119 (2015). www.insideindonesia.org/keeping-women-and-babies-healthy-within-an-unequal-system-2.

Djalal, Zaidir. *Prof. Dr. W. Z. Yohannes*. Jakarta: Mutiara, 1978.

Djohan, Bahder, 'Gerakan Pemuda Membawa Perobahan Mental'. In *45 Tahun Sumpah Pemuda*, edited by Subagio Reksodipuro, 171–75. Jakarta: Gunung Agung, 1974.

'Segi-Segi Sosial Politik dalam Perkembangan Dunia Kedoktoran Indonesia'. In *125 Tahun Pendidikan Dokter di Indonesia 1851–1976*, edited by M. A. Hanafiah, Bahder Djohan, and Surono, 77–84. Jakarta: Fakultas Kedoktoran Universitas Indonesia, 1976.

Bahder Johan: Pengabdi Kemanusian. Jakarta: Gunung Agung, 1980.

Doel, H. W. van den. 'Indianisatie en Ambtenarensalarissen'. *Tijdschrift voor Geschiedenis* 100, no. 4 (1987): 556–79.

Douglas, Stephen A. *Political Socialization and Student Activism in Indonesia*. Chicago: University of Illinois Press, 1970.

Drooglever, Pieter Joost. *De Vaderlandse Club, 1929–1942: Totoks en de Indische Politiek*. Franeker: Wever, 1980.

Duara, Prasenjit. 'The Discourse of Civilization and Pan-Asianism'. *Journal of World History* 12, no. 1 (2001): 99–130.

'Asia Redux: Conceptualizing a Region for Our Times'. *Journal of Asian Studies* 69, no. 4 (2010): 963–83.

Elson, R. E. *Suharto: A Political Biography*. Cambridge: Cambridge University Press, 2001.

'Constructing the Nation: Ethnicity, Race, Modernity and Citizenship in Early Indonesian Thought'. *Asian Ethnicity* 6, no. 3 (2005): 145–60.

The Idea of Indonesia: A History. Cambridge: Cambridge University Press, 2008.

Ernst & Young. *Ripe for Investment: The Indonesian Health Care Industry Post Introduction of Universal Health Coverage*. London: Ernst & Young Global Limited, 2015.

Eryudhawan, Bambang, ed. *100 Tahun Kebangkitan Nasional: Jejak Boedi Oetomo, Peristiwa, Tokoh dan Tempat*. Jakarta: Badan Pelestarian Pusaka Indonesia, 2009.

Escobar, Arturo. *Encountering Development: The Making and Unmaking of the Third World*. 2nd edn. Princeton, NJ: Princeton University Press, 2012.

Ettling, John. *The Germ of Laziness: Rockefeller Philanthropy and Public Health in the New South*. Cambridge, MA: Harvard University Press, 1981.

Farley, John. *To Cast Out Disease: A History of the International Health Division of the Rockefeller Foundation (1913–1951)*. New York: Oxford University Press, 2004.

Farmer, Paul, Jim Yong Kim, Arthur Kleinman, and Matthew Basilico, eds. *Reimagining Global Health: An Introduction*. Berkeley: California University Press, 2013.

Fasseur, Cees. *De Indologen: Ambtenaren Voor de Oost, 1825–1950*. Amsterdam: Bert Bakker, 1993.

'Cornerstone or Stumbling Block: Racial Classification and the Late Colonial State in Indonesia'. In *The Late Colonial State in Indonesia: Political and Economic Foundations of the Netherlands East Indies, 1880–1942*, edited by Robert Cribb, 31–56. Leiden: KITLV Press, 1994.

'Colonial Dilemma: Van Vollenhoven and the Struggle between Adat Law and Western Law in Indonesia'. In *The Revival of Tradition in Indonesian Politics: The Deployment of Adat from Colonialism to Indigenism*, edited by Jamie S. Davidson and David Henley, 50–67. London, New York: Routledge, 2007.

Feith, Herbert. *The Decline of Constitutional Democracy in Indonesia*. Jakarta: Equinox, 2007.

Feith, Herbert and Lance Castles, eds. *Indonesian Political Thinking, 1945–1965*. Jakarta: Equinox, 2007.

Ferguson, James. *The Anti-Politics Machine: Development, Depoliticization, and Bureaucratic Power in Lesotho*. Minneapolis: University of Minnesota Press, 1994.

Ferzacca, Steven. 'Mediations of Health and the Development of a Nation: Late Suharto, Late Modernity'. In *Liberalizing, Feminizing and Popularizing Health Communications in Asia*, edited by Liew Kai Khiun, 15–42. Farnham, MA: Ashgate, 2012.

Formichi, Chiara. *Islam and the Making of the Nation: Kartosuwiryo and Political Islam in Twentieth-Century Indonesia*. Leiden: KITLV Press, 2012.

Fox, Renée C. *Essays in Medical Sociology: Journeys into the Field*. New Brunswick, NJ: Transaction, 1988.

   Experiment Perilous: Physicians and Patients Facing the Unknown. New Brunswick, NJ: Transaction, 1998.

Fraassen, C.F. van and P. Jobse, eds. *Bronnen betreffende de Midden-Molukken 1900–1942*. 4 vols. The Hague: Instituut voor Nederlandse Geschiedenis, 1997.

Friend, Theodore. *Indonesian Destinies*. Cambridge, MA: Belknap Press of Harvard University Press, 2003.

Gellner, Ernest. *Nationalism*. New York: New York University Press, 1997.

   Nations and Nationalism. 2nd edn. Ithaca, NY: Cornell University Press, 2006.

Glissenaar, Frans. *D. D.: Het Leven van E. F. E. Douwes Dekker*. Hilversum: Verloren, 1999.

Goss, Andrew. *The Floracrats: State-Sponsored Science and the Failure of the Enlightenment in Indonesia*. Madison: University of Wisconsin Press, 2011.

Gotō, Ken'ichi. 'Cooperation, Submission, and Resistance of Indigenous Elites of Southeast Asia in the Wartime Empire'. In *The Japanese Wartime Empire, 1931–1945*, edited by Peter Duus, Ramon Hawley Myers, and Mark R. Peattie, 274–301. Princeton, NJ: Princeton University Press, 1996.

   Tensions of Empire: Japan and Southeast Asia in the Colonial and Postcolonial World. Singapore: Singapore University Press, 2003.

Gouda, Frances. *Dutch Culture Overseas: Colonial Practice in the Netherlands Indies, 1900–1942*. Amsterdam: Amsterdam University Press, 1995.

   'Good Mothers, Medeas, or Jezebels: Feminine Imagery in Colonial and Anticolonial Rhetoric in the Dutch East Indies, 1900–1942'. In *Domesticating the Empire: Race, Gender, and Family Life in French and Dutch Colonialism*, edited by Julia Clancy-Smith and Frances Gouda, 236–54. Charlottesville: University Press of Virginia, 1998.

Grant, Bruce. *Indonesia*. 3rd edn. Melbourne: Melbourne University Press, 1996.

Graves, Elizabeth E. *The Minangkabau Response to Dutch Colonial Rule in the Nineteenth Century*. Ithaca, NY: Cornell Modern Indonesia Project, 1981.

Greene, Jeremy, Marguerite Thorp Basilico, Heidi Kim, and Paul Farmer. 'Colonial Medicine and Its Legacies'. In *Reimagining Global Health: An Introduction*, edited by Paul Farmer, Jim Yong Kim, Arthur Kleinman, and Matthew Basilico, 33–73. Berkeley: California University Press, 2013.

Groeneboer, K. *Weg tot het Westen: Het Nederlands Voor Indië 1600–1950: Een Taalpolitieke Geschiedenis*. Leiden: KITLV Press, 1993.

Guénel, Annick. 'The 1937 Bandung Conference on Rural Hygiene: Toward a New Vision of Healthcare?' In *Global Movements, Local Concerns: Medicine and Health in Southeast Asia*, edited by Laurence Monnais and Harold J. Cook, 62–80. Singapore: National University of Singapore Press, 2012.

Haliman, Arif and Glen Williams. 'Can People Move Bureaucratic Mountains?: Developing Primary Health Care in Rural Indonesia'. *Social Science & Medicine* 17, no. 19 (1983): 1449–55.

Hanafiah, Mohammad Ali. 'Sepuluh Tahun dalam Asrama STOVIA'. In *125 Tahun Pendidikan Dokter di Indonesia 1851–1976*, edited by M. A. Hanafiah, Bahder Djohan, and Surono, 97–112. Jakarta: Fakultas Kedoktoran Universitas Indonesia, 1976.

77 Tahun Riwayat Hidup. Jakarta: Author, 1977.

Harrison, Mark. *Climates and Constitutions: Health, Race, Environment and British Imperialism in India, 1600–1850*. New Delhi: Oxford University Press, 1999.

Headrick, Daniel R. *The Tools of Empire: Technology and European Imperialism in the Nineteenth Century*. New York: Oxford University Press, 1981.

Henley, David. 'Nationalism and Regionalism in Colonial Indonesia: The Case of Minahasa'. *Indonesia*, no. 55 (1993): 91–112.

Nationalism and Regionalism in a Colonial Context: Minahasa in the Dutch East Indies. Leiden: KITLV Press, 1996.

Heering, Bob. *Soekarno: Founding Father of Indonesia, 1901–1945*. Leiden: KITLV Press, 2002.

Heryanto, Ariel. *Language of Development and Development of Language: The Case of Indonesia*. Canberra: Australian National University, Research School of Pacific and Asian Studies, 1995.

Hesselink, Liesbeth. 'The Unbearable Absence of Parasols: The Formidable Weight of a Colonial Java Status Symbol'. *IIAS Newsletter*, no. 45 (2007): 26.

Healers on the Colonial Market: Native Doctors and Midwives in the Dutch East Indies. Leiden: KITLV Press, 2011.

Heywood, Peter and Nida P. Harahap. 'Health Facilities at the District Level in Indonesia'. *Australia and New Zealand Health Policy* 6, no. 13 (2009): 1–11. www.anzhealthpolicy.com/content/6/1/13.

Hill, Hal. *Indonesia's New Order: The Dynamics of Socio-Economic Transformation*. Sydney: Allen & Unwin, 1994.

Hodges, Sarah. 'The Global Menace'. *Social History of Medicine* 25, no. 3 (2012): 719–28.

Hoesein, Rushdy. *Terobosan Sukarno dalam Perundingan*. Jakarta: Kompas, 2010.

Hoogervorst, Tom and Henk Schulte Nordholt. 'Urban Middle Classes in Colonial Java (1900–1942): Images and Language'. *Bijdragen tot de Taal-, Land- en Volkenkunde* 173 (2017): 442–74.

Hovinga, Henk. 'End of a Forgotten Drama: The Reception and Repatriation of *Rōmusha* after the Japanese Capitulation'. In *Asian Labor in the Wartime Japanese Empire: Unknown Histories*, edited by Paul H. Kratoska, 197–212. Singapore: Singapore University Press, 2006.

Hughes, John. *The End of Sukarno: A Coup That Misfired, a Purge That Ran Wild*. Singapore: Archipelago, 2002 [1967].

Hull, Terence H. 'Fertility Decline in the New Order Period: The Evolution of Population Policy, 1965–90'. In *Indonesia's New Order: The Dynamics of Socio-Economic Transformation*, edited by Hal Hill, 123–45. Sydney: Allen & Unwin, 1994.

Looking Back to the Hygiene Study Ward: A Brief Guide to the Literature. Canberra: Australian National University, Research School of Social Sciences, 1995.

'The Political Framework for Family Planning in Indonesia: Three Decades of Development'. In *Two Is Enough: Family Planning in Indonesia under the New Order, 1968–1998*, edited by Firman Lubis and Anke Niehof, 57–81. Leiden: KITLV Press, 2003.

'Conflict and Collaboration in Public Health: The Rockefeller Foundation and the Dutch Colonial Government in Indonesia'. In *Public Health in Asia and the Pacific: Historical and Comparative Perspectives*, edited by Milton Lewis and Kerrie L. MacPherson, 139–52. New York: Routledge, 2007.

Hull, Terence H. and Valerie J. Hull. 'From Family Planning to Reproductive Health Care: A Brief History'. In *People, Population, and Policy in Indonesia*, edited by Terence H. Hull, 1–69. Singapore: Equinox for ISEAS, 2005.

Iliffe, John. *East African Doctors: A History of the Modern Profession*. Cambridge: Cambridge University Press, 1998.

Ingleson, John. *Perhimpunan Indonesia and the Indonesian Nationalist Movement, 1923–1928*. Melbourne: Centre of Southeast Asian Studies, Monash University, 1975.

Road to Exile: The Indonesian Nationalist Movement 1927–1934. Singapore: Heinemann, 1979.

In Search of Justice: Workers and Unions in Colonial Java, 1908–1926. Singapore: Oxford University Press, 1986.

'Sutomo, the Indonesian Study Club and Organised Labour in Late Colonial Surabaya'. *Journal of Southeast Asian Studies* 39, no. 1 (2008): 31–57.

Irna, H. N. and Hadi Soewito, eds. *BAPERPI: Badan Perwakilan Peladjar Peladjar Indonesia, Cikini 71*. Jakarta: Yayasan Tjikini 71, 1990.

Irwin, Rachel. 'Indonesia, H5N1, and Global Health Diplomacy'. *Global Health Governance* 3, no. 2 (2010). http://blogs.shu.edu/ghg/files/2011/11/Irwin_Indonesia-H5N1-and-Global-Health-Diplomacy_Spring-2010.pdf.

Joint Committee on Reducing Maternal and Neonatal Mortality in Indonesia. *Reducing Maternal and Neonatal Mortality in Indonesia: Saving Lives, Saving the Future*. Washington, DC: National Academy of Sciences, 2013.

Kahin, George McTurnan. *Nationalism and Revolution in Indonesia*. Ithaca, NY: Cornell University Press, 1952.

'In Memoriam: Mohamad Roem (1908–1983)'. *Indonesia*, no. 37 (1984): 134–38.

Kanahele, George Sanford. 'The Japanese Occupation of Indonesia: Prelude to Independence'. PhD, Cornell University, 1967.

Kaptein, Nico J. G. 'Southeast Asian Debates and Middle East Inspiration: European Dress in Minangkabau at the Beginning of the 20th Century'. In *Southeast Asia and the Middle East: Islam, Movement, and the Longue Durée*, edited by Eric Tagliacozzo, 176–95. Singapore: National University of Singapore Press, 2009.

Kardarmadja, M. Soenjata. *Prof. Dr. Wilhelmus Zakarias Johannes*. Jakarta: Departemen Pendidikan dan Kebudayaan, 1985.

Karimoeddin, T. 'Pendidikan Dokter Jaman Pendudukan Jepang (Ika Dai Gaku)'. In *125 Tahun Pendidikan Dokter di Indonesia 1851–1976*, edited by M. A. Hanafiah, Bahder Djohan, and Surono, 26–32. Jakarta: Fakultas Kedoktoran Universitas Indonesia, 1976.

Karma, Mara. *Ibnu Sutowo Mengemban Misi Revolusi: Sebagai Dokter, Tentara, Pejuang Minyak Bumi*. Jakarta: Pustaka Sinar Harapan, 2001.

Kartodirdjo, Sartono, Marwati Djoened Poesponegoro, and Nugroho Notosusanto. *Zaman Jepang dan Zaman Republik Indonesia, 1942–1998*. Sejarah Nasional Indonesia, Vol. 6. Jakarta: Balai Pustaka, 2008.

Kennedy, Dane. 'The Perils of the Midday Sun: Climatic Anxieties in the Colonial Tropics'. In *Imperialism and the Natural World*, edited by John M. MacKenzie, 118–40. Manchester: Manchester University Press, 1990.

Keppy, Herman. *Tussen Ambon en Amsterdam*. Amsterdam: Conserve, 2004.

'Beschaamt de Minahassa Niet'. In *Pendek: Korte Verhalen over Indische Levens*, edited by Herman Keppy, 75–80. Amsterdam: West, 2013.

Khiun, Liew Kai. 'Wats and Worms: The Activities of the Rockefeller Foundation's International Health Board in Southeast Asia (1913–1940)'. In *Global Movements, Local Concerns: Medicine and Health in Southeast Asia*, edited by Laurence Monnais and Harold J. Cook, 43–61. Singapore: Singapore University Press, 2012.

Klinken, Gerry van. *Minorities, Modernity and the Emerging Nation: Christians in Indonesia, a Biographical Approach*. Leiden: KITLV Press, 2003.

Koch, D. M. G. *Om de Vrijheid: De Nationalistische Beweging in Indonesië*. Jakarta: Jajasan Pembangunan Djakarta, 1946.

Verantwoording: Een Halve Eeuw in Indonesië. The Hague/Bandung: Van Hoeve, 1956.

Batig Slot: Figuren uit het Oude Indië. Amsterdam: De Brug/Djambatan, 1960.

'Rd. Dr. Soetomo'. In *Batig Slot: Figuren uit het Oude Indië*, 138–45. Amsterdam: De Brug/Djambatan, 1960.

'Dr. Tjipto Mangoenkoesoemo'. In *Batig Slot: Figuren uit het Oude Indië*, edited by D.M.G. Koch, 146–53. Amsterdam: De Brug/Djambatan, 1960.

Koentjaraningrat, Raden Mas and H. W. Bachtiar. 'Higher Education in the Social Sciences in Indonesia'. In *The Social Sciences in Indonesia*, edited by R. M. Koentjaraningrat, 1–42. Jakarta: LIPI, 1975.

Koestedjo, Raden. *Inilah Jalan Hikupku*. Jakarta: Rosda Jayaputra, 1996.

Köllmann, Nathalie and Corrie van Veggel. 'Posyandu: Theory and Practice'. In *Health Care in Java: Past and Present*, edited by Peter Boomgaard, Rosalia Sciortino, and Ines Smyth, 95–110. Leiden: KITLV Press, 1996.

Koning, Juliette. 'Family Planning Acceptance in a Rural Central Javanese Village'. In *Health Care in Java: Past and Present*, edited by Peter Boomgaard, Rosalia Sciortino, and Ines Smyth, 147–69. Leiden: KITLV Press, 1996.

Korver, A. P. E. *Sarekat Islam, 1912–1916: Opkomst, Bloei en Structuur van Indonesië's Eerste Massabeweging*. Amsterdam: Historisch Seminarium, Universiteit van Amsterdam, 1982.

Kratoska, Paul. *Food Supplies and the Japanese Occupation in South-East Asia* New York: St. Martins, 1998.

Kristiansen, Stein and Purwo Santoso. 'Surviving Decentralisation?: Impacts of Regional Autonomy on Health Service Provision in Indonesia'. *Health Policy* 77 (2006): 247–59.

Kurasawa, Aiko. 'Propaganda Media on Java under the Japanese, 1942–1945'. *Indonesia*, no. 44 (1987): 59–116.

Kurniati, A., E. Rosskam, M. M. Afzal, T. B. Suryowinoto, and A. G. Mukti. 'Strengthening Indonesia's Health Workforce through Partnerships'. *Public Health* 129 (2015): 1138–49.

Laffan, Michael F. *Islamic Nationhood and Colonial Indonesia: The Umma below the Winds*. London: Routledge, 2007.

    The Making of Indonesian Islam: Orientalism and the Narration of a Sufi Past. Princeton, NJ: Princeton University Press, 2011.

Lakoff, Andrew. 'Two Regimes of Global Health'. *Humanity: An International Journal of Human Rights, Humanitarianism, and Development* 1, no. 1 (2010): 59–79.

Lakoff, Andrew and Stephen J. Collier. *Biosecurity Interventions: Global Health and Security in Question*. New York: Columbia University Press, 2008.

Laporan Perkembangan Pendidikan Dokter pada Fakultas Kedoktoran Universitas Indonesia Djakarta. Jakarta: Fakultas Kedoktoran Universitas Indonesia, 1960.

Latham, Michael E. *Modernization as Ideology: American Social Science and 'Nation Building' in the Kennedy Era*. Durham: University of North Carolina Press, 2000.

    The Right Kind of Revolution: Modernization, Development, and U.S. Foreign Policy from the Cold War to the Present. Ithaca, NY: Cornell University Press, 2010.

Lauw, Gabrielle M. 'De Dokter Djawa School te Batavia (1850–1875)'. *Spiegel Historiael: Maandblad voor Geschiedenis en Archeologie* 23, no. 2 (1988): 75–79.

Lee, Christopher J. *Making a World after Empire: The Bandung Moment and Its Political Afterlives*. Athens: Ohio University Press, 2010.

Lee, Doreen. 'Images of Youth: On the Iconography of History and Protest in Indonesia'. *History and Anthropology* 22, no. 3 (2011): 307–36.

Legge, J. D. *Sukarno: A Political Biography* London: Allan Lane, 1972.

    Intellectuals and Nationalism in Indonesia: A Study of the Following Recruited by Sutan Sjahrir in Occupation Jakarta. Ithaca, NY: Southeast Asia Program, Cornell University, 1988.

Leirissa, R. Z. *Kewarganegaraan yang Bertanggungjawab: Mengenang Dr. J. Leimena*. Jakarta: Gunung Mulia, 1995.

Lewis, Martin Deming. 'One Hundred Million Frenchmen: The "Assimilation" Theory in French Colonial Policy'. *Comparative Studies in Society and History* 4, no. 2 (1962): 129–53.

Li, Tania Murray. *The Will to Improve: Governmentality, Development, and the Practice of Politics*. Durham, NC: Duke University Press, 2007.

Limpach, Rémy. *De Brandende Kampongs van Generaal Spoor*. Amsterdam: Boom, 2016.

Litsios, Socrates. 'Malaria Control, the Cold War, and the Postwar Reorganization of International Assistance'. *Medical Anthropology* 17, no. 3 (1997): 255–78.

    'The Christian Medical Commission and the Development of the World Health Organization's Primary Health Care Approach'. *American Journal of Public Health* 94, no. 11 (2004): 1884–93.

    'The Long and Difficult Road to Alma Ata: A Personal Reflection'. *International Journal of Health Services* 32 (2002): 709–32.

Livingstone, David N. 'Tropical Climate and Moral Hygiene: The Anatomy of a Victorian Debate'. *British Journal for the History of Science* 32, no. 1 (1999): 93–110.

Lo, Ming-Cheng M. *Doctors within Borders: Profession, Ethnicity, and Modernity in Colonial Taiwan*. Berkeley: University of California Press, 2002.

Locher-Scholten, Elsbeth. *Ethiek in Fragmenten: Vijf Studies over Koloniaal Denken en Doen van Nederlanders in de Indonesische Archipel, 1877–1942*. Utrecht: H&S, 1981.

Lowe, Celia. 'Preparing Indonesia: H5N1 Influenza through the Lens of Global Health'. *Indonesia*, no. 90 (2010): 147–70.

'Viral Clouds: Becoming H5N1 in Indonesia'. *Cultural Anthropology* 25, no. 4 (2010): 625–49.

Lubis, Firman. 'History and Structure of the National Family Planning Program'. In *Two Is Enough: Family Planning in Indonesia under the New Order, 1968–1998*, edited by Firman Lubis and Anke Niehof, 31–55. Leiden: KITLV Press, 2003.

Jakarta 1960-an: Kenangan Semasa Mahasiswa. Jakarta: Masup, 2008.

Jakarta 1970-an: Kenangan Sebagai Dosen. Jakarta: Masup, 2010.

Lubis, Firman and Anke Niehof, eds. *Two Is Enough: Family Planning in Indonesia under the New Order, 1968–1998*. Leiden: KITLV Press, 2003.

Luttikhuis, Bart. 'Beyond Race: Constructions of "Europeanness" in Late-Colonial Legal Practice in the Dutch East Indies'. *European Review of History* 20, no. 4 (2013): 539–58.

'Negotiating Modernity: Europeanness in Late Colonial Indonesia, 1910–1942'. Dissertation, European University Institute, 2014.

Luttikhuis, Bart and A. Dirk Moses, eds. *Colonial Counterinsurgency and Mass Violence: The Dutch Empire in Indonesia*. London: Routledge, 2014.

MacLeod, Roy. 'Introduction'. In *Disease, Medicine, and Empire: Perspectives on Western Medicine and the Experience of European Expansion*, edited by Roy MacLeod and Milton Lewis, 1–18. London: Routledge, 1988.

Madjiah, Matia. *Kisah Seorang Dokter Gerilya: Dalam Revolusi Kemerdekaan di Banten*. Jakarta: Sinar Harapan, 1986.

Mangunwidodo, Soebaryo. *Dr. K. R. T. Radjiman Wediodiningrat: Perjalanan Seorang Putra Bangsa 1879–1952*. Jakarta: Yayasan Dr. K. R. T. Radjiman Wediodiningrat, 1994.

Mark, Ethan. 'Suharto's New Order Remembers Japan's New Order: Oral Accounts from Indonesia'. In *Representing the Japanese Occupation of Indonesia: Personal Testimonies and Public Images in Indonesia, Japan, and the Netherlands*, edited by Remco Raben, 72–84. Zwolle: Waanders, 1999.

'Appealing to Asia: Nation, Culture, and the Problem of Imperial Modernity in Japanese-Occupied Java, 1942–1945'. PhD thesis, Columbia University, 2003.

'"Asia's" Transwar Lineage: Nationalism, Marxism, and "Greater Asia" in an Indonesian Inflection'. *Journal of Asian Studies* 65, no. 3 (2006): 461–93.

'The Perils of Co-Prosperity: Takeda Rintaro, Occupied Southeast Asia, and the Seductions of Postcolonial Empire'. *American Historical Review* 119, no. 4 (2014): 1184–206.

Martosewojo, Soejono. 'Risalah Pembentukan Djakarta Ika Dai Gaku'. In *125 Tahun Pendidikan Dokter di Indonesia 1851–1976*, edited by M. A. Hanafiah, Bahder Djohan, and Surono, 33–34. Jakarta: Fakultas Kedoktoran Universitas Indonesia, 1976.

Martosewojo, Soejono, Eri Soedewo, Sarnanto, Taufik Abdullah, and Idris Siregar. *Mahasiswa '45, Prapatan 10: Pengabdiannya*. Bandung: Patma, 1984.

Mashad, Dhurorudin. *Tahun Penuh Perjuangan: Soedjono Djoened Poesponegoro, Menteri Riset Pertama di Indonesia*. Jakarta: Lembaga Ilmu Pengetahuan Indonesia, 2008.

McCoy, Alfred W. 'Introduction'. In *Southeast Asia under Japanese Occupation*, 1–13. New Haven, CT: Yale University Southeast Asia Studies, 1980.

McDonald, Hamish. *Suharto's Indonesia*. Melbourne: Fontana, 1980.

McGilvray, James C. *The Quest for Health and Wholeness*. Tübingen: German Institute for Medical Missions, 1981.

McGregor, Katherine E. *History in Uniform: Military Ideology and the Construction of Indonesia's Past*. Singapore: National University of Singapore Press, 2007.

McMillan, Richard. *The British Occupation of Indonesia: 1945–1946: Britain, The Netherlands and the Indonesian Revolution*. New York: Routledge, 2005.

Merton, Robert K., George G. Reader and Patricia L. Kendall. *The Student-Physician: Introductory Studies in the Sociology of Medical Education*. Cambridge, MA: Harvard University Press for the Commonwealth Fund, 1957.

Messer, Adam. 'Effects of the Indonesian National Revolution and Transfer of Power on the Scientific Establishment'. *Indonesia*, no. 58 (1994): 41–68.

Mesters, Han. 'J. L. Hydrick in the Netherlands Indies: An American View of Dutch Public Health Policy'. In *Health Care in Java: Past and Present*, edited by Peter Boomgaard, Rosalia Sciortino, and Ines Smyth, 51–62. Leiden: KITLV Press, 1996.

Miert, Hans van. *Een Koel Hoofd en een Warm Hart: Nationalisme, Javanisme en Jeugdbeweging in Nederlands-Indië, 1918–1930*. Amsterdam: Bataafsche Leeuw, 1995.

Mohamad, Kartono. 'Family Planning'. In *Indonesia in the Soeharto Years: Issues, Incidents and Images*, edited by John H. McGlynn, Oscar Motuloh, Suzanne Charlé, Jeffrey Hadler, Bambang Bujono, Margaret Glade Agusta, and Gedsiri Suhartono, 132–34. Jakarta: Lontar, 2007.

Monnais, Laurence and Hans Pols. 'Health and Disease in the Colonies: Medicine in the Age of Empire'. In *The Routledge History of Western Empires*, edited by Robert Aldrich and Kirsten McKenzie, 270–84. New York: Routledge, 2014.

Moon, Suzanne. 'Takeoff or self-sufficiency: Ideologies of development in Indonesia, 1957–1961'. *Technology and Culture* 39, no. 2 (1998): 187–213.

    Technology and Technical Idealism: A History of Development in the Netherlands East Indies. Leiden: CNWS, 2007.

Mrázek, Rudolf, *Sjahrir: Politics and Exile in Indonesia*. Ithaca, NY: Southeast Asia Program, Cornell University, 1994.

    'Indonesian Dandy: The Politics of Clothes in the Late Colonial Period, 1893–1942'. In *Outward Appearances: Dressing State and Society in Indonesia*, edited by Henk Schulte Nordholt, 117–50. Leiden: KITLV Press, 1997.

    A Certain Age: Colonial Jakarta through the Memories of Its Intellectuals. Durham, NC: Duke University Press, 2010.

Murakami, Saki. 'Call for Doctors!: Medical Provision and the State during Indonesian Decolonisation, 1930s–1950s'. In *Cars, Conduits, and Kampongs: The Modernization of the Indonesian City, 1920–1960*, edited by Freek Colombijn and Joost Coté, 29–62. Leiden: Brill, 2005.

Murray, R. Thomas. *A Chronicle of Indonesian Higher Education: The First Half Century, 1920–1970*. Singapore: Chopmen, 1973.

Nagazumi, Akira. *The Dawn of Indonesian Nationalism: The Early Years of the Budi Utomo, 1908–1918*. Tokyo: Institute of Developing Economies, 1972.

Nalenan, Ruben and Iskandar Gani. *Dr. A. K. Gani: Pejuang Berwawasan Sipil dan Militer*. Jakarta: Yayasan Indonesianologi, 1990.

Naysmith, Scott. 'Disease Control in Democratic Indonesia'. *Inside Indonesia*, no. 111 (2013). www.insideindonesia.org/disease-control-in-democratic-indonesia-2.

Neelakantan, Vivek. 'Eradicating Smallpox in Indonesia: The Archipelagic Challenge'. *Health and History* 12, no. 1 (2010): 61–87.

'Health and Medicine in Soekarno Era Indonesia: Social Medicine, Public Health and Medical Education, 1949 to 1967'. PhD thesis, University of Sydney, 2014.

'The Campaign against the Big Four Endemic Diseases and Indonesia's Engagement with the WHO during the Cold War 1950s'. In *Public Health and National Reconstruction in Post-War Asia: International Influences, Local Transformations*, edited by Liping Bu and Ka-che Yip, 154–74. London: Routledge, 2015.

Science, Public Health and Nation-Building in Soekarno-Era Indonesia. Newcastle upon Tyne: Cambridge Scholars, 2017.

Neill, Deborah. *Networks in Tropical Medicine: Internationalism, Colonialism, and the Rise of a Medical Specialty, 1890–1930*. Stanford, CA: Stanford University Press, 2012.

Newland, Kathleen and Kamala Chandrakirana Soedjatmoko, eds. *Transforming Humanity: The Visionary Writings of Soedjatmoko*. West Hartford, CT: Kumarian Press, 1994.

Niehof, Anke and Firman Lubis. 'Family Planning in Practice: Cases from the Field'. In *Two Is Enough: Family Planning in Indonesia under the New Order, 1968–1998*, edited by Firman Lubis and Anke Niehof, 119–50. Leiden: KITLV Press, 2003.

Niel, Robert van. *The Emergence of the Modern Indonesian Elite*. The Hague: Van Hoeve, 1960.

Nikijuluw, Victor P. H. and Erlita Rachman, eds. *Sang Upuleru: Mengenang 100 Tahun Prof. Dr. Gerrit Augustinus Siwabessy (1914–2014)*. Jakarta: Gramedia, 2014.

Nourse, Jennifer. 'The Meaning of Dukun and Allure of Sufi Healers: How Persian Cosmopolitans Transformed Malay-Indonesian History'. *Journal of Southeast Asian Studies* 44, no. 3 (2013): 400–22.

Nugraha, Iskandar P. *Teosofi, Nasionalisme and Elite Modern Indonesia*. Jakarta: Kommunitas Bambu, 2011.

Nursam, M. *Pergumulan Seorang Intelektual: Biografi Soedjatmoko*. Jakarta: Gramedia Pustaka Utama, 2002.

Prof. Dr. Dr. Moh. Saleh Mangundiningrat: Potret Cendekiawan Jawa. Jakarta: SUN, 2006.

Oostindie, Gert. *Soldaat in Indonesië, 1945–1950*. Amsterdam: Prometheus, 2015.

Oppenheimer, Joshua. *The Act of Killing*. Copenhagen: Final Cut for Real, 2012.

The Look of Silence. Copenhagen: Final Cut for Real, 2014.

Packard, Randall M. 'Malaria Dreams: Postwar Visions of Health and Development in the Third World'. *Medical Anthropology* 17, no. 3 (1997): 279–96.

The Making of a Tropical Disease: A Short History of Malaria. Baltimore, MD: Johns Hopkins University Press, 2007.

Padmodiwiryo, Suhario 'Kecik'. *Memoar Hario Kecik: Autobiografi Seorang Mahasiswa Prajurit*. Jakarta: Yayasan Obor Indonesia, 1995.
  Student Soldiers: A Memoir of the Battle That Sparked Indonesia's National Revolution. Jakarta: Yayasan Pustaka Obor Indonesia, 2015.
Pisani, Elizabeth. *The Wisdom of Whores: Bureaucrats, Brothels and the Business of AIDS*. New York: Norton, 2009.
  Indonesia Etc.: Exploring the Improbable Nation. London: Granta, 2014.
Poesponegoro, Marwati Djoened and Nugroho Notosusanto. *Zaman Kebangkitan Nasional dan Masa Hindia Belanda*. Sejarah Nasional Indonesia, Vol. 5. Jakarta: Balai Pustaka, 2008.
Poeze, Harry A. *In het Land van de Overheerser I: Indonesiërs in Nederland, 1600–1950*. Dordrecht: FORIS, 1986.
  'Early Indonesian Emancipation: Abdul Rivai, Van Heutsz and the Bintang Hindia'. *Bijdragen tot de Taal-, Land- en Volkenkunde* 145, no. 1 (1989): 87–106.
Pols, Hans. 'Anomie in the Metropolis: The City in American Sociology and Psychiatry'. *Osiris*, no. 18 (2003): 194–211.
  'European Botanists and Physicians, Indigenous Herbal Medicine in the Dutch East Indies, and Colonial Networks of Mediation'. *East Asian Science, Technology, and Society: An International Journal* 3, no. 2–3 (2009): 173–208.
  'The Totem Vanishes, the Hordes Revolt: A Psychoanalytic Interpretation of the Indonesian Struggle for Independence'. In *Globalizing the Unconscious: Psychoanalysis, Colonial Trauma, Sovereignties*, edited by Warwick H. Anderson, Deborah Jenson, and Richard Keller, 141–65. Durham, NC: Duke University Press, 2011.
  'Notes from Batavia, the European's Graveyard: The 19th Century Debate on Acclimatization in the Dutch East Indies'. *Journal of the History of Medicine and Allied Sciences* 67, no. 1 (2012): 120–48.
  'Indo-Europeans in the Dutch East Indies: An Indo-European Analysis of a Paradoxical Colonial Category'. In *Health and Difference: Rendering Human Variation in Colonial Engagements*, edited by Alexandra Widmer and Veronika Lipphardt, 205–23. Oxford: Berghahn Books, 2016.
Porter, Natalie. 'Risky Zoographies: The Limits of Place in Avian Flu Management'. *Environmental Humanities* 1 (2012): 103–21.
Post, Peter, William H. Frederick, Iris Heidebrink, and Shigeru Sato, eds. *The Encyclopedia of Indonesia in the Pacific War*. Leiden: Brill, 2010.
Post, Peter and Elly Touwen-Bouwsma. 'Introduction'. In *Japan, Indonesia, and the War: Myths and Realities*, 1–13. Leiden: KITLV Press, 1997.
Pour, Julius. *Doorstoot naar Djokja: Pertikaian Pemimpin Sipil-Militer*. Jakarta: Kompas, 2009.
Prakash, Gyan. *Another Reason: Science and the Imagination of Modern India*. Princeton, NJ: Princeton University Press, 1999.
Protschky, Susie. 'Race, Class, and Gender: Debates over the Character of Social Hierarchies in the Netherlands Indies, circa 1600–1942'. *Bijdragen tot de Taal-, Land- en Volkenkunde* 167, no. 4 (2011): 543–56.
Purdey, Jemma. *From Vienna to Yogyakarta: The Life of Herb Feith*. Sydney: University of New South Wales Press, 2011.
Putjuk, Hari Fitri. 'Indonesia's Family Planning Program: From Stagnation to Revitalization'. *Devex International Development News* (25 September 2015).

Raben, Remco. 'Indonesian *Rōmusha* and Coolies under Naval Administration: The Eastern Archipelago, 1942–45'. In *Asian Labor in the Wartime Japanese Empire: Unknown Histories*, edited by Paul H. Kratoska, 197–212. Singapore: Singapore University Press, 2006.

Raillon, François. *Les Étudiants Indonésiens et L'ordre Nouveau: Politique et Idéologie du Mahasiswa Indonesia, 1966–1974*. Paris: Editions de la Maison des Sciences de l'Homme, 1984.

Ramadhan K. H. *Ibnu Sutowo: Saatnya Saya Bercerita!* Jakarta: National Press Club, 2008.

Redfield, Peter. *Life in Crisis: The Ethical Journey of Doctors without Borders*. Berkeley: University of California Press, 2013.

Reid, Anthony. *The Indonesian National Revolution, 1945–1950*. Hawthorn: Longman, 1974.

   The Blood of the People: Revolution and the End of Traditional Rule in Northern Sumatra. New York: Oxford University Press, 1979.

   'The Identity of "Sumatra" in History'. In *Cultures and Societies of North Sumatra*, edited by R. Carle, 25–42. Berlin: Dietrich Reimer, 1987.

   'Sumatran Bataks: From Statelessness to Indonesian Diaspora', in *Imperial Alchemy: Nationalism and Political Identity in Southeast Asia*, edited by Anthony Reid, 145–86. Cambridge: Cambridge University Press, 2009.

   'Why Not Federalism?' In *To Nation by Revolution: Indonesia in the 20th Century*, 208–28. Singapore: National University of Singapore Press, 2011.

Rex, Mortimer. *Indonesian Communism under Sukarno: Ideology and Politics, 1959–1965*. Ithaca, NY: Cornell University Press, 1974.

Reyes, Raquel A.G. *Love, Passion and Patriotism: Sexuality and the Philippine Propaganda Movement, 1882–1892*. Seattle: University of Washington Press, 2008.

Richards, Robert. *Darwin and the Emergence of Evolutionary Theories of Mind and Behavior*. Chicago: University of Chicago Press, 1987.

Ricklefs, M. C. *A History of Modern Indonesia: c. 1200 to the Present*. 3rd edn. Stanford, CA: Stanford University Press, 2001.

Rifai, Bachtiar and Koesnadi Hardjasoemantri. *Perguruan Tinggi di Indonesia*. Jakarta: Departemen Perguruan Tinggi dan Ilmu Pengetahuan, 1965.

Roem, Mohamad. 'Tradisi Berpolitik'. In *45 Tahun Sumpah Pemuda*, edited by Yayasan Gedung-Gedung Bersejarah Jakarta, 243–52. Jakarta: Gunung Agung, 1974.

Rogaski, Ruth. *Hygienic Modernity: Meanings of Health and Disease in Treaty-Port China*. Berkeley: University of California Press, 2004.

Roosa, John. *Pretext for Mass Murder: The September 30th Movement and Suharto's Coup D'état in Indonesia*. Madison: University of Wisconsin Press, 2006.

Rosenberg, Charles E. and Janet Golden, eds. *Framing Disease: Studies in Cultural History, Health and Medicine in American Society*. New Brunswick, NJ: Rutgers University Press, 1992.

Rosser, Andrew. 'Realising Free Health Care for the Poor in Indonesia: The Politics of Illegal Fees'. *Journal of Contemporary Asia* 42, no. 2 (2012): 255–75.

Rosser, Andrew and Ian Wilson. 'Democratic Decentralisation and Pro-Poor Policy Reform in Indonesia: The Politics of Health Insurance for the Poor in Jembrana and Tabanan'. *Asian Journal of Social Science* 40 (2012): 608–34.

Sadowsky, Jonathan. 'Psychiatry and Colonial Ideology in Nigeria'. *Bulletin of the History of Medicine* 71, no. 1 (1997): 94–111.

Safwan, Mardanas. *Riwajat Hidup dan Pengabdian Prof. Dr. Sutomo Cokronegoro*. Jakarta: Lembaga Sejarah dan Antropologi, 1972.

Saito, Ayami. 'The Development of *Posyandu*: Historical and Institutional Aspects'. In *Critical and Radical Geographies of the Social, the Spatial and the Political*, edited by Toshio Mizuuchi, 80–97. Osaka: Department of Geography, Osaka City University, 2006.

Sandiantoro. *Jejak Jiwa: Di Listasan Zaman (1913–2013): Mengenang yang Silam, Meretas Masa Depan*. Surabaya: Peringatan 1 Abad Pendidikan Dokter di Surabaya, 2013.

Santosa, Paulus Hidayat. 'Participation from Below in Hierarchical Bureaucracies: The Unsolved Dilemma in Indonesian Primary Health Care'. In *The Hidden Crisis in Development: Development Bureaucracies*, edited by Philip Quarles van Ufford, Dirk Kruijt, and Theodore Downing, 211–22. Tokyo: United Nations University, 1988.

Santoso, Slamet Imam and Boen S. Oemarjati. *Warna-Warni Pengalaman Hidup*. Jakarta: Penerbit Universitas Indonesia, 1992.

Sastroamijoyo, Ali. *Milestones on My Journey: The Memoirs of Ali Sastroamijoyo, Indonesian Patriot and Political Leader* Brisbane: University of Queensland Press, 1979.

Sato, Shigeru. '"Economic Soldiers" in Java: Indonesian Laborers Mobilized for Agricultural Projects'. In *Asian Labor in the Wartime Japanese Empire: Unknown Histories*, edited by Paul H. Kratoska, 129–51. Singapore: Singapore University Press, 2006.

'Indonesia 1939–1942: Prelude to the Japanese Occupation'. *Journal of Southeast Asian Studies* 37, no. 2 (2006): 225–48.

'Forced Labourers and Their Resistance in Java under Japanese Military Rule, 1942–1945'. In *Resisting Bondage in Indian Ocean Africa and Asia*, edited by Edward A. Alpers, Gwyn Campbell, and Michael Salman, 82–95. New York: Routledge, 2007.

Satrio. *Perjuangan dan Pengabdian: Mosaik Kenangan Prof. Dr. Satrio, 1916–1986*. Jakarta: Arsip Nasional Republik Indonesia, 1986.

Scherer, Savitri Prastiti. 'Harmony and Dissonance: Early Nationalist Thought on Java'. MA thesis, Cornell University, 1975.

'Soetomo and Trade Unionism'. *Indonesia*, no. 24 (1977): 27–38.

Schneider, William H. *Rockefeller Philanthropy and Modern Biomedicine: International Initiatives from World War I to the Cold War*. Bloomington: Indiana University Press, 2002.

Schulte Nordholt, Henk. 'Modernity and Cultural Citizenship in the Netherlands Indies: An Illustrated Hypothesis'. *Journal of Southeast Asian Studies* 42, no. 3 (2011): 435–57.

'Modernity and Middle Classes in the Netherlands Indies: Cultivating Cultural Citizenship'. In *Photography, Modernity and the Governed in Late-Colonial Indonesia*, edited by Susie Protschky, 223–54. Amsterdam: Amsterdam University Press, 2015.

Sciortino, Rosalia. *Care-Takers of Cure: An Anthropological Study of Health Centre Nurses in Rural Central Java*. Yogyakarta: Gadjah Mada University Press, 1995.

'Rural Nurses and Doctors: The Discrepancy between Western Concepts and Javanese Practices'. In *Health Care in Java: Past and Present*, edited by Peter Boomgaard, Rosalia Sciortino, and Ines Smyth, 111–28. Leiden: KITLV Press, 1996.

Scott, David. *Conscripts of Modernity: The Tragedy of Colonial Enlightenment*. Durham, NC: Duke University Press, 2004.

Scott, James C. *Seeing Like a State: How Certain Schemes to Improve the Human Condition Have Failed*. New Haven, CT: Yale University Press, 1998.

Sears, Laurie J. 'Intellectuals, Theosophy and Failed Narratives of the Nation in Late Colonial Java'. In *A Companion to Postcolonial Studies*, edited by Henry Schwarz and Sangeeta Ray, 333–59. London: Blackwell, 2004.

Sejarah Kesehatan Nasional Indonesia. 3 vols. Jakarta: Departement Kesehatan RI, 2009.

Seth, Suman. 'Colonial History and Postcolonial Science Studies'. *Radical History Review*, no. 127 (2017): 63–85.

Shepherd, Christopher. *Development and the Environment Politics Unmasked: Authority, Participation and Equity in East Timor*. New York: Routledge, 2013.

Shields, Linda and Lucia Endang Hartati. 'Primary Care in Indonesia'. *Journal of Child Health Care* 10, no. 1 (2006): 4–8.

Shiraishi, Takashi. *An Age in Motion: Popular Radicalism in Java, 1912–1926*. Ithaca, NY: Cornell University Press, 1990.

Siddharta, Amanda. 'Healthcare within Borders'. *Tempo (English)* (3 May 2015): 64–66.

Siegel, James T. *Fetish, Recognition, Revolution*. Princeton, NJ: Princeton University Press, 1997.

Silean, Victor, Jerry Rudolf Sirait, Yanedi Jagau, Abraham Simatupang, Marojahan Doloksaribu, John Pieris, Nikson Gans Lalu, and Midian Saragi. *Dr. Johannes Leimena: Negarawan Sejati dan Politisi Berhati Nurani*. Jakarta: Gunung Mulia, 2007.

Simpson, Bradley R. *Economists with Guns: Authoritarian Development and U.S.– Indonesian Relations, 1960–1968*. Stanford, CA: Stanford University Press, 2008.

Siwabessy, G. A. *Upuleru: Memoar Dr. G. A. Siwabessy*. Jakarta: Gunung Agung, 1979.

Smith, Bruce L. *Indonesian-American Cooperation in Higher Education*. East Lansing: Institute of Research on Overseas Programs, Michigan State University, 1960.

Smith, Catherine. 'Traveling for a Cure'. *Inside Indonesia*, no. 111 (2013). www .insideindonesia.org/traveling-for-a-cure-2.

Smocovitis, Vassiliki Betty. 'Desperately Seeking Quinine'. *American Chemical Society* 6, no. 5 (2003): 57–58.

Smyth, Ines. 'Maternal Mortality and Family Planning in Indonesia'. In *Health Care in Java: Past and Present*, edited by Peter Boomgaard, Rosalia Sciortino, and Ines Smyth, 131–45. Leiden: KITLV Press, 1996.

Soedarpo, Mien. *Reminiscences of the Past*. 2nd edn. 2 vols. Jakarta: Ngrumat Bondo Utomo, 2005.

Soedewo, Mang Eri. *A Freedom Fighter: My Life with Eri-San*. Jakarta: Kata Hasta Pustaka, 2008.

Soedjatmoko. *Asia di Mata Soedjatmoko*. Jakarta: Kompas, 2010.

Soeharto, Pitut and A. Zainoel Ihsan, eds. *Maju Setapak: Kumpulan Tulisan Asli Tokoh-Tokoh Jong Java, Jong Sumatranen Bond, Jong Bataks Bond dll*, Vol. 3. Jakarta: Aksara Jayasakti, 1981.

Soeharto, Raden. *Saksi Sejarah Mengikuti Perjuangan Dwitunggal*. Jakarta: Gunung Agung, 1982.

Soeprono, Raden. *Selangkah Tapak di Tiga Jaman: Mahasiswa Pejuang Kedoktoran*. Jakarta: IDI, 1997.

Somadikarta, S., Tri Wahyuning M. Irsyam, and Boen S. Oemarjati. *Tahun Emas Universitas Indonesia*. Jakarta: Universitas Indonesia, 2000.

Steijlen, Fridus. *RMS, van Ideaal tot Symbool: Moluks Nationalisme in Nederland, 1951–1994*. Amsterdam: Spinhuis, 1996.

Stein, Eric Andrew. 'Vital Times: Power, Public Health, and Memory in Rural Java'. PhD, University of Michigan, 2005.

   'Colonial Theatres of Proof: Representation and Laughter in 1930s Rockefeller Foundation Hygiene Cinema in Java'. *Health and History* 8, no. 2 (2006): 14–44.

   'Hygiene and Decolonization: The Rockefeller Foundation and Indonesian Nationalism, 1933–1958'. In *Science, Public Health, and the State in Modern Asia*, edited by Liping Bu, Darwin H. Stapleton, and Ka-Che Yip, 51–70: New York: Routledge, 2012.

Stoler, Ann Laura. *Carnal Knowledge and Imperial Power: Race and the Intimate in Colonial Rule*. Berkeley: University of California Press, 2002.

   'On Degrees of Imperial Sovereignty'. *Public Culture* 18, no. 1 (2006): 125–46.

Stone, Richard. 'Righting a 65-Year-Old Wrong'. *Science* 329 (2 July 2010): 30–31.

Strassler, Karen. *Refracted Visions: Popular Photography and National Modernity in Java*. Durham, NC: Duke University Press, 2010.

Stutje, Klaas. 'Indonesian Identities Abroad: International Engagement of Colonial Students in the Netherlands, 1908–1931'. *BMGN: Low Countries Historical Review* 128, no. 1 (2013): 151–72.

Subagyo, Wisnu. *Dr. Mohamad Amir: Karya dan Pengabdiannya*. Jakarta: Departemen Pendidikan dan Kebudayaan, 1986.

Sunario. *Perhimpunan Indonesia dan Peranannja dalam Perdjuangan Kemerdekaan Kita*. Djakarta: Departemen Pendidikan dan Kebudajaan, 1970.

Suryadinata, Leo. 'Indonesian Nationalism and the Pre-War Youth Movement: A Reexamination'. *Journal of Southeast Asian Studies* 9, no. 1 (1978): 99–114.

Suryanegara, Achmad Mansur. *Api Sejarah: Buku yang Akan Mengubah Drastis Pandangan Anda tentang Sejarah Indonesia*. Bandung: Salamadani Pustaka Semesta, 2009.

Sutaryo. *Sejarah Fakultas Kedoktoran UGM – Rumah Sakit UGM/RSUP Dr. Sardjito*. Yogyakarta: Puspagama, 2016.

Sutherland, Heather. *The Making of a Bureaucratic Elite: The Colonial Transformation of the Javanese Priyayi*. Singapore: Heinemann Asia 1979.

Tan, See Seng and Amitav Acharya, eds. *Bandung Revisited: The Legacy of the 1955 Asian-African Conference for International Order*. Singapore: National University of Singapore Press, 2008.

Taylor, Jean Gelman. 'Costume and Gender in Colonial Java, 1800–1940'. In *Outward Appearances: Dressing State and Society in Indonesia*, edited by Henk Schulte Nordholt, 85–116. Leiden: KITLV Press, 1997.

Taylor, Norman. *Cinchona in Java: The Story of Quinine*. New York: Greenberg, 1945.

Taylor, Rex and Annelie Rieger. 'Rudolf Virchow on the Typhus Epidemic in Upper Silesia: An Introduction and Translation'. *Sociology of Health and Illness* 6, no. 2 (1984): 201–17.

Toer, Pramoedya Ananta. *The Fugitive*. Translated by Willem Samuel. Harmondsworth: Penguin, 1990.

Tollenaere, H. A. O. *The Politics of Divine Wisdom: Theosophy and Labour, National, and Women's Movements in Indonesia and South Asia, 1875–1947*. Nijmegen: Katholieke Universiteit Nijmegen, 1996.

Tomes, Nancy. *The Gospel of Germs: Men, Women, and the Microbe in American Life*. Cambridge, MA: Harvard University Press, 1998.

Touwen-Bouwsma, Elly. 'The Indonesian Nationalists and the Japanese "Liberation" of Indonesia: Visions and Reactions'. *Journal of Southeast Asian Studies* 27, no. 1 (1996): 1–18.

Tsing, Anna Lowenhaupt. *Friction: An Ethnography of Global Connection*. Princeton, NJ: Princeton University Press, 2005.

Tsuchiya, Kenji. *Democracy and Leadership: The Rise of the Taman Siswa Movement in Indonesia*. Translated by Peter Hawkes. Honolulu: University of Hawaii Press, 1987.

Turner, Mark, Owen Podger, Maria Sumardjono, and Wayan K. Tirthaysa. *Decentralisation in Indonesia: Redesigning the State*. Canberra: Asia Pacific Press, 2003.

Van der Veur, Paul W. *The Lion and the Gadfly: Dutch Colonialism and the Spirit of E. F. E. Douwes Dekker*. Leiden: KITLV Press, 2006.

Van der Wal, S. L. *De Volksraad en de Staatkundige Ontwikkeling van Nederlands-Indië: Een Bronnenpublicatie*. 2 vols. Groningen: Wolters, 1964–65.

Van Dijk, Kees. 'Sarongs, Jubbahs, and Trousers: Appearance as a Means of Distinction and Discrimination'. In *Outward Appearances: Dressing State and Society in Indonesia*, edited by Henk Schulte Nordholt, 39–83. Leiden: KITLV Press, 1997.

The Netherlands Indies and the Great War, 1914–1918. Leiden: KITLV Press, 2007.

Van Doorn, J. J. A. and W. J. Hendrix. *Ontsporing van Geweld: Het Nederlands-Indonesisch Conflict*. Zutphen: Walburg, 2012.

Van Liempt, Ad. *Nederland Valt aan: Op Weg naar Oorlog met Indonesië, 1947*. Amsterdam: Balans, 2012.

Van Miert, Hans. 'The "Land of the Future": The Jong Sumatranen Bond (1917–1930) and Its Image of the Nation'. *Modern Asian Studies* 30, no. 3 (1996): 591–616.

Vanvugt, Ewald. *Een Propagandist van het Zuiverste Water: H. F. Tillema (1870–1952) en de Fotografie van Tempo Doeloe*. Amsterdam: Mets, 1993.

Vaughan, Megan. *Curing Their Ills: Colonial Power and African Illness*. Stanford, CA: Stanford University Press, 1991.

Verhave, Jan Peter. *The Moses of Malaria: Nicolaas H. Swellengrebel (1885–1970) Abroad and at Home*. Rotterdam: Erasmus Publishing, 2011.

Vickers, Adrian. *A History of Modern Indonesia*. Cambridge: Cambridge University Press, 2013.

Vuyk, Beb. 'De Laatste Waardigheid'. In *Verzameld Werk*, edited by Beb Vuyk, 446–61. Amsterdam: Querido, 1972.

Waitzkin, Howard. *Medicine and Public Health at the End of Empire*. New York: Routledge, 2015.

Warwick, Donald P. 'The Indonesian Family Planning Program: Government Influence and Client Choice'. *Population and Development Review* 12, no. 3 (1986): 453–90.

Wasisto, Broto. 'Pembangunan Kesehatan di Indonesia: Masalah dan Prospeknya'. *Prisma* 6 (1990): 36–53.

Webster, Paul C. 'Indonesia Makes Maternal Health a National Priority'. *Lancet* 380 (8 December 2012): 1981–82.

'Indonesia: Stratified Health the Norm'. *Canadian Medical Association Journal* 185, no. 2 (5 February 2013): E99–E100.

'Indonesia: The Midwife and Maternal Mortality Miasma'. *Canadian Medical Association Journal* 185, no. 2 (2013): E95–E96.

Weindling, Paul, ed. *International Health Organizations and Movements, 1918–1939.* New York: Cambridge University Press, 1995.

Wendland, Claire. *A Heart for the Work: Journeys through an African Medical School.* Chicago: University of Chicago Press, 2010.

Widohariadi and Bambang Permono. *Peringatan 70 Tahun Pendidikan Dokter di Surabaya.* Surabaya: Gideon, 1983.

Peringatan 90 Tahun Pendidikan Dokter di Surabaya. Surabaya: Fakultas Kedoktoran Universitas Airlingga, 2003.

Williams, Glen and Satoto. 'Socio-Political Constraints on Primary Health Care: A Case Study from Java'. *Development Dialogue* 1 (1980): 85–101.

Wiryosukarto, Amir Hamzah. *Wawasan Politik Seorang Muslim Patriot: Kumpulan Karangan.* Jakarta: YP2LPM, 1984.

Worboys, Michael. *Spreading Germs: Disease Theories, and Medical Practice in Britain, 1865–1900.* New York: Cambridge University Press, 2000.

Yang, Timothy. 'Selling an Imperial Dream: Japanese Pharmaceuticals, National Power, and the Science of Quinine Self-Sufficiency'. *East Asian Science, Technology, and Medicine* 6 (2012): 101–25.

Index